The Science of Well-Being

Social Indicators Research Series

Volume 37

General Editor:

ALEX C. MICHALOS
University of Northern British Columbia,
Prince George, Canada

Editors:

ED DIENER
University of Illinois, Champaign, U.S.A.

WOLFGANG GLATZER
J.W. Goethe University, Frankfurt am Main, Germany

TORBJORN MOUM
University of Oslo, Norway

MIRJAM A.G. SPRANGERS
University of Amsterdam, The Netherlands

JOACHIM VOGEL
Central Bureau of Statistics, Stockholm, Sweden

RUUT VEENHOVEN
Erasmus University, Rotterdam, The Netherlands

This new series aims to provide a public forum for single treatises and collections of papers on social indicators research that are too long to be published in our journal Social Indicators Research. Like the journal, the book series deals with statistical assessments of the quality of life from a broad perspective. It welcomes the research on a wide variety of substantive areas, including health, crime, housing, education, family life, leisure activities, transportation, mobility, economics, work, religion and environmental issues. These areas of research will focus on the impact of key issues such as health on the overall quality of life and vice versa. An international review board, consisting of Ruut Veenhoven, Joachim Vogel, Ed Diener, Torbjorn Moum, Mirjam A.G. Sprangers and Wolfgang Glatzer, will ensure the high quality of the series as a whole.

For futher volumes:
http://www.springer.com/series/6548

Ed Diener
Editor

The Science of Well-Being

The Collected Works of Ed Diener

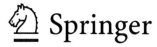 Springer

Editor
Prof. Ed Diener
University of Illinois
Dept. Psychology
603 E. Daniel St.
Champaign IL 61820
USA
ediener@uiuc.edu

ISSN 1387-6570
ISBN 978-90-481-2349-0   e-ISBN 978-90-481-2350-6
DOI 10.1007/978-90-481-2350-6
Springer Dordrecht Heidelberg London New York

Library of Congress Control Number: 2009926874

Cover design: Boekhorst Design BV

Printed on acid-free paper

Springer is part of Springer Science+Business Media (www.springer.com)

Contents

Contributors

Robert Biswas-Diener Center for Applied Positive Psychology, robert@cappeu.org

Ed Diener Department of Psychology, University of Illinois, Urbana-Champaign, Champaign, IL 61820, USA, ediener@uiuc.edu

Pelin Kesebir University of Illinois, Urbana-Champaign, Champaign, IL 61820, USA, kesebir@uiuc.edu

Richard E. Lucas Department of Psychology, Michigan State University, East Lansing, MI 48824, USA, lucasri@msu.edu

Shigehiro Oishi Department of Psychology, University of Virginia, Charlottesville, VA 22904, soishi@virginia.edu

Christie Napa Scollon School of Social Sciences, Singapore Management University, Singapore 178903, cscollon@smu.edu.sg

Martin E.P. Seligman Department of Psychology, University of Pennsylvania, Philadelphia, PA 19104, USA, seligman@psych.upenn.edu

William Tov School of Social Sciences, Singapore Management University, Singapore 178903, williamtov@smu.edu.sg

Endorsements

Over the past several decades Professor Diener has contributed more than any other psychologist to the rigorous research of subjective well-being. The collection of this work in this series is going to be of invaluable help to anyone interested in the study of happiness, life-satisfaction, and the emerging discipline of positive psychology

Mihaly Csikszentmihalyi, Professor of Psychology and Management, Claremont Graduate University

---

Ed Diener, the Jedi Master of the world's happiness researchers, has inspired and informed all of us who have studied and written about happiness. His life's work epitomizes a humanly significant psychological science. How wonderful to have his pioneering writings collected and preserved for future students of human well-being, and for practitioners and social policy makers who are working to promote human flourishing.

David G. Myers, Hope College, and author, *The Pursuit of Happiness*

Ed Diener's work on life satisfaction – theory and research – has been ground-breaking. Having his collected works available will be a great boon to psychologists and policy-makers alike.

Christopher Peterson, Professor of Psychology, University of Michigan

---

By looking at happiness and well-being in many different cultures and societies, from East to West, from New York City to Calcutta slums, and beyond, Ed Diener has forever transformed the field of culture in psychology. Filled with bold theoretical insights and rigorous and, yet, imaginative empirical studies, this volume will be absolutely indispensable for all social and behavioral scientists interested in transformative power of culture on human psychology.

Shinobu Kitayama, Professor and Director of the Culture and Cognition Program, University of Michigan

---

Ed Diener is one of the most productive psychologists in the world working in the field of perceived quality of life or, as he prefers, subjective wellbeing. He has served the profession as a researcher, writer, teacher, officer in professional organizations, editor of leading journals, a member of the editorial board of still more journals as well as a member of the board of the Social Indicators Research Book Series. As an admirer of his work and a good friend, I have learned a lot from him, from his students, his relatives and collaborators. The idea of producing a collection of his works came to me as a result of spending a great deal of time trying to keep up with his work. What a wonderful public and professional service it would be, I thought, as well as a time-saver for me, if we could get a substantial number of his works assembled in one collection. In these three volumes we have not only a fine selection of past works but a good number of new ones as well. So, it is with considerable delight that I write these lines to thank Ed and to lend my support to this important publication.

Alex C. Michalos, Ph.D., F.R.S.C., Chancellor, Director, Institute for Social Research and Evaluation, Professor Emeritus, Political Science, University of Northern British Columbia

Editor's note concerning source publications

Diener: Subjective Well-Being: *Psychological Bulletin*, 95/3 (1984), American Psychological Association

Kesebir & Diener: In Pursuit of Happiness: Empirical Answers to Philosophical Questions, *Perspectives on Psychological Science*, 3/2 (2008), Wiley-Blackwell Publishing

Diener & Lucas: Personality and Subjective Well-Being, (O.P. John, R.W. Robins, L.A. Pervin) *Handbook of Personality, Third Edition: Theory and research*, 2008, Guilford Press

Diener, Lucas, & Scollon: Beyond the Hedonic Treadmill: Revising the Adaptation Theory of Well-Being, *American Psychologist*, 61/4 (2006), American Psychological Association

Diener & Biswas-Diener: Will Money Increase Subjective Well-Being?, *Social Indicators Research*, 57/2 (2002), Springer SBM

Tov & Diener: The Well-Being of Nations: Linking Together Trust, Cooperation, and Democracy, Cooperation, (B.A. Sullivan, M. Snyder, J.L. Sullivan): *The Political Psychology of Effective Human Interaction*, 2008, Wiley-Blackwell Publishing

Oishi, Diener, & Lucas: The Optimum Level of Well-Being: Can People Be Too Happy?, *Perspectives on Psychological Science*, 2/4 (2007), Wiley-Blackwell Publishing

Diener & Seligman: Beyond Money: Toward an Economy of Well-Being, *Psychological Science in the Public Interest*, 5/1 (2004), Wiley-Blackwell Publishing

Introduction—The Science of Well-Being: Reviews and Theoretical Articles by Ed Diener

Ed Diener

Developing the Science of Well-Being

Since the time of the ancient Greeks, and even before that, people have wondered about the nature of "the good life." What is it that makes life desirable? What determines a high quality of life? One answer to these questions is that a person feels and thinks his or her life is desirable regardless of how others see it. This phenomenon has come to be called *subjective well-being*, which refers to the fact that the person subjectively believes his or her life is desirable, pleasant, and good. Throughout history different philosophers have placed varying weight on the subjective definition of the good life, some arguing that the most desirable life can be defined by a list of characteristics such as virtue, and others suggesting that pleasurable feelings are the essence of the good life. Even when pleasant feelings were the focus, some argued that the best approach was an educated hedonism, whereas others argued that stoicism was the best policy. Only in the last several decades have scholars of the good life turned to the empirical methods of science.

For a review of various philosophical views of happiness, the reader is referred to Tatarkiewicz (1976), Haybron (2008), Kesebir and Diener (2008), and McMahon (2006). Once scientists began to study subjective well-being, they focused less on trying to decide whether it is, in fact, the most desirable of all states, which was usually considered to be a philosophical question beyond science. Instead, they emphasized understanding the antecedents and consequences of subjective well-being, assuming that it was good regardless of whether it was the highest good. Thus, the question was no longer whether happiness is the *summum bonum*, the highest good, but what causes this state and whether it produces outcomes that are seen as desirable.

During the first half of the 20th century, a few scientists studied happiness, typically conducting surveys on people's moods. However, after 1960 several large-scale surveys of happiness emerged, some sampling the average happiness in entire

E. Diener (✉)
Department of Psychology, University of Illinois, Urbana-Champaign, Champaign, IL 61820, USA; The Gallup Organization
e-mail: ediener@uiuc.edu

E. Diener (ed.), *The Science of Well-Being: The Collected Works of Ed Diener*, Social Indicators Research Series 37, DOI 10.1007/978-90-481-2350-6_1,
© Springer Science+Business Media B.V. 2009

1

nations (e.g. Cantril, 1965; Gallup, 1976). Overall, this work was focused on trying to broadly describe who is happy. In a review of this work, Warner Wilson (1967) described the happy person as a "young, healthy, well-educated, well-paid, extroverted, optimistic, worry-free, religious, married person with high self-esteem, high job morale, modest aspirations, of either sex and of a wide range of intelligence" (p. 294). However, scholars also began to notice that "happiness" is not a single thing, but can be broken down into its constituent elements. For example, Bradburn and Caplovitz (1965) conducted large surveys that led them to the distinction between "positive affect" and "negative affect," which they found not to be bipolar opposites as had been assumed. Bradburn and Caplovitz found that the two types of affect formed separate dimensions and were caused by different factors.

Large surveys of happiness were often based on the sociological tradition, and therefore emphasized the causal role of demographic factors such as income, sex, education, marital status, and age as the correlates of well-being. At the same time, others worked in a tradition stemming from personality psychology. For example, Wessman and Ricks (1966) collected intensive data on Harvard students, studying their moods on a daily basis. In contrast to the survey studies, this classic research focused on internal factors related to psychological dynamics, such as defense mechanisms and personality traits.

One reason that sociologists and other behavioral scientists began studying happiness was to assess how well societies were performing, with the assumption that happiness levels reflect whether a nation is meeting human needs. Thus, measures of well-being would provide social indicators much like crime, income, and education statistics that would monitor the progress of nations. If modern countries were to make progress, they needed measures against which to gauge it, and subjective well-being was argued to be one such measure. However, many anthropologists and sociologists questioned the idea that "happiness" would reflect true human progress. One argument was that the nature of "happiness" varies so substantially across societies that they cannot be compared with respect to it.

Another objection to using measures of well-being to gauge societal progress was the theory that people will adapt to the circumstances of their societies so that eventually all people will be equivalent in terms of happiness. Moreover, the very nature of happiness as an outcome was criticized on the grounds that it is a western idea that should not be imposed on other cultures. In Volumes 38 and 39 of this series, I will discuss in more depth issues such as cultural differences in the nature and causes of happiness. One important issue is thus the degree to which measures of subjective well-being reflect the progress of societies.

I have been studying well-being for the past several decades. In this volume, I trace my thinking and research over the 25-year period from 1984 to 2008. In the articles in Volume 37, I describe several of the questions about happiness raised by thinkers over thousands of years, and I also address questions that seem to have arisen only recently. In both cases I review what scientific studies can tell us about the answers to these questions. Throughout this book I hope to show that "happiness" is even more deeply reflective of the well-being of societies than the utilitarian philosophers had imagined.

Major Theoretical Questions

Theories about subjective well-being have grown over the past several decades, but have been refined only slowly as adequate data have been compiled to test them. We can characterize the theories describing happiness along several dimensions. The first dimension is whether the theory places the locus of happiness in external conditions such as income and status, as many sociological theories do, or within the attitudes and temperament of the individual, as many psychological theories do. Some have maintained that people adapt to all circumstances over time, so that only individual personality matters for producing happiness, whereas others believe that economic and other societal factors are the dominant forces in producing well-being. Throughout my writings there is a mix of both the internal and external factors that influence well-being.

A second dimension that characterizes scholarship on well-being is the issue of whether the factors affecting well-being are relative or absolute. That is, are there standards used by people at all times and places in judging their lives and in reacting to events? Or are standards dependent on what other people possess, on expectations, and on adaptation levels based on past circumstances? Again, there is evidence supporting the role of both universal and relative standards. People around the globe are probably influenced by common factors such as friendship versus loneliness, but even these universal influences on happiness are probably subject to some degree of comparison depending on what the person is used to and what others have. However, some factors might be much more comparative than other influences, as Hsee, Yang, Li, and Shen (in press) have described.

A third and related issue is the degree to which the influences on happiness are inborn and universal or are learned, based on the goals and values of the culture and of individuals. Here, the focus on the particularistic influences on happiness is not so much comparative standards, but whether people's varied values and goals result in a variety of different causes of happiness. In a sense, this is similar to relative standards, except that goals and values become the standards in this case. One issue in the debate over this dimension is whether people's specific goals differ, or whether there are some abstract elements in common that lie behind these different specific goals. For instance, the elderly might seek a shiny Mercedes, while children might seek a shiny bicycle, but they may both be motivated by the desire for a means of transportation of which they can be proud. Thus, whether the causes of happiness are universal or specific might depend in part on the level of abstraction of the causes being studied.

The fourth important dimension in the scholarship of well-being is how subjective well-being is defined—ranging from global judgments of life to momentary feelings of pleasure and well-being. At one end of the spectrum, scholars have argued for the importance of global judgments of life such as life satisfaction, which are made when an individual evaluates his or her life taken as a whole. At the other end of the spectrum are the feelings of pleasure versus pain, and positivity versus negativity, that are felt at specific times and reflect a momentary assessment of how things are going. Kahneman (1999) argued that assessments of moments aggregated across time amount to "objective happiness," whereas philosophers such as Sumner (1995) propose that global evaluations of life are the bedrock of true well-being. I have argued that both ends of the spectrum should be of interest to scholars, but that we ought to be careful to differentiate them in our discussions of "happiness." Issues related to this dimension, defining and measuring well-being, are covered in Volume 39.

The final dimension regarding scholarship on well-being is the issue of whether a happy state is functional or dysfunctional, or simply neutral in terms of effective functioning. While emotion researchers might argue that our emotions, both pleasant and unpleasant, evolved to help us adapt, and are therefore all equally desirable in appropriate circumstances, well-being researchers assume that positive emotions are desirable and negative emotions are undesirable. Only very recently has the debate over the adaptive value of well-being begun to emerge. In 2005, Sonja Lyubomirsky, Laura King, and I published a review article in *Psychological Bulletin*, which concluded that happy people are more successful in health, social relationships, and work. In this volume, I present evidence suggesting that happy people are more likely to be pro-peace and cooperative in their attitudes. However, the idea that happy people are always more successful might be oversimplified, and the truth is likely to be more intricate. In the concluding chapter of this volume, I discuss this important issue in more detail.

The Articles in this Volume

In the present volume, the articles reprinted relate in important ways to each of the dimensions described above. Thus, the articles in this volume cover a range of important debates in the field of subjective well-being. In the 1984 *Psychological Bulletin* article, which popularized the field among psychologists, I describe findings on both the internal and external causes of happiness, and also outline the relativistic theories of well-being. A major feature of this article was to differentiate several forms of subjective well-being. It is important to note that the answers we find to the debates about the causes and consequences of "happiness" might depend on the types of well-being we examine, although this possibility has thus far received too little attention in the field. My 1984 article has become a citation classic, with over 1,400 citations by 2008. This citation count represents about 1/10th of the total 14,500 citations to my work. This article points to several of the major conceptual approaches to understanding well-being, such as telic theories, and it also reviewed the major conclusions at that time about demographic and personality variables. Since that article, the number of scholarly publications on subjective well-being has multiplied many times. From 1980 to 1985, there were 2,152 publications on the topics of life satisfaction, happiness and well-being, whereas 20 years later in the period of 2000–2005, there were 35,069 studies—a 17-fold increase! This rate of increase greatly outpaced the growth of publications in psychology, suggesting that subjective well-being had become a vibrant and growing area of science. The number of studies on negative states, such as depression, were still greater than the studies on well-being, but the gap had closed considerably.

Kesebir and Diener (2008) present a current overview of findings in the field in light of the questions raised by philosophers over the ages. What have we learned about the "big questions" of scholars prior to the scientific study of the area? The Kesebir and Diener article gives a broad overview of progress in the field, discussing the answers we have learned to questions posed by the ancient Greeks and other philosophers of the past. The great thinkers of old wondered about many of the issues that we inquire about today regarding well-being, and Kesebir and Diener reveal that we are now able to at least partially answer their questions. Whereas the Greeks usually relied on intuition and casual observation to form opinions about well-being, we now have the advantage of understanding the scientific method, and this has accelerated obtaining valid answers to the insightful questions raised by the earlier scholars.

The next articles in the volume are relevant to the internal versus external debate about the causes of well-being. The Diener and Lucas (2008) paper reviews how personality is related to well-being, and how these effects compare to the size of situational, or "bottom-up," effects. It corrects the misconception that environmental influences, the "bottom-up" effects, on well-being are necessarily small. In the *American Psychologist* article by Diener, Lucas, and Scollon (2006), we describe the importance of adaptation, but show how this idea must be modified to conform to the findings that adaptation is often incomplete, thus allowing for life circumstances to have a long-lasting impact on well-being. The findings in this area are important in showing that people often adapt to conditions to some degree, but frequently do not adapt completely. Importantly, individuals seem to adapt to different degrees. Thus, the findings not only show that both internal and external factors influence well-being, but also raise the important issue of what causes the differences in adaptation.

One of the major trends in the field over the decades has been to examine external factors, often demographic variables, which characterize people and influence their well-being. Income and wealth have been a major focus of study for both theoretical and practical reasons. At the practical level, scholars wonder whether increases in the wealth of nations increases well-being, thus addressing the question of whether economic development is a good thing. At the theoretical level, income is an important resource that helps people acquire goods and services from others. In the Diener and Biswas-Diener (2002) review that I authored with my son Robert, we explore the current data that are relevant to the question: "Will money make us happy?". Substantial amounts of data exist at both the individual and national levels relating to this question. Although levels of income are correlated with higher subjective well-being at both the individual and national levels, this pattern becomes more intricate when one examines it in detail. Furthermore, the available evidence on longitudinal income changes has not yet been sufficient to yield agreement about the relation between income change and changes in well-being, perhaps because this relationship is not simple and linear.

Income is usually considered to be an external resource that can improve a person's well-being, but it is also a resource that can originate from that individual's well-being. Happy people might earn more money on average than unhappy people. Income effects moving in both causal directions suggest that the external–internal dichotomy is not so clear-cut, and that there is a complex interplay between the two. In conclusion, the data reviewed in the articles in this section make a strong case for the importance of both internal and external inputs to people's subjective well-being and suggest that what I called in 1984 the "bottom-up" versus "top-down" approaches to subjective well-being (SWB) are both essential to our understanding and are more intermixed than is often recognized.

The next set of articles in this volume address the emerging discussion of when, where, and how much "happiness" is good for effective functioning. Surprisingly, the question of whether feelings of well-being are beneficial has only recently received scholarly attention. "Happiness" hitherto has been seen as an end state that people seek for its own sake. In other words, having feelings of well-being is seen as a goal in itself, and is often seen as the final goal for which all other goals are sought. However, in another tradition within psychology, the function of emotions in guiding behavior has been emphasized. The focus of emotion theorists has been on how positive and negative emotions aid adaptation to the environment, and ultimately reproduction and survival. In this tradition, negative emotions are seen as being often beneficial.

The split between emotion theorists and well-being scholars raises the clear question: If negative emotions are often adaptive, are frequent feelings of happiness beneficial? Not only can we examine the desirability of feelings in terms of whether people seek them because they feel good, but we can also analyze whether they help people to succeed in life. Success can be defined in this case in terms of helping people achieve the goals they value, such as health, good social relationships, and money. Are happy people better or worse at achieving these goals, or might unhappy people better achieve valued goals?

In 2005, Lyubomirsky, King, and Diener reviewed evidence suggesting that people high in feelings of well-being are more likely to be successful in a variety of life domains, including health and longevity, work and income, and rewarding social relationships. The article by Tov and Diener (2008) shows that happy people are not just likely to be personally successful, but are good citizens in that they value democracy, and are more likely to be trusting and cooperative compared to less happy people.

In the next article in this section, researchers in our laboratory show that it might be possible to have too much of a good thing. Shigehiro Oishi, myself, and Richard Lucas (2007) argue that people do not have to be at the top of well-being scales to function well, and that some experience of negative emotions is probably necessary to success. We show, for example, that on some tasks and in some situations, people who are somewhat below the top of the scale are most successful in terms of achievement behavior at work and school. We do not suggest that there is some perfect level of well-being for effective functioning in all circumstances because the optimal level probably differs depending on the person and situation. We do suggest, however, that the search for lasting intense positive emotions might be an impossible task that is not helpful to effective functioning. Thus, we attempt to marry the tradition in emotion research that points to the potential value of negative emotions to the research tradition in subjective well-being that implies that positive emotions are to be preferred to the negative.

It could be that although momentary emotions can be beneficial to effective functioning, chronic negative emotions are often detrimental. However, this hypothesis has not been rigorously tested. It is almost certainly true that high levels of happiness are not beneficial in all circumstances, and that unhappiness is not always detrimental to effective adaptation. The truth is undoubtedly complex, and one of the most important tasks for the future is to rigorously explore this uncharted territory.

The next article in this volume, "Beyond Money: Toward an Economy of Well-Being" by myself and Martin E. P. Seligman (2004), proposes that we need national accounts to measure the well-being of societies, and to ensure that policy makers consider more than just economic progress as they formulate their nations' policies. Finally, in the concluding chapter I point to what I see as the most important directions for future research. I describe the studies that I believe add little value to existing knowledge, in the hopes that aspiring researchers will devote their energies to research that will truly further important knowledge. All too often investigators do quick and convenient studies that add little to our scientific understanding, and their efforts could be better spent on more sophisticated issues. It is my hope that this volume will increase the speed of progress in our understanding of well-being.

Strengths and Weaknesses of the Field

The field of subjective well-being has strengths that are also weaknesses. One of these is that it is a highly interdisciplinary field with scholars from philosophy, psychology, economics, sociology, and other related disciplines all working together. This is a strength because it brings many perspectives, questions, and methods to bear on the topic, and greatly enriches the field. On the other hand, this can be a weakness in that interdisciplinary fields are rarely core areas within specific disciplines, and, therefore, they do not attract the legions of graduate students and grant funds that are drawn to questions that are addressed primarily from within a single discipline. The core areas of disciplines draw the most interest within them, and, consequently, an interdisciplinary area such as subjective well-being is likely to be a smaller "boutique-area" within any one discipline such as psychology. Another problem that interdisciplinary study brings is that researchers are often ignorant of relevant work conducted in other disciplines. Citations reveal this ignorance, with scholars generally citing those in their own discipline and rarely citing others. We need to overcome this tendency by more carefully searching for relevant work outside of our own discipline.

A related strength and weakness is that subjective well-being has a strong tradition in broad survey sciences such as sociology, but also roots in the intense study of individuals and internal psychological dynamics. While survey researchers ask broad questions of huge populations about how "happy" or "satisfied" they are, those working within a personality tradition tend to eschew large surveys in favor of the intensive study of individual persons, collecting large amounts of data on each respondent. For example, while survey researchers might ask whether people in general adapt to unemployment over time, as reflected in their responses to well-being questions, personality psychologists might ask who adapts and who does not adapt and what psychological processes predict this. While this diversity of approaches brings a richness to the field, it also can represent a challenge. Researchers in the two traditions may talk past each other, or may just not talk to each other at all. They often publish in separate journals and ignore the work of the other tradition. When they do communicate, they may be perplexed about how to integrate the two approaches.

Yet another strength and weakness is that subjective well-being is a field that is of great interest to journalists and lay persons. For example, many researchers in the field of subjective well-being are contacted by the media with questions about happiness. People are inherently interested in the area because it is so relevant to their lives. This is a strength because it means that scientific findings on happiness might be put to use in everyday life, which is certainly the hope of many researchers. On the other hand, the intense interest of the media in this area means that results are often presented before definitive conclusions can be drawn, and often in oversimplified ways. Journalists are often interested in more information than scholars can validly provide, and there is pressure to give them what they want. Thus, the field is continually pushed beyond the limits of its understanding by the keen interest of the public. A related problem stemming from the popularity of the field is that there are a large number of books devoted to well-being, and these are hungrily devoured by the public. Unfortunately, it is difficult for lay people to separate conclusions based on science and sound scholarship from those that are based on mere conjecture, or even worse, on hokum and superstition. Moreover, it is difficult to convey the fact that most of our conclusions are tentative and circumscribed.

Advancing the Field

Several developments have immensely helped the science of well-being. Ruut Veenhoven in the Netherlands created the World Database of Happiness, and posted on his website valuable information such as the results of surveys of the subjective well-being of nations. Along with myself and Alex Michalos, Veenhoven also created the *Journal of Happiness Studies*, which publishes scholarly works in this area. In terms of surveys, several large scale assessments of nations have been initiated, collecting representative samples from countries—the Gallup World Poll and the World Values Survey are noteworthy. In addition, large-scale longitudinal studies have been put in place in nations such as Germany (the German Socioeconomic Panel) and the United Kingdom (the British Household Panel); they include measures of well-being and have been a boon to answering scientific questions about well-being.

Because better data are now available, certain popular theories have been altered. For example, longitudinal studies over long periods of time and examining a variety of life circumstances have shown that people adapt to some degree to most circumstances, but that the adaptation to some conditions is often only partial. These findings contradict the strong form of adaptation labeled the "hedonic treadmill" by Brickman and Campbell (1971). For example, studies following individuals over many years showed that they do not completely adapt to conditions, such as widowhood, unemployment, or extreme disability, or that they take many years to do so. Similarly, the findings cast doubt on a strong form of the "set-point" theory of happiness (Lykken, 1999), which suggested that virtually all long-term differences in well-being are due to inborn temperamental differences between people. In longitudinal studies, researchers found that sometimes people change in their long-term subjective well-being, and occasionally change by substantial amounts. Thus, several hypotheses that had a powerful influence on the field for many years were altered by new and better data. My hope is that this volume will inspire researchers to collect more rigorous types of data that will rapidly refine our theories of well-being.

References

Bradburn, N. M., & Caplovitz, D. (1965). *Report on happiness*. Chicago: Aldine.

Brickman, P., & Campbell, D. T. (1971). Hedonic relativism and planning the food society. In M. H. Appley (Ed.), *Adaptation-level theory.* (pp. 287–305). New York: Academic Press.

Cantril, H. (1965). *The pattern of human concerns*. New Brunswick, NJ: Rutgers University Press.

Diener, E. (1984). Subjective well-being. *Psychological Bulletin, 95*, 542–575.

Diener, E., & Biswas-Diener, R. (2002). Will money increase subjective well-being? A literature review and guide to needed research. *Social Indicators Research, 57*, 119–169.

Diener, E., & Lucas, R. (2008). Personality and subjective well-being. In O. John, R. Robins, & L. Pervin (Eds.), *Handbook of personality* (3rd ed.). New York: Guilford.

Diener, E., Lucas, R., & Scollon, C. N. (2006). Beyond the hedonic treadmill: Revising the adaptation theory of well-being. *American Psychologist, 61*, 305–314.

Diener, E., & Seligman, M. E. P. (2004). Beyond money: Toward an economy of well-being. *Psychological Science in the Public Interest, 5*, 1–31.

Gallup, G. H. (1976). Human needs and satisfactions: A global survey. *Public Opinion Quarterly, 40*, 459–467.

Haybron, D. M. (2008). *The pursuit of unhappiness: The elusive psychology of well-being*. Oxford, UK: Oxford University Press.

Hsee, C. K., Yang, Y., Li, N., & Shen, L. (in press). Wealth, warmth and wellbeing: Whether happiness is relative or absolute depends on whether it is about money, acquisition or consumption. *Journal of Marketing Research*.

Kahneman, D. (1999). Objective happiness. In D. Kahneman, E. Diener, & N. Schwarz (Eds.), *Well-being: The foundations of hedonic psychology.* (pp. 3–25). New York: Russell Sage Foundation.

Kesebir, P., & Diener, E. (2008). In pursuit of happiness: Empirical answers to philosophical questions. *Perspectives on Psychological Science, 3*, 117–125.

Lykken, D. (1999). *Happiness: What studies on twins show us about nature, nurture, and the happiness set point*. New York: Golden Books.

Lyubomirsky, S., King, L., & Diener, E. (2005). The benefits of frequent positive affect: Does happiness lead to success? *Psychological Bulletin, 131*, 803–855.

McMahon, D. M. (2006). *Happiness: A history*. New York: Atlantic Monthly Press.

Oishi, S., Diener, E., & Lucas, R. E. (2007). Optimal level of well-being: Can people be too happy? *Perspectives on Psychological Science, 2*, 346–360.

Sumner, L. W. (1995). The subjectivity of welfare. *Ethics, 105*, 764–790.

Tatarkiewicz, W. (1976). *Analysis of happiness*. Warsaw: Polish Scientific Publishers.

Tov, W., & Diener, E. (2008). The well-being of nations: Linking together trust, cooperation, and democracy. In B. A. Sullivan, M. Snyder, & J. L. Sullivan (Eds.), *Cooperation: The political psychology of effective human interaction*. Malden, MA: Blackwell Publishing.

Wessman, A. E., & Ricks, D. F. (1966). *Mood and personality*. New York: Holt, Rinehart and Winston.

Wilson, W. (1967). Correlates of avowed happiness. *Psychological Bulletin, 67*, 294–406.

Subjective Well-Being

Perceived quality of life

Ed Diener

Abstract The literature on subjective well-being (SWB), including happiness, life satisfaction, and positive affect, is reviewed in three areas: measurement, causal factors, and theory. Psychometric data on single-item and multi-item subjective well-being scales are presented, and the measures are compared. Measuring various components of subjective well-being is discussed. In terms of causal influences, research findings on the demographic correlates of SWB are evaluated, as well as the findings on other influences such as health, social contact, activity, and personality. A number of theoretical approaches to happiness are presented and discussed: telic theories, associationistic models, activity theories, judgment approaches, and top-down versus bottom-up conceptions.

Throughout history philosophers considered happiness to be the highest good and ultimate motivation for human action. Yet for decades psychologists largely ignored positive subjective well-being, although human unhappiness was explored in depth. In the last decade behavioral and social scientists have corrected this situation, and theoretical and empirical work is emerging at an increasingly faster pace. In 1973 *Psychological Abstracts International* began listing happiness as an index term, and in 1974 the journal *Social Indicators Research* was founded, with a large number of articles devoted to subjective well-being (SWB). For a comprehensive bibliography of the burgeoning SWB literature, see Diener and Griffin (in press). Excellent reviews of the history and philosophy of happiness and related terms are available (Chekola, 1975; Culberson, 1977; Jones, 1953; Tatarkiewicz, 1976; Wessman, 1957; and Wilson, 1960).

The literature on SWB is concerned with how and why people experience their lives in positive ways, including both cognitive judgments and affective reactions. As such, it covers studies that have used such diverse terms as happiness, satisfaction, morale, and positive affect. Wilson's (1967) review of this emergent area contained two broad conclusions. First, Wilson wrote that those with the most advantages were happiest. He concluded that the "happy person emerges as a young,

E. Diener (✉)
Department of Psychology, University of Illinois, 603 East Daniel, Champaign, ILL 61820, USA

E. Diener (ed.), *The Science of Well-Being: The Collected Works of Ed Diener*, Social Indicators Research Series 37, DOI 10.1007/978-90-481-2350-6_2,
© Springer Science+Business Media B.V. 2009

11

healthy, well-educated, well-paid, extroverted, optimistic, worry-free, religious, married person with high self-esteem, high job morale, modest aspirations, of either sex and of a wide range of intelligence" (p. 294). Wilson's second major conclusion was that little theoretical progress in understanding happiness has been made in the two millennia since the time of the Greek philosophers.

Over 700 studies have been published since Wilson's review. Are his conclusions still valid? In the first section of this article, recent work on measuring and conceptualizing SWB is reviewed. However, the majority of the emerging literature has examined demographic and other external correlates of SWB. Several of Wilson's conclusions are called into question by these findings. For example, as is discussed in upcoming sections, later research did not indicate a substantial correlation between health and happiness or between age and happiness. More importantly, the variance accounted for by the demographic factors is not large. This has led to an increasing number of studies on psychological causes of happiness. An overview of the large literature on the correlates of SWB is given in the second major section of this review. Because the area of subjective well-being can no longer be reviewed in depth in a single article, the reader is also referred to other major works (Andrews & Withey, 1976; Bradburn, 1969; Campbell, Converse, & Rodgers, 1976). Theoretical work on well-being has not progressed as rapidly since Wilson's review, although there are several notable theoretic–empiric advances. Several major theoretical questions related to subjective well-being are discussed in the last section of this review. Perhaps the most important advance since Wilson's review is in defining and measuring happiness. This advance is crucial because the ability to measure SWB is necessary to scientific understanding. In addition, work on measurement is helping to provide clearer definitions of the components of subjective well-being.

Defining and Measuring Subjective Well-Being

Definitions of Subjective Well-Being

Many philosophers and social scientists have concerned themselves with defining happiness or well-being. Definitions of well-being and happiness can be grouped into three categories.

First, well-being has been defined by external criteria such as virtue or holiness. Coan (1977) reviewed the varying conceptions of the ideal condition that have held sway in different cultures and eras. In normative definitions happiness is not thought of as a subjective state, but rather as possessing some desirable quality. Such definitions are normative because they define what is desirable. Thus, when Aristotle wrote that eudaemonia is gained mainly by leading a virtuous life, he did not mean that virtue leads to feelings of joy. Rather, Aristotle was prescribing virtue as the normative standard against which people's lives can be judged. Therefore, eudaemonia is not happiness in the modern senses of the word, but a desirable state judged from a particular value framework. The criterion for happiness of this type is not the actor's subjective judgment, but the value framework of the observer. A related meaning of happiness given by Tatarkiewicz (1976) is success, which must be defined relative to some standard.

Second, social scientists have focused on the question of what leads people to evaluate their lives in positive terms. This definition of subjective well-being has come to be labeled life satisfaction and relies on the standards of the respondent to determine what is the good life. Although well-being from a subjective perspective has become a popular idea in the last century, this concept can be traced back several millennia. For example, Marcus Aurelius wrote that "no man is happy who does not think himself so." Shin and Johnson (1978) have defined this form of happiness as "a global assessment of a person's quality of life according to his own chosen criteria" (p. 478). Andrews and Withey (1976) found that over 99% of their respondents had previously made such an assessment of their lives. A related set of definitions of happiness is that it is the harmonious satisfaction of one's desires and goals (Chekola, 1975). If one is concerned with the person's assessment of this, then it clearly falls within the realm of subjective well-being and is an idea related to satisfaction.

A third meaning of happiness comes closest to the way the term is used in everyday discourse—as denoting a preponderance of positive affect over negative affect (Bradburn, 1969). This definition of subjective well-being thus stresses pleasant emotional experience. This may mean either that the person is experiencing mostly pleasant emotions during this period of life or that the person is predisposed to such emotions, whether or not he or she is currently experiencing them.

Satisfaction with life and positive affect are both studied by subjective well-being researchers. How these two components relate to one another is an empirical question, not one of definition. Unfortunately, terms like happiness that have been used frequently in daily discourse will necessarily have fuzzy and somewhat different meanings. Nevertheless, as measurement and other work proceeds, the most scientifically useful concepts will be those that can be measured and show, within a theoretical framework, interesting relationships to other variables.

The area of subjective well-being has three hallmarks. First, it is subjective. According to Campbell (1976), it resides within the experience of the individual. Notably absent from definitions of SWB are necessary objective conditions such as health, comfort, virtue, or wealth (Kammann, 1983). Although such conditions are seen as potential influences on SWB, they are not seen as an inherent and necessary part of it.

Second, subjective well-being includes positive measures. It is not just the absence of negative factors, as is true of most measures of mental health. However, the relationship between positive and negative indices is not completely understood.

Third, the subjective well-being measures typically include a global assessment of all aspects of a person's life. Although affect or satisfaction within a certain domain may be assessed, the emphasis is usually placed on an integrated judgment of the person's life. Nonetheless, measures may cover a period ranging from a few weeks to one's entire life. There is no a priori way to decide what time period is best. Rather, researchers must uncover the correlates of SWB within the varying time frames.

Numerous scales have been designed to measure both the affective and cognitive satisfaction components of well-being. This review does not cover momentary mood scales, depression, or other inventories designed exclusively to measure dysfunction or lack of well-being.

Single-Item Measures

Because subjective well-being has been of central importance to those interested in measuring the quality of life (Campbell, 1976), it is not surprising that several of the most frequently used measures are single-item survey questions (see Table 1). Despite the obvious advantages of brevity, single-item scales have been criticized on a number of grounds (e.g., McKennell, 1974). With reliance on a single item, the variance due to the specific wording of the item cannot be averaged out. Because it is impossible to obtain estimates of internal consistency, usually the only estimate of reliability for these scales is temporal reliability, in which it is difficult to separate true change from measurement error. Single-item scales tend to be less reliable over time than multi-item scales, although the temporal reliability of the single item measures has been moderately high (Stock, Okun, Stock, Haring, & Witter, 1982). For example, a 2-year reliability for Cantril's ladder was 0.65 (Palmore & Kivett, 1977), 15-min reliabilities for the Delighted–Terrible (D–T) satisfaction scale averaged 0.66, and a 6-month reliability was 0.40 for the D–T measure.

One major source of evidence for the validity of the scales is their convergence with other SWB measures (Andrews & Withey, 1976). On the basis of convergent validity data, Andrews and Withey estimated that their D–T measure contains 65% valid variance. The convergent validities reported by Andrews and Withey and others in this area are usually based, unfortunately, only on very similar measures (i.e., self-report). However, the items are sometimes administered in an oral survey and sometimes in a written questionnaire. The single-item scales usually correlate as we would expect with external variables such as self-efficacy, marriage, and standard of living (Andrews & Withey, 1976). Larsen, Emmons, and Diener (1983) also reported evidence on the validity of these measures. Their average convergence with other well-being measures was close to $r = 0.40$. They assessed construct validity by measuring the correlations with positive affective scales (e.g., Tellegen's Well-Being Scale) and negative affective scales (e.g., neuroticism). The average construct validity correlations with eight other scales were all close to 0.35. They also examined validity based on a criterion: mood reported daily over a 6- to 10-week period. The criterion validities for the three scales were close to 0.34. Finally, the measures did not seem to be highly contaminated by social desirability.

Despite the evidence for moderate reliability and validity, these measures suffer from several faults. Scores tend to be skewed, with most responses falling in the happy categories (Andrews & Withey, 1976). Acquiescence is a potential problem because the item is always scored in one direction. Finally, the scales cannot hope to cover all aspects of SWB, but must rely on subjects' integration of these in arriving at a single response. The single-item scales do not offer a finely differentiated view of a person's subjective well-being. Evidence will be reviewed that suggests that SWB is composed of several components, and it must be remembered that information on these components is lost when single-item scales are used. Nevertheless, the validity and reliability of these scales suggest that they are adequate if a very brief measure of global well-being is required.

Multi-Item Scales

Geriatric SWB scales. Several multi-item scales have emerged that are designed specifically for older respondents (see Table 1) and a discussion of them is provided by George and Bearon (1980), Conte and Salamon (1982), and Larson (1978). Because many of the items on these scales make specific reference to age and time of life, the scales tend to be unsuitable for young and middle-aged respondents. Another characteristic of the geriatric scales is that well-being factors are included that are not, strictly speaking, measures of subjective well-being (George, 1979; Larson, 1978). Nevertheless, these scales do appear to be heavily laden with content related to the respondents' affect and to a cognitive evaluation of their lives. This is supported by the fact that the scales show substantial convergent validity (Forrester, 1980; Lohmann, 1977; Moriwaki, 1974; Paintal, 1978) despite the varying labels applied to their subscales. Lohmann reported an average convergence of the geriatric scales of 0.65, with the Philadelphia Geriatric Center Scale seeming to perform the best. Kozma and Stones (1980, 1982) reported high internal consistency and test–retest reliability figures for the Memorial University of Newfoundland Scale of Happiness (MUNSH). Although the scales were designed to measure somewhat different factors, their high convergent validity suggests a strong underlying common source of variance related to subjective well-being. The fact that the geriatric scales measure an underlying construct of subjective well-being is also attested to by the internal consistency of these tests (e.g., Kozma & Stones, 1980; Larson, 1978; Lawton, 1972, 1975; Wood, Wylie, & Sheafor, 1969). Researchers have also examined the correlation of the geriatric measures with ratings of happiness made by professionals (Lawton, 1972; Neugarten, Havighurst, & Tobin, 1961; Wood et al., 1969). The measures have shown impressive correlations of about 0.55 with the ratings. Although a number of factor analytic studies have been conducted on various scales (e.g., Dobson, Powers, Keith, & Goudy, 1979; Hoyt & Creech, 1983), analyses of individual items have rarely been presented (Adams, 1969). Little is known about the extent to which the scales are influenced by acquiescence, social desirability, and artifacts. Some geriatric morale scales seem to contain a strong ideological factor (Cumming, Dean, & Newell, 1958). In sum, the geriatric scales do a satisfactory job in measuring well-being of older persons, although more empirical work is necessary. These measures converge and correlate as one would

Table 1 Subjective well-being scales

Study	Scales	Description
Cantril (1965)	Self-Anchoring Ladder (single item)	A nine-rung ladder is anchored at the top with "best life for you" and at the bottom with "worst possible life for you." Respondent marks one rung
Gurin, Veroff and Feld (1960)	Gurin Scale (single item)	To a question about how things are these days, respondent chooses among "very happy," "pretty happy," and "not too happy"
Andrews and Withey (1976)	Delighted-Terrible Scale (single item)	To a question about "how happy you feel about how happy you are," the respondent selects one of seven responses ranging from "delighted" to "terrible"
Lawton (1975)	PGCMS (multi-item, geriatric)	17-item scale measures lonely dissatisfaction, agitation, and attitude toward one's aging
Morris and Sherwood (1975)	PGC-M (multi-item, geriatric)	Revision of the original PGCMS
Neugarten, Havighurst and Tobin (1961)	LSI (multi-item, geriatric)	Factors measured include zest vs. apathy, resolution, fortitude, and congruence between desired and achieved goals
Wood, Wylie, and Sheafor (1969)	LSI-Z (multi-item, geriatric)	13-item revision of the LSI
Kozma and Stones (1980)	MUNSH (multi-item, geriatric)	24-item scale measures positive and negative affect and experiences
Tellegen (1979)	Differential Personality Questionnaire—Well-Being subscale (multi-item, general use)	21-item subscale of an omnibus personality inventory measures a combination of positive affect, positive attitudes, and optimism
Campbell et al. (1976)	Index of General Affect (multi-item, general use)	Subjects rate their lives on eight semantic differential scales such as enjoyable–miserable
Underwood and Framing (1980)	Mood Survey (multi-item, general use)	Two subscales measure hedonic level and hedonic variability or reactivity (16 items)
Dupuy (1978)	General Well-Being Schedule (multi-item, general use)	Seven specific aspects of well-being are assessed: life satisfaction, health concerns, depressed mood, person–environment fit, coping, energy, level, and stress
Fordyce (1978)	Self-Description Inventory (multi-item, general use)	Several subscales are included: achieved personal happiness, happy personality, happiness values and attitudes, and happy life-style. Two forms are available that correlate 0.95
Bradburn (1969)	Affect Balance Scale	10 items designed to measure both positive and negative affect
Fordyce (1977b)	Happiness Measures	Asks respondents to estimate the percent of time they are happy, unhappy, and neutral. Also includes an 11-choice scale on which respondents rate overall happiness
Kammann and Flett (1983)	Affectometer	Measures the frequency of positive and negative affect
Larsen (1983)	Affect Intensity Measure	Measures the typical strength or intensity of a person's affective responses
Diener, Emmons, Larsen, and Griffin (1983)	Satisfaction with Life Scale	Measures general life satisfaction and is suitable for all ages, from adolescents to adults

Note: PGCMS = Philadelphia Geriatric Center Morale Scale; LSI = Life Satisfaction Index; MUNSH = Memorial University of Newfoundland Scale of Happiness.

expect with external factors. A question that has not been adequately assessed for any of the SWB measures is that of discriminative validity (Dobson et al., 1979; Klemmack, Carlson, & Edwards, 1974).

Whether an investigator uses these measures or others that can be used on all populations will depend on the purpose of the study. These measures contain specific content in which investigators working in the geriatric area may be interested. However, use of these scales makes it difficult to compare findings across samples using differing age groups. In addition, there are scales reviewed later that are designed to measure general dimensions of SWB for all persons; these scales provide information on several general well-being dimensions that are not specifically assessed in most geriatric scales. In selecting a measure, an investigator must decide whether the specific content of these scales directed at the elderly is a more desirable feature than gaining knowledge of SWB dimensions.

General scales. The multi-item scales designed for general use are presented in Table 1. Data on these scales are available from the sources listed in the table and from Larsen, Emmons, and Diener (1983).

The Structure of Subjective Well-Being

The creation of multi-item scales raises the important question about the structure of SWB. If one is interested in satisfaction with specific domains of life (e.g., satisfaction with work, marriage, or clothes), a multifaceted picture may emerge. The particular structure of judged satisfaction with specific domains of one's life undoubtedly depends on the culture and the way one's life is structured. In support of this, N. E. Cutler (1979) found that the structure of domain satisfaction varied for different age groups. Although no universal structure of domain satisfactions may emerge, perhaps a similar structure will be found for many cultures and groups because of their similarity (Andrews & Inglehart, 1979; Usui, Keil, & Phillips, 1983). One important finding is that the domains that are closest and most immediate to people's personal lives are those that most influence SWB (Andrews & Withey, 1976; Campbell et al., 1976).

Despite the lack of generality we may find in the organization of satisfaction with life domains, a general structure of SWB may still exist. However, this structure is based on the experience of well-being. Andrews and Withey (1976) have found three general components of subjective well-being: life satisfaction judgments, positive affect, and negative affect. As we will see, the near independence of positive and negative affect has been uncovered in numerous studies using varying methodologies, thus suggesting that these might be two independent components of subjective well-being. However, the possible independence of negative and positive affect has become controversial. The relation between the third component, the evaluative or judgmental one, and affect has not been as thoroughly researched.

In the 1960s Bradburn developed a scale to measure emotional well-being (1969; Bradburn & Caplovitz, 1965) and found that positive and negative affect items were relatively independent of one another. Bradburn proposed that happiness is composed of two separable components—positive affect and negative affect. In support of this, it has been found that although the positive and negative affect scales were virtually uncorrelated with each other, they each showed independent and incremental correlations with a global well-being item (Beiser, 1974; Bradburn, 1969; Moriwaki, 1974). Bradburn hypothesized that happiness is really a global judgment people make by comparing their negative affect with their positive affect. Thus, his Affect Balance Scale (ABS) score is derived by subtracting the sum of negative items from the sum of positive ones. Bradburn's positive affect scale asks whether the respondents, during the few weeks prior, have felt, for example, proud because someone complimented them on something they had done and pleased about having accomplished something. The negative affect scale asks, for example, if the respondents have felt upset because someone criticized them and depressed or very unhappy.

Bradburn's conclusion that positive and negative affect are independent supported the long-standing argument of the humanists that psychologists focus too exclusively on the negative. Humanistic psychologists such as Rogers and Maslow have maintained that concern with psychopathology ignores the positive aspects of life, and Bradburn's proposal supports the idea that absence of negative affect is not the same as the presence of positive affect. Thus, according to Bradburn's findings, attempts to enhance life must both reduce negative affect and increase positive affect. Bradburn's conclusion is supported by the frequent finding that positive and negative affect correlate with different variables (e.g., Bradburn, 1969; Cherlin & Reeder, 1975; Costa & McCrae, 1980; Diener & Emmons, in press; Harding, 1982; Warr, 1978). However, there are data that show that the differential correlations are moderated by other variables and that cross-over effects do occur (Reich & Zautra, 1983; Zautra, 1983; Zautra & Reich, 1983).

Bradburn's statement that positive and negative affect are independent sparked a controversy in the field. His conclusion was challenged on a number of grounds, the chief one being the scales used. Critics contended that the relative independence of the two types of affect may have been due to a number of weaknesses in the Bradburn measure (Brenner, 1975; Kozma & Stones, 1980; Larsen, Diener, & Emmons, 1983a). Some of the weaknesses of Bradburn's scale are: (a) the positive affect items more strongly reflect arousal content, (b) there is much specific non-affective content in the items, (c) the simple occurrence of feelings is measured, not their intensity or frequency, and (d) the scale may suffer from acquiescence-response bias as well as ceiling and floor effects. All of these potential problems could serve to lower the correlation between positive and negative affect. Thus, although Bradburn's finding has been replicated numerous times with varying populations in studies using his scale (e.g., Harding, 1982; Moriwaki, 1974; Perry & Warr, 1980; Warr, 1978), the conclusion remained suspect because of possible limitations in the basic measuring instrument. However, the independence of positive and negative affect has now been confirmed using other measures and methodologies. Zevon and Tellegen (1982) and Bryant and Veroff (1982) offered evidence to support the dual nature of affective well-being. Diener and Emmons (in press) also have offered extensive evidence for the independence of negative and positive affect. They sampled affect, not at a single point in time, but over varying periods of time from moments to weeks. They measured the degree to which subjects felt particular positive and negative emotions (e.g., joy, anger, and depression), but did not restrict the emotions to particular situations as occurs in many of Bradburn's items. In addition, they compared correlations based on between- and within-subject data. Their major finding was that positive and negative affect are negatively correlated at particular moments in time, but that the correlation between the two decreases as the time interval increases. Thus, when one considers a period of weeks (or longer) in a person's life, the average levels of positive and negative affect one experiences are independent, even though experiencing the two simultaneously is unlikely. Average levels of affect refer to a combination of how frequently each emotion is felt in combination with how intensely it is usually felt.

Thus, there is extensive evidence showing that average levels of positive and negative affect are independent, even when very different measuring instruments are used. However, critics and doubts remain. Intuitively, it seems that because the two types of affect suppress one another, the more frequently a person feels one type, the less frequently that person feels the other. In addition, several investigators found results that directly contradict the idea that the two types of affect are independent. Kammann, Christie, Irwin, and Dixon (1979) and Kammann, Farry, and Herbison (1982) found with their Affectometer scale that positive and negative affect correlate an average of −0.58. Brenner (1975), using several positive and negative affect scales, also found strong negative correlations averaging −0.62 between the two types of affect. Most damaging of all to the Bradburn hypothesis is that when his scale is reworded in terms of frequency of occurrence of the feelings, a strong inverse correlation emerges between positive and negative affect (Warr, Barter, & Brownbridge, 1983).

Thus, there are studies that replicate Bradburn's findings, and there are results that directly contradict his own. Diener and Emmons (in press) finding that the independence of the two types of affect depends on the time period does not totally resolve the confusion because Brenner, Kammann, and Warr et al. found lack of independence even though periods longer than a day were considered. In addition, there are basic theoretical reasons why positive and negative affect should vary inversely (Brenner, 1975).

In order to explain the past contradictory findings, Diener, Larsen, Levine, and Emmons (in press) proposed that only mean levels of affect over longer time spans such as weeks or more are statistically independent. These mean levels result from two separable components: the frequency of the type of affect and the intensity of affect. In terms of frequency, positive and negative affect are strongly inversely correlated. The more frequently a person feels one affect, the less frequently the person feels the other affect. This is consistent with Diener and Emmons' finding showing that people rarely experience strong negative and positive affect at the same time, which suggests that the two vary inversely in frequency. However, because the two are inversely related in duration in people's lives, they must covary in terms of intensity in order for mean levels to be independent. This is exactly what Diener et al. (in press) have found in a series of studies—that across persons the intensity of positive and negative affect correlates positively in the neighborhood of $r = +0.70$. Because duration of positive affect and intensity of affect appear to be uncorrelated and combine in an additive way to produce mean affect, the resulting influence of the two over time, when persons are considered, is to make mean levels of positive and negative affect uncorrelated.

The theory of Diener et al. (in press) makes clear the relationship of positive and negative affect that has become so controversial. First, positive and negative affect are not independent at particular moments in time. Each type of affect clearly tends to suppress the other, although the mechanism by which this occurs is not yet clearly understood. Second, because of the suppressive mechanism, the two types of affect are not independent in terms of their frequency of occurrence, that is, the more a person feels positive or negative affect, the less that person will feel the other. Finally, when one measures average levels of positive and negative affect over longer time periods, they show a low correlation with each other because mean levels are a result of both frequency and intensity. Thus, their positive relationship in terms of intensity across persons cancels their inverse relationship in terms of frequency. In support of this, Diener et al. (in press) found that when emotional intensity was partialed out of the relationship between average levels of positive and negative affect, the correlation between them became strongly negative.

How does this approach explain Brenner and Kammann's failure to find independence of the two types of affect even though they studied longer time periods? When one examines their scales, the answer is obvious—they measured the frequency of positive and negative affect, not average levels. Their questions dealt with how often respondents experience various sorts of affect, but intensity is not a part of these scales. Thus, whenever one uses a scale that taps frequency of affect, positive and negative affect will be strongly inversely correlated. If one uses a scale that has both intensity and frequency items, one is more nearly measuring mean levels of affect, and the results are likely to show near independence between positive and negative affect. Finally, if one uses a scale such as the Affective Intensity Measure (AIM; Larsen, 1983) that assesses only emotional intensity, one will find that positive and negative affect correlate strongly in the positive direction. The distinction between frequency and intensity clears up the contradictory and confusing results in this area, and virtually all results, both from emotion researchers and from those working in the SWB area, fall into place with this conceptualization. Nevertheless, there could be some actual independence of positive and negative affect in that certain variables might influence average levels of one but not the other.

One of the shortcomings of the single-item measures is their inability to assess separately the various dimensions of well-being. Despite these shortcomings, the choice of measures always deals with cost and benefit in terms of the purposes of the study. If a survey must be extremely brief or only the grossest indication of subjective well-being is needed for the purposes of the study, a single global measure is defensible. When more time is available, multiple-item scales of well-being can be used that measure the separate components of well-being.

Scales for measuring components. Several scales are available for measuring the separate components of frequency and intensity. The data of Larsen et al. (1983a) on the first part of the Fordyce Happiness Measure indicate that this scale is quite similar to Andrew and Withey's (1976) D-T scale and reflects both cognitive satisfaction and affective content. In some cases, however, it has yielded higher correlations than the D-T scale, perhaps because it has more steps or because each step has more labels. The 11-point Fordyce item showed the strongest correlations with daily affect and life satisfaction of any measure assessed, and thus should receive more wide-spread use. The positive affect frequency estimates in Fordyce's scale were found to have validities equal or superior to those found for the Bradburn scale (Larsen et al., 1983a). Fordyce reported a 2-week reliability of 0.86 and a 4-month reliability of 0.67 for his combined scale. Thus, it appears that this is a suitably short instrument that can yield an estimate of the duration of positive and negative affect. Nevertheless, the Fordyce scale has not been thoroughly investigated and may suffer some of the liabilities of scales with very few items.

Given the favorable data on Kammann and Flett's (1983) Affectometer, it deserves to be a widely used measure of the frequency of positive and negative affect. The high level of internal homogeneity suggests that the scale does indeed measure the unitary frequency of positive affect dimension. It had a very high convergence with other SWB scales (an average of 0.70).

The second dimension of affective well-being—intensity—can be measured by the AIM created by Larsen (1983). He has shown that this scale possesses a strong first factor and correlates highly with the intensity of daily affect and of affect at emotional times. Larsen et al. (1983a) found that the Affective Intensity Measure showed low correlations with other measures of subjective well-being which tend to reflect duration of positive affect. However, the AIM did correlate with Underwood and Framing's (1980) variability subscale that reflects the changeableness of a person's moods. When used alone, the AIM identified those persons who experience emotion in a strong way. The items ask about how strongly various emotions are usually felt on those occasions when they are experienced. In combination with a duration of positive affect measure, the AIM can yield a more specific picture of the person's affective life. Those high in duration of positive affect and high in intensity of affect will exhibit an exuberant, joyful affective life, whereas those high in duration of positive affect but low in intensity of affect will usually experience contentment and serenity. Those who are high in duration of negative affect and high in intensity of affect will often experience depression or other strong negative emotions, and persons who are high in duration of positive affect and low in intensity of affect will be better characterized as melancholic or mildly unhappy most of the time. Larsen, Diener, and Emmons (1983b) have shown that personality differences in affective intensity are not merely due to situational or event differences between persons. Thus, some internal process must be responsible for individual differences in affective intensity.

Some investigators may not be interested in the intensity, frequency, or duration of positive affect and desire a direct measure of mean levels of the two types of affect. Bradburn's scale may be used, but it has deficiencies. Kozma and

Stones' (1980) MUNSH is a promising alternative designed to measure positive and negative affect, although many of the items are directed toward older persons. Thus, there is not yet a general-use scale for measuring average levels of positive and negative affect that has strong psychometric properties.

The third dimension of subjective well-being identified by Andrews and Withey (1976) is life satisfaction. This component is a cognitive judgmental evaluation of one's life. As such, it may be indirectly influenced by affect but is not itself a direct measure of emotion. There are data to indicate differences in affective and cognitive SWB reports and in their correlates (Beiser, 1974; Campbell et al., 1976; Kushman & Lane, 1980). Although several measures for the elderly are designated life satisfaction scales, they contain many elements besides a life satisfaction judgment (e.g., fortitude). Diener, Emmons, Larsen, and Griffin (1983) have developed the Satisfaction with Life Scale with items measuring persons' global satisfaction with their lives. All items show high-factor loadings on a single common factor, and the scale has a very high alpha and test-retest reliability (Larsen et al., 1983a).

Measurement Issues

Several issues related to measuring SWB remain. First, to what extent is the measurement influenced by momentary mood at the time of completing the scale? Few investigators in this area want their scales simply to measure current affect, and many scales carry explicit time frames (e.g., these days or the past few weeks). Nevertheless, there is evidence that momentary mood influences subjects' responses to SWB questions (Schwarz & Clore, 1983). Schwarz and Clore found that momentary affective states (e.g., those produced by the weather) influenced happiness and satisfaction judgments. This finding is consistent with memory research (e.g., Natale & Hantas, 1982), which shows that people tend to recall past events that are consonant with their current affect. In addition, T. W. Smith (1979) reported evidence suggesting that SWB scales are influenced by the questions immediately preceding their administration. Despite the influence that current mood can have on SWB measures, Kammann (1983) and Kammann et al. (1979) presented evidence indicating that this does not substantially distort multi-item scores. Another way to approach this issue is to examine temporal reliabilities of the instruments because these correlations partly reflect the degree that mood at the moment is introducing instabilities into the scores. The substantial temporal reliabilities of the multi-item SWB measures indicate that they are not greatly influenced by the mood at the moment of responding. Taken together, the data of Schwarz and Clore and the long-term reliability data suggest that both current mood and long-term affect are reflected in SWB measures.

Happiness can to some extent be considered both a trait and a state. The trait is a predisposition to experience certain levels of affect. Such a trait should be measured as independently from current mood as possible. It is an empirical question to what extent such a hypothesized trait is temporally stable and cross-situationally consistent. Diener and Larsen (in press) found substantial amounts of cross-situational consistency and temporal stability in mean levels of person affect. Life satisfaction was the most consistent and stable variable of the many on which they reported. However, when emotion at particular moments (rather than average levels over time) are examined, it is evident that people are, not unexpectedly, much less stable and consistent. In addition to these findings, one can plot the decay curves of the reliabiities of the SWB instruments and thereby estimate the short-term influences. Unfortunately, only a few reliabilities beyond 6 months have been reported thus far. The long-term reliabilities show values ranging from 0.55 to 0.70. Therefore, it can be estimated that the percentage of variance in the happiness measures that is due to person factors is between 30 and 49. It cannot be estimated from these figures the degree to which SWB is due to personality or to the stability of conditions in the respondents' lives. Because stable environmental factors are probably responsible to some extent for the stability of SWB, it is clear that internal person factors do not control a majority of the variance in happiness. Thus, the reliabilities point to some portion of happiness being due to personality, but also accentuate the importance of life circumstances. The best measure in terms of time covered and stability will depend on the particular theoretical questions that the investigator wishes to study (Bradburn, 1969).

A second issue concerns the validity of the self-report nature of these measures. Conscious distortion and response artifacts are always a concern. Perhaps more troubling is the possibility that persons may at some level be unhappy but for some reason label themselves as being happy. This problem is exacerbated by the ambiguity in words such as happy. In addition, a researcher need not believe in the unconscious to think that in some cultures, groups, or individuals it may be thought of as normative to be happy, and therefore persons may label themselves as happy without due regard for their experiences. Thus far, the evidence is encouraging regarding the self-report scales.

None of the scales shows high social desirability effects.[1] Usually the correlation with lie scales and social desirability scale is about 0.20 (Larsen et al., 1983a). Most measures are balanced in terms of response direction so that acquiescence is not a problem. The scales usually correlate as expected with personality measures and show high convergent validity. In addition, the scales correlate as expected with non-self-report data, for example with demographic variables. Weinstein (1982) found that self-reported happiness was strongly related to an unobtrusive measure of smiling and laughing in an interview. Another encouraging finding is that the scales correlate moderately with happiness ratings made about respondents by others. A tally of five studies using peer reports shows an average correlation of 0.39, whereas seven studies using ratings made by the researchers, staff, or other experts show an average correlation of 0.52. Kozma and Stones (1983) report an intriguing finding

---

[1] Although social desirability may have little influence on the rank ordering of individuals, there is evidence that this factor can have an overall main effect on scores. Sudman, Greeley, and Pinto (1967) found that respondents reported more happiness when they were given the Gurin et al. (1960) scale in an interview than when they took it in a self-administered questionnaire.

showing that expert ratings correlate more strongly with negative than with positive affect.

Thus, the SWB measures seem to contain substantial amounts of valid variance. However, this does not imply that some distortions do not occur. The topic of distortion, bias, and encoding of SWB is a valuable direction for future research. Thus, although there is certainly sufficient validity in the measures to build theories of SWB, one part of these theories should be how these subjective reports are formed (including various forms of distortion). Theories of encoding one's affect should be integrated with the bottom-up versus top-down approaches to happiness that are discussed later.

Measurement Conclusion

One can be encouraged by the state of measurement of subjective well-being. Most measures correlate moderately with each other and have adequate temporal reliability and internal consistency. In addition, well-being scales show interesting theoretical relationships with other variables. The global concept of happiness (Brenner, 1975) is being replaced by researchers with more specific and well-defined concepts, and measuring instruments are being developed concurrently with the theoretical advances.

Although many of the multi-item scales have shown promising results initially, they have yet to be adequately tested. Now that a number of scales are available, psychometric testing and refinement are critical. Andrews and Withey's (1976) LIS-REL-based approach can serve as a model in testing the amount of variance due to various method and content sources. Additional psychometric properties need to be explored such as response interval sizes, sensitivity to change, factor purity, and discriminant validity. In addition, investigators need to understand the scale properties (e.g., sensitivity and skewness) within their particular sample of subjects because differences in correlational findings between studies are probably often attributable to such factors. Researchers should explore the time period that is reflected in the scales and how the encoding of self-related material influences scores on these measures. Finally, validation of the scales is needed in terms of external non-self-report criteria such as interviewer ratings, peer ratings, facial coding, and other nonverbal measures. In order to test rigorously the validity of the subjective well-being scales, measures are needed that rely on dissimilar methods (e.g., not all self-report).

Influences on Subjective Well-Being

Philosophers and writers have hypothesized numerous causes of happiness. Rousseau placed the source of happiness in a good bank account, a good cook, and good digestion; Thoreau, his follower, wrote that happiness comes from activity. Psychological causes of happiness were often emphasized by early writers such as the Stoics. Fielding implied through his character, Tom Jones, that a sanguine temperament was more important than external blessings. The ascetics maintained that attitudes and activities that reflect detachment from the world lead to well-being. Unfortunately, only a few of the potential influences on happiness have been tested empirically.

A review of some of the major research areas related to causes of happiness follows. The purpose of this review is to provide an introduction to the literature by providing readers with an overview of some of the more consistent or theoretically intriguing findings. Some of the major questions that remain unresolved are also discussed. Due to space limitations, this review does not cover a number of important topics; the reader is referred to the following reports for more detailed discussion: Kimmel, Price, and Walker (1978) on retirement; Campbell et al. (1976), Dicken and Lloyd (1981), Mitchell (1976), and Schneider (1975) on place of residence; Wright (1978) on housewifery; London, Crandall, and Seals (1977), Mancini and Orthner (1980), Miller (1980), and Riddick (1980) on leisure; T. W. Smith (1979) on trends over time and seasons; Campbell et al. (1976) and Mathes and Kahn (1975) on physical attractiveness; Dixon and Johnson (1980) and Gershon, Bunney, Lecksman, Van Erwegh, and DeBauche (1976) on the heritability of mood.

Subjective Satisfaction

This review of the SWB correlates focuses on objective conditions. However, researchers have gathered information on subjective correlates as well (e.g., on the covariation of satisfaction with different domains and life satisfaction). Satisfaction judgments tend to correlate higher with SWB than do objective conditions, and this probably occurs for two reasons. First, they often share method variance with the SWB measure that tends to inflate the correlations. Second, the subjective judgments appear closer in the causal chain to SWB because objective conditions will usually be mediated by subjective processes. It is informative to compare the satisfaction with various domains and overall life satisfaction (Campbell, 1981). The highest correlation was with satisfaction with self (0.55), suggesting that people must have self-esteem to be satisfied with their lives. Satisfaction with standard of living and with family life were also highly correlated with life satisfaction, whereas the correlation for satisfaction with work was moderate (0.37), and satisfaction with health and community were somewhat lower (0.29). In creating theoretical models of SWB, scientists need to articulate the degree to which subjective satisfaction is a necessary precursor of life satisfaction and positive affect. Certain theories (e.g., classical conditioning) suggest that there could be a direct connection between objective external conditions and happiness without any mediation by conscious subjective satisfaction with that area. In addition, the top-down approach described later suggests that subjective domain satisfactions derive from, rather than cause, overall subjective well-being.

Income

There is an overwhelming amount of evidence that shows a positive relationship between income and SWB within countries (e.g., Larson, 1978). This relationship exists even when other variables such as education are controlled. As might be expected, satisfaction with income is also related to happiness (Braun, 1977; Campbell et al., 1976). In addition to those studies reviewed by Larson, many others have found objective income to be related to SWB (e.g., Alston, Lowe, & Wrigley, 1974; Andrews & Withey, 1976; Bortner & Hultsch, 1970; Clemente & Sauer, 1976a; Freudiger, 1980; Kimmel et al., 1978; Mancini & Orthner, 1980; Riddick, 1980). Although the effect of income is often small when other factors are controlled, these other factors may be ones through which income could produce its effects (e.g., better health). Easterlin (1974) reviewed 30 crosssectional studies conducted within countries. In every study, wealthier persons were happier than poorer persons in that country, and this effect was often strong.

However, when one turns to other types of data, an interesting picture emerges. Although persons in wealthier countries report higher SWB than persons in poorer countries (Easterlin, 1974; Gallup, 1976–1977; Silver, 1980), this effect may be weaker than within-country differences, although a rigorous analysis of effect sizes has not been reported. Japan is not much happier than India, and Latin American countries are in some respects happier than European countries. However, the data over time are most revealing. They indicate that as real income increases within a country, people do not necessarily report more happiness. Data over time are available from the U.S. for the years 1946 through 1978 (Campbell, 1981; Easterlin, 1974). During that period, real income in the U.S. rose dramatically (even after taxes and inflation), but there was absolutely no increase in average reports of happiness. In every year the surveys were taken, wealthier persons were on the average happier than poorer persons, but there was no increase in happiness over the years in either the high-, average-, or low-income groups. Indeed, the data reported by Campbell suggest a general downward drift in happiness from 1957 to 1978 in all but the lowest income quartile. This pattern occurred during a period of tremendous economic growth. These data suggest the possibility that the influence of income is largely relative; it is not the absolute level of goods and services that a person can afford. People who are wealthier than others tend to be happier, but as the overall level of income rises, happiness does not necessarily rise with it.

Because it does not appear that absolute levels of income are critical to happiness, there are several plausible, but unexplored, hypotheses as to why persons with higher incomes within a country are happier than those with lower incomes.

First, income has an effect only at extreme levels of poverty, but once the basic needs are met, income is no longer influential (Freedman, 1978). This hypothesis seems to be contradicted by the U.S. data which show similar levels of happiness for poor persons in 1946 and in 1970, even though basic needs were met to a much greater extent in the latter period. However, the data of Campbell et al. (1976) indicate that income had less effect within the United States in 1978 than in 1957, raising the possibility that the United States was reaching a plateau for the effect of income.

Second, factors such as status and power that covary with income may be responsible for the effect of income on SWB. However, these are relative within a society and therefore do not increase as real income increases.

Third, a related explanation is that the effect of income is direct, but depends on social comparison. People may only know how satisfied they should be by comparing their situation with that of others.

Finally, it is possible that income has not only direct benefits, but also some disutilities that tend to balance the positive effects. For example, higher incomes over time may also be related to increased pollution, congestion, stress, or other negative influences that may prevent SWB from rising with income. However, this explanation does not explain the tendency for wealthier countries to have happier inhabitants.

Given the concern for economic development throughout the world, the questions concerning income and happiness are immensely important ones. We now need research into the processes that control this relationship. Data over time from countries besides the U.S. need to be examined, as well as longitudinal data on individuals. In addition, questions about income distributions, not just mean levels, are probably quite important. Seidman and Rapkin (1983) have shown that although the prevalence of mental illness increases in economic downturns, this effect is greatest in heterogeneous communities in which recession does not affect everyone equally. Similarly, Morawetz (1977) has shown that a community with less equal incomes was less happy than a community with more equal incomes. The findings of Liang, Kahana, and Doherty (1980) suggest that feelings of distributive justice and relative deprivation mediate the effect of income. These studies suggest that it is not only purchasing power or mean levels of income that are important, but the overall distribution of income, including the range and skew, that influences SWB.

Other Demographic Variables

Age. Early studies found that young people were happier than old (Bradburn & Caplovitz, 1965; Gurin et al., 1960; Kuhlen, 1948; Wessman, 1957). In relatively recent years, however, a number of researchers have found virtually no age effects (Alston et al., 1974; Andrews & Withey, 1976; Cameron, 1975; Sauer, 1977; Spreitzer & Snyder, 1974), and several more have found a positive correlation between age and satisfaction (Bortner & Hultsch, 1970; Cantril, 1965; Clemente & Sauer, 1976a; Medley, 1980). Braun (1977) found that younger respondents reported stronger levels of both positive and negative affect, but that older subjects reported greater levels of overall happiness. Given the confusing nature of the findings, Adams (1971) wrote that "the inconsistency of findings in regards to chronological age indicates that it is, at best, a very gross index of group characteristics" (p. 67). In support of this, a meta-analysis of studies conducted prior to

1980 revealed that the correlation between age and SWB was near zero, regard-less of whether other variables were controlled (Stock, Okun, Haring, & Witter, 1983).

There are a number of considerations to keep in mind when trying to understand these findings. First, some studies such as those reviewed by Larson (1978) use nar-row age ranges, so that the correlations only reflect the ups and downs within those years. Second, most studies have not controlled for other factors that tend to covary with age (Cameron, 1975). Third, the large-scale studies have been cross-sectional, not longitudinal, and therefore may reflect cohort differences, not age differences (Knapp, 1976). Finally, the differences may reflect differences in the constructs being measured. Campbell et al. (1976) reported that satisfaction and their Index of General Well-Being correlated positively with age, whereas reports of being very happy decreased with age. Campbell et al. (1976) found that older persons reported greater satisfaction in every domain except health. Most results show a slow rise in satisfaction with age, but it seems that positive and negative affect are experienced more intensely by the young (Diener et al., in press). Thus, young persons appear to experience higher levels of joy, but older persons tend to judge their lives in more positive ways. In recent years investigators have begun to focus not so much on age per se but on life cycle patterns (e.g., Estes & Wilensky, 1978; Harry, 1976; Medley, 1980). Life stages are examined that create characteristic demands and rewards for persons.

Gender. Although women report more negative affect, they also seem to expe-rience greater joys (Braun, 1977; Cameron, 1975; Gurin et al., 1960), so that little difference in global happiness or satisfaction is usually found between the sexes (Andrews & Withey, 1976; Campbell et al., 1976; Goodstein, Zautra, & Goodhart, 1982; Gurin et al., 1960; Olsen, 1980; Palmore & Kivett, 1977; Sauer, 1977; Tose-land & Rasch, 1979–1980). Nevertheless, two studies have reported a modest inter-action with age. It appears that younger women are happier than younger men, and older women are less happy than older men (Medley, 1980; Spreitzer & Snyder, 1974). Although the crossover appears to occur around age 45, the difference between the sexes is never great.

Race. Blacks have usually been found to be lower on SWB than whites in the U.S. (Alston et al., 1974; Andrews & Withey, 1976; Bortner & Hultsch, 1970; Bradburn, 1969; Freudiger, 1980; Wessman, 1957), although this effect has not been found universally (Messer, 1968). Because blacks and whites in general differ on age, education, income, marital status, and urbanicity, it is important to control for these factors if one wants to know if race per se has an effect. When this is done, an effect is still found, but it seems to depend on the gender and age of subjects (Campbell et al., 1976; Clemente & Sauer, 1976b; Spreitzer & Snyder, 1974). It appears that, aside from factors such as urbanicity and lower income, being black carries additional factors that lower SWB, but only for certain groups of blacks. Indeed, Campbell et al. (1976) concluded that older blacks in their national sample were happier than older whites. Thus, whereas on the average being black may lead to slightly lower SWB, this conclusion must be clearly qualified by other factors, In addition, the predictors of SWB may differ for blacks and whites (Sauer, 1977).

Campbell et al. (1976) showed that, although blacks reported less happiness than whites from 1957 through 1972, both showed comparable decreases in happiness during this period. However, Gibbs (1973) has analyzed data from 1946 to 1966 and found that elite blacks (more educated, higher income, higher status) decreased sharply in their happiness during this period, whereas there was no comparable decline among white elites. Thus, despite apparent political advances made by blacks in the U.S. in the decades following World War II, there was no concomitant increase in happiness. Indeed, the blacks who might have most benefitted from increased equality were those who became most unhappy. In contrast, black farm workers reported high levels of happiness throughout this period. One hypothesis is that, with the political awakening of more educated blacks, their aspirations and hopes exceeded the gains that were actually made.

One caution is in order concerning the race, education, and other data related to specific subgroups in national samples. The subsamples of these groups are often quite small (e.g., 10–30 persons) and thus the conclusions are quite tentative.

Employment. Campbell et al. (1976) found that unemployed people were the unhappiest group, even when income differences were controlled. This suggests that unemployment has a devastating impact on the SWB for many persons that goes beyond the obvious financial difficulties involved. Catalano and Dooley (1977) have shown that regional unemployment rates are strong longitudinal predictors of mood. Bradburn reported evidence that unemployment influences the well-being of both men and women. However, it does not appear that homemakers are less happy than those who work in salaried jobs (Wright, 1978). Job satisfaction appears to be related to SWB. However, this literature is voluminous, and the reader is referred to several excellent sources: Cohn (1979), Near, Rice, and Hunt (1978, 1980), Rice, Near, and Hunt (1979, 1980), Weaver (1978).

Education. Campbell's (1981) data suggest that education had an influence on SWB in the U.S. during 1957–1978. However, the effects of education on SWB do not appear to be strong (Palmore, 1979; Palmore & Luikart, 1972) and seem to interact with other variables such as income (Bradburn & Caplovitz, 1965). Several studies have found that there is no significant effect when other factors are controlled (Clemente & Sauer, 1976a; Spreitzer & Snyder, 1974; Toseland & Rasch, 1979–1980), and several studies have indicated more positive effects for women (Freudiger, 1980; Glenn & Weaver, 1981b; Mitchell, 1976). After suggesting that education has some positive influence, Glenn and Weaver cautioned that "the estimated effects on males of all levels of education and of college on both sexes are especially likely to be disappointing" (p. 34). Campbell's (1981) analysis suggests that although education may serve as a resource for the person, it may also raise aspirations and alert the person to alternative types of life.

Religion. Because religiosity has been operationalized in different ways, it is unsurprising that the findings are mixed. Religious faith, importance of religion, and religious traditionalism generally relate positively to SWB (Cameron, Titus, Kostin, & Kostin, 1973; Cantril, 1965; Wilson, 1960), although Cameron (1975) found that religiosity correlated inversely with positive moods. Most studies on church attendance and participation in religious groups show positive relations to

SWB (Clemente & Sauer, 1976a; S. J. Cutler, 1976; Edwards & Klemmack, 1973; Freudiger, 1980; McClure & Loden, 1982), although others have found no relationship (Ray, 1979; Toseland & Rasch, 1979–1980). It should be noted that Campbell et al. (1976) incorrectly analyzed their data on religiosity, and this error was corrected by Hadaway (1978), who concluded that religion is one potential resource in people's lives. Spreitzer and Snyder (1974) found that religion had a significant effect on those under age 65 but, surprisingly, not on older respondents. Although it appears that religious belief and participation may positively influence SWB, many questions remain unanswered. What factors interact with religion, and what types of faith and participation are related in what ways to SWB? If other factors that covary with religiosity (e.g., race, income, location of residence) are controlled for, is the effect enhanced or diminished? If some persons seek out religion during trying times, does it have a positive impact? In other words, when and why is religion related to SWB?

Marriage and family. Although several studies have failed to find statistically significant effects on SWB for marriage (e.g., Bortner & Hultsch, 1970; Sauer, 1977; Spreitzer & Snyder, 1974; Toseland & Rasch, 1979–1980), virtually all relationships are positive (e.g., Larson, 1978). A number of large-scale studies indicate that married persons report greater SWB than any category of unmarried persons (Andrews & Withey, 1976; Glenn, 1975). Glenn reported that although married women may report greater stress symptoms than unmarried women, they also report greater satisfactions. Glenn and Weaver (1979) found that marriage was the strongest predictor of SWB even when education, income, and occupational status were controlled. Because the effects for marriage are positive but not always strong, investigators should explore factors that may interact with marriage, such as race (Freudiger, 1980; Mitchell, 1976). The ultimate goal should be to understand the underlying processes that mediate the effects of marriage. Along this line, Glenn (1981) has found that previous divorce is not related to the happiness of persons who are remarried. This suggests that marriage has an effect on SWB, and it is not simply a selection factor of happier people getting or staying married. When one turns from the objective fact of marriage to the importance of marital satisfaction on global happiness, the conclusion is that marriage and family satisfaction is one of the most important predictors of SWB (Campbell et al., 1976; Glenn & Weaver, 1979, 1981a). Indeed, family and marriage satisfaction was the strongest predictor of SWB in many studies (e.g., Freudiger, 1980; Michalos, 1980; Toseland & Rasch, 1979–1980). When parenthood and SWB are studied together, the results are not so sanguine. Most studies find either negligible or negative effects of having children on SWB (Andrews & Withey, 1976; Glenn & McLanahan, 1981; Glenn & Weaver, 1979).

Behavior and Outcomes

Social contact. Wilson (1967) concluded that extraverted individuals are happier, and evidence since then has corroborated this conclusion, although differences from introverts may be small. However, this does not necessarily mean that social contact improves SWB. It could be that extraverted or sociable individuals are happier persons without any effect of social activity per se. Many studies have found a correlation between satisfaction with friends or other subjective measures (e.g., loneliness) and SWB (Anderson, 1977; Campbell et al., 1976; Falkman, 1973; Liang et al., 1980; Mitchell, 1976; Rhodes, 1980). However, a large number of studies have also found positive correlations between various objective measures of social activity and various SWB measures (Beiser, 1974; Campbell et al., 1976; Edwards & Klemmack, 1973; Knapp, 1976; Markides & Martin, 1979; Olsen, 1980; Palmore & Luikart, 1972; Rhodes, 1980; Toseland & Rasch, 1979–1980; VanCoevering, 1974; Zeglen 1977). A program to increase happiness (Fordyce, 1977a, 1983) strongly recommends social contact as a way to improve SWB, and the program has proven effective. In addition, longitudinal studies have found that increases or decreases in social contact are accompanied by concurrent changes in SWB (Bradburn, 1969; Graney, 1975). A direct influence on happiness has been found for social participation even when factors such as health and SES are controlled (e.g., Bradburn, 1969). Okun, Stock, Haring, and Witter (in press-b) reported a meta-analysis of 115 sources that examined the relationship between social activity and SWB. Although they estimated that social activity predicted only 2–4% of the variance in SWB, an effect remained even when other variables were controlled. Effect sizes were larger for formal than for informal social activities.

Despite all the positive evidence previously cited, there are studies that found no relationship between social participation and happiness (Hasak, 1978; Liang et al., 1980; Palmore & Kivett, 1977; Sauer, 1977; Solomowitz, 1979). Some studies have found that the relationship disappears when other factors such as health are controlled (Bull & Aucoin, 1975; S. J. Cutler, 1973; Smith & Lipman, 1972). The mixed evidence indicates that the issue may be more complex than originally thought and that there are a number of studies that support this conclusion. Phillips (1967) found that the effect of social participation on SWB depended on one's education, and Smith and Lipman (1972) found that it depended on the constraint of the setting. Hasak (1978) found that it depended on a person's need for interaction, and Palys and Little (1983) found that the number of persons around is not important, although the degree to which they are integrated into one's social network was influential. These findings point out the need for more sophisticated theory and research designs.

The studies reviewed here suggest that it is not merely that extraverts are happier, but that social contact itself is somehow related to SWB. However, the direction of influence is uncertain. It could be that when people are happier, they are more sociable. It could be, as Bradburn suggested, that there is a bidirectional influence between sociability and happiness, but as yet no experimental studies have been attempted that could pinpoint the causal direction. Consequently, at this point it is not certain whether being happy is the causal condition that comes prior to social contact.

Another important consideration is the personality of the respondent because people undoubtedly have different needs for social contact. In support of this idea,

Diener, Larsen, and Emmons (in press) reported that extraverts are happier than introverts in social settings. They also reported evidence supporting Bradburn's finding that social participation influences positive but not negative affect. Thus, the absolute amount of social contact in relation to personality should be studied.

The type and quality of social contact differs from study to study, but has not been systematically analyzed. Studies have variously measured number of friends, number of close friends or confidants, amount of social contact, whether the social contact is freely chosen (Diener et al., in press), and so forth. The findings of Mancini and Orthner (1980) support the idea that some social contact is related to happiness (e.g., with friends), but that other contact is not (e.g., with relatives). In conclusion, social contact is often related to SWB, but the parameters that affect this relationship are not well understood. Although Bradburn (1969) offered evidence for the intriguing idea that novelty was one critical component in social contact, few other psychological analyses have emerged in the ensuing years. At this point data is needed on the types of contact, various individual difference parameters, and data that can provide insight on the path of influence between sociality and SWB. More importantly, theoretical ideas indicating when and why social contact increases SWB are needed.

An intense form of friendship—love—has been related to SWB in a number of studies. Not only is love rated as one of the most important factors (Anderson, 1977; Freedman, 1978), but satisfaction with one's love life is a strong predictor of life satisfaction (Emmons, Larsen, Levine, & Diener, 1983). Forrester (1980) found that having a love relationship was a significant predictor of life satisfaction, and Gordon (1975) found that love was the most important resource for happiness. As with social contact, researchers should now turn to more fine-grained questions about when and why love is related to happiness.

Life events. Life events have shown a consistent, but modest, relationship to SWB (e.g., Kammann, 1982; Miller, 1980). However, several things should be noted. First, evidence suggests that good and bad events are independent in the lives of individuals (Warr et al., 1983) and that good events are related to positive affect and bad events to negative affect (Reich & Zautra, 1981; Warr et al., 1983; Zautra & Reich, 1980). However, there is also evidence that one's ability to take action or control events is related to the impact they have (Guttmann, 1978; Reich & Zautra, 1981); therefore, even pleasant events can perhaps lessen SWB if they lead to a feeling of lack of control. What is needed at this point is a clearer system of classifying events. Past research has shown that whether the event is controllable is an important factor, and other aspects of events will certainly be found to be important moderating variables. An understanding of the impact of large-scale events and of the cumulative impact of smaller daily events is needed. A conceptual framework is important in this area. Whether lack of positive reinforcement in one's life causes depression (Lewinsohn & MacPhillamy, 1974) is still a matter of debate (Sweeney, Schaeffer, & Golin, 1982).

Activities. Activities tend to be behavioral, whereas events tend to be outcomes. Activity theory has played a central role in gerontology, popularizing the idea that active involvement causes happiness. The research that is based mainly on elderly samples tends to support activity theory (Beiser, 1974; Markides & Martin, 1979; Palmore, 1979; Palmore & Kivett, 1977; Ray, 1979; Riddick, 1980; Sauer, 1977). Graney (1975) and Maddox (1963) found that longitudinal changes in activity are accompanied by concurrent changes in SWB. Nevertheless, there are a number of null findings (Hoyt, Kaiser, Peters, & Babchuk, 1980; Lemon, Bengston, & Peterson, 1972; Olsen, 1980; Pierce, 1981; Wolk & Telleen, 1976), and when other factors such as health and SES are controlled, the activity–SWB relationship may disappear (Bull & Aucoin, 1975; S. J. Cutler, 1973). Kozma and Stones (1978) and S. J. Cutler (1976) found that some activities are good predictors of SWB and others are not. Schaffer (1977) demonstrated that the relation between activity and SWB depended on the respondent's personality. Given the breadth and vagueness of the concept of activity, it is not surprising that the findings have been mixed. The concept of activity can apply to such diverse things as social contacts, physical activities, hobbies, and participation in formal organizations. In view of this diversity, Lemon et al. (1972) and Hoyt et al. (1980) criticized activity theory and called for more articulated and formalized theorizing. Involvement in certain types of activities certainly must enhance SWB, but as yet we have little understanding of the parameters that influence this relationship.

Personality

Personality is suggested as an influence on happiness by the long-popular belief that temperament is more important to subjective well-being than are the number of a person's external blessings (Tatarkiewicz, 1976). This reasoning is indirectly supported by the fact that individual demographic variables rarely account for more than a few percent of the variance in SWB, and taken together probably do not account for much more than 15% of the variance. In fact, Andrews and Withey (1976) gave a figure less than 10% of the variance in SWB accounted for by all the demographics they assessed. A number of studies have appeared in recent years that examine the influence of personality on SWB. Because these studies are usually conducted with fewer broadly representative samples than those that examine demographic factors, the conclusions should only be given credence if the results are replicated across a number of studies with varying types of samples. When one accepts this criterion, several personality variables show consistent relationships to SWB.

High self-esteem is one of the strongest predictors of SWB. Many studies have found a relationship between self-esteem and SWB (Anderson, 1977; Czaja, 1975; Drumgoole, 1981; Ginandes, 1977; Higgins, 1978; Kozma & Stones, 1978; Peterson, 1975; Pomerantz, 1978; Reid & Ziegler, 1980; VanCoevering, 1974; Wilson, 1960), although this effect has been weak or complex in several studies (Reid & Ziegler, 1977; Wessman & Ricks, 1966; Wolk & Telleen, 1976). Campbell et al. (1976) found that satisfaction with the self showed the highest correlation with life satisfaction of any variable. An intriguing finding is that self-esteem drops during periods of unhappiness (Laxer, 1964; Wessman & Ricks, 1966). This indicates that the relationship between mood and self-esteem may be bidirectional, and an important question is why self-esteem drops when people are unhappy.

Another personality trait that has been consistently related to happiness is internality, a tendency to attribute outcomes to oneself rather than to external causes. This variable, usually assessed by Rotter's Locus of Control scale, has been found to relate to SWB in a number of populations (Baker, 1977; Brandt, 1980; Sundre, 1978). Nevertheless, one might wonder whether there would be certain environments or cultures in which externality would lead to higher SWB. If the events happening to a person were negative (e.g., failure), it might be better to attribute them to outside forces. Similarly, if one lives in an environment in which there is little freedom, an external orientation may be related to happiness, and this conclusion is supported by the findings of Felton and Kahana (1974). A variable that is related to internality is the degree of perceived choice or control in a person's life, and this has consistently covaried with happiness (Eisenberg, 1981; Knippa, 1979; Morganti, Nehrke, & Hulicka, 1980; Reid & Ziegler, 1980). When subjects rate their efficacy, personal resources, or competence, these also relate to SWB (Bortner & Hultsch, 1970; Campbell et al., 1976; Noberini, 1977; Rux, 1977). However, the direction of causality is very uncertain between internality and happiness. It may be that people with an external locus of control are that way due to unfortunate life circumstances which also lead to unhappiness. Similarly, people who have more control over their lives may also live in more fortunate circumstances.

Extraversion and related constructs such as sensation seeking and sociability have been found to covary with SWB (Gorman, 1972; Joshi, 1964; H. C. Smith, 1961; Tolor, 1978). However, our own findings reveal that it is the sociability aspect of extraversion that correlates with positive mood, not the impulsivity component (Emmons & Diener, 1983). Costa and McCrae (1980) found that extraversion correlates with positive affect, whereas neuroticism is related to negative affect. Others also found that neuroticism (Cameron, 1975; Hartmann, 1934) is related to unhappiness. Costa and McCrae suggest that extraversion and neuroticism are two basic dimensions of personality that lead to positive affect and negative affect, respectively.

Intelligence is a personality variable that would be expected to relate strongly to SWB because it is a highly valued resource in this society. However, it appears that intelligence as measured by IQ tests is not related to happiness (Hartmann, 1934; Palmore, 1979; Palmore & Luikart, 1972; Sigelman, 1981; Watson, 1930; Wilson, 1960). Although several investigators found positive effects for intelligence (Campbell et al., 1976; Jasper, 1930; Washburne, 1941), others found a negative relation (Fellows, 1956). Because the studies thus far are based on narrow samples and none are representative of the general population, the results remain extremely tentative. Nonetheless, it is strange that intelligence should ever correlate negatively with happiness in persons such as college students for whom it should be rewarded. If there is no overall relationship between intelligence and SWB in a broadly based sample, this result would seem to contradict the general finding that resources have some relationship to SWB, and thus might indicate the possibility that there is some process tied to intelligence that also serves to decrease SWB. It could be that intelligence also brings greater aspirations, desire for achievement, or awareness of alternatives.

Recently an extremely popular personality dimension has been androgyny, a trait that implies a person is not highly sex typed as either masculine or feminine, but exhibits characteristics of both. Wish (1977) found that sex typed women (but not men) were more satisfied. However, other investigators have not found that androgynous individuals experience greater SWB (Allen-Kee, 1980; DeGuire, 1974; O'Sullivan, 1980).

It is interesting that Hasak (1978) found a totally different set of personality predictors for men and women. This finding raises the question: Are individuals with certain types of personalities happier only within the confines of a particular cultural milieu because their traits are those that are rewarded? This may not be true for traits that concern internal reactions such as self-esteem, optimism, or neuroticism—these may have a universal relationship to happiness. But what about traits such as aggressiveness? Although the question of trait by environment interactions has been little explored, Diener et al. (in press) found some support for the idea that individuals experience more SWB when they are in situations that are congruent with their personalities, although this effect did not appear to be strong. For example, although those who were high in need for achievement were happier in work situations compared with those who were low in need, the main effect for situation was stronger—all groups were happier when involved in recreation. It is quite possible that persons living for long periods in environments that are congruent with their personalities may experience greater happiness.

A great deal more research in personality is required. For example, it is unclear if factors such as optimism or positive outlook cause or follow from events. Longitudinal and perhaps laboratory experimental studies will be needed to understand the process that connects factors such as optimism and self-esteem to positive affect.

Biological Influences

A substantial number of studies show a relatively sizable relationship between self-rated health and SWB (e.g., Edwards & Klemmack, 1973; Larson, 1978; Markides & Martin, 1979; Near et al., 1978; Ray, 1979; Riddick, 1980; Spreitzer & Snyder, 1974; Toseland & Rasch, 1979–1980; Wessman, 1957; Wilson, 1960; Zeglen, 1977), and this effect remains when other variables such as SES and age are controlled (Clemente & Sauer, 1976a; Freudiger, 1980; Larson, 1978). Campbell et al. (1976) found that although health was rated by subjects as the most important factor in happiness, satisfaction with health was actually only the eighth strongest predictor of life satisfaction. Although some investigators (Mancini & Orthner, 1980; Miller, 1980) found a strong zero-order correlation between health and SWB, they found that when other factors such as leisure activities were covaried, the effect was nonsignificant. This indicates that part of the influence of health on SWB is not simply the direct effect on how people feel physically, but also on what their health allows them to do. However, Bultena and Oyler (1971) found an effect for health even when differences in social interaction were taken into account. A number of studies have used more objective measures of health such as disease checklists (Bultena & Oyler, 1971; Larson, 1978; Liang et al., 1980; Mancini & Orthner, 1980). Although physicians' ratings also tend to correlate with SWB (Palmore & Luikart, 1972), they usually do so at a lower level (Larson, 1978; Maddox, 1963; Suchman, Phillips, & Strieb, 1958). A meta-analysis of studies on health and SWB revealed a consistent moderate correlation of about 0.32 between them, with virtually all findings being significant (Okun, Stock, Haring, & Witter, in press-a). The relationship between health and SWB was stronger for women and stronger when subjective measures of health were used.

It appears that subjective health shows a strong relationship to happiness, and that objective health has a weak, but still significant, relationship to SWB (Zautra & Hempel, 1983). Nevertheless, several warnings are in order. Miller (1980) reported that health influenced satisfaction only cross-sectionally, not longitudinally. This finding raises questions about the process and causal direction by which health and satisfaction are related (Zautra & Hempel, 1983). Thus, the degree to which objective health is related to SWB is uncertain, although it is clearly less than subjective health. In order to understand the underlying processes involved, much more research is needed that examines both subjective and objective measures and the degree of relationship when other factors are controlled. Although it appears that objective health is related to happiness, it is surprising that this relationship is so weak. Kammann and Campbell (1982) found that lay persons strongly believe that happiness is closely allied with good health.

Several other seemingly biological factors have been related to SWB. Poor sleep has been related to SWB. Poor sleep has been related to unhappiness (Barry & Bousfield, 1935; Bousfield, 1938, 1942; Roth, Kramer, & Roehrs, 1976; Sherman, 1980; VanCoevering, 1974; Wiltsey, 1967). One might question the direction of causality here, because it is likely that distressed persons do not sleep as well. Nevertheless, because interruption of REM seems to influence psychological well-being adversely, it seems probable that the influence could be bidirectional. Exercise has also been related to higher mood (Morris & Husman, 1978; Reffruschini, 1978; Tredway, 1978), although well-controlled experimental work is still lacking on this topic. Finally, seasonal variations in mood have been found (Andrews & Withey, 1976; Bradburn, 1969; T. W. Smith, 1979; Springer & Roslow, 1935), although it is not clear whether these influences are biological in origin. Weather has been found to influence mood (e.g., Barnston, 1975; Catalano & Dooley, 1977; Schwarz & Clore, 1983), although this may not be a long-term effect.

It is clear that at some level hormonal and other biological events must mediate mood and SWB. These findings and theories are beyond the scope of this review. It should be noted, however, that biological mediation does not invalidate theories that are at a different level of analysis such as the psychological or sociological levels.

Conclusion

Importance of influences. A number of investigators have noted with dismay the small proportion of variance that can be accounted for with demographic variables. This has led some to look elsewhere for more potent variables, to fields such as personality or attitudes. However, in these fields a parallel finding often emerges—no single trait accounts for much of the variance in behavior. Thus, it seems likely that subjective well-being will not be accounted for by a handful of potent variables, because of the immense number of factors that can influence it. Variables from the weather to beliefs to interactions between personality and environment will probably play a part, and it is unrealistic that any one will be prepotent. Nevertheless, moving away from specifics to more abstract concepts in the realm of theory (e.g., goals), stronger relationships may be found. However, SWB is probably determined by a large number of factors that can be conceptualized at several levels of analysis, and it is perhaps unrealistic to hope that a few variables will be of overwhelming importance.

Limits of the influence studies. Virtually all of the studies on the influences on happiness suffer from certain common shortcomings. There are few experimental, quasi-experimental, or even longitudinal studies, and thus the direction of causality is impossible to determine in most cases. It is usually possible to argue that the putative causal variable could actually be caused by SWB. For example, health or social contact might result from happiness as well as cause it. This points out a much neglected question: What are the effects of happiness? For example, Wilson and Matheny (1983) found that positive emotional tone covaried with sustained attention, and Weinstein (1982) found that the performance of happy people is enhanced more by positive changes in incentives. An important activity for future research is to map more completely the effects of positive affect.

Curvilinear and interactional effects are often not examined in this literature. One large difficulty is trying to separate the effects of different variables that are intercorrelated. One can examine the unique variance predicted by each variable, but the common variance is often the largest portion of variance accounted for. In most studies, there is no satisfactory way to apportion the effects of this common variance. Although regression is often used to do so, the device of simply apportioning the common variance to the strongest predictor is usually not defensible. Researchers need longitudinal and quasi-experimental data in which potential causal variables fluctuate somewhat independently in order to separate their influences. Another element that is usually lacking in most areas is a theoretical structure to guide empirical work. It is true that theory should proceed from carefully collected data. However, theory and empirical data have a two-way influence, and theory is necessary in order to know what types of data should be collected.

Recommendations. Much progress has been made since Wilson's (1967) review. At this point there is an idea of how many variables are correlated with SWB. However, there is a great need for more sophisticated methodologies. A better understanding is needed of parameters that influence the relationships, the directions of influence between variables, and how the different influences interact. There are unexplored potential causes of SWB (e.g., inheritance, social networks, and life-style). In addition, an understanding of how the variables influence the separate components of SWB is needed. In sum, methodologies that allow a deeper under-standing of how variables influence SWB and more adequate theorizing to guide empirical work are essential.

Theory

Wilson (1967) stated that little theoretical progress in understanding happiness had been made since the time of the ancient Greeks. Although several notable theoret-ical advances have occurred in the last decade, progress is still limited. A closer connection between theory and research is sorely needed. This review focuses on some of the more provocative psychological theories related to happiness, but does not describe biological (including heritability) or sociological theories.

Telic Theories

Telic or endpoint theories of subjective well-being maintain that happiness is gained when some state, such as a goal or need, is reached. One theoretical postulate offered by Wilson (1960) is that the "satisfaction of needs causes happiness and conversely, the persistence of unfulfilled needs causes unhappiness" (p. 71). Much of the re-search on SWB seems to have been based on an implicit model related to needs and goals. The degree of resources presumably related to needs and desires is assessed and correlated with SWB. However, specific theoretical formulations are rare in this work.

Many philosophers were concerned with questions related to telic theories. For example, they asked whether happiness is gained by satisfying one's desires or by suppressing them. Whereas hedonistic philosophers have recommended fulfillment of desires, ascetics have recommended the annihilation of desire. Which desires or goals are most important, and what balance should be struck between different types of desires? Are certain desires deleterious to happiness? Perhaps one of the most important questions is whether happiness comes from already having one's desires fulfilled, from having recently achieved a desire, or from the process of moving toward desired objects. As Scitovsky (1976) stated, "being on the way to those goals and struggling to achieve them are more satisfying than is the actual attainment of the goals" (p. 62).

Alternative telic theories derive from different origins of the striving. In need theories, there are certain inborn or learned needs that the person seeks to fulfill. The person may or may not be aware of these needs. Nevertheless, it is postulated that happiness will follow from their fullfilment. In contrast, goal theories are based on specific desires of which the person is aware. The person is consciously seeking certain goals, and happiness results when they are reached (Michalos, 1980). Goals and needs are related in that underlying needs may lead to specific goals. A person may also have certain values that lead to specific goals. Needs may be universal, such as those postulated by Maslow, or they may differ markedly from individual to individual such as those proposed by Murray. There is widespread agreement that the fulfillment of needs, goals, and desires is somehow related to happiness.

Maslow proposed a universal hierarchy of needs that emerges in the same order in all persons. Individuals should experience SWB if they are fulfilling the needs at their particular levels, although it is also possible that happiness might be higher for those at higher levels of the need hierarchy. Research findings on Maslow's theory are not encouraging (e.g., Lawler & Suttle, 1972; Wahba & Bridwell, 1976), so more work is needed before applying the theory to happiness. Murray postulated a large number of needs varying in their origin. People differ greatly in these needs (e.g., for achievement of affiliation). Diener et al. (in press) found some support for the idea that people experience happiness when their particular needs are fulfilled. Their approach to happiness was based upon person-environment fit—the idea that people are happy when they are in situations that match their personalities.

A number of universal human needs (e.g., for efficacy, self-approval, and understanding) have been proposed. If these are truly universal needs, then their fulfillment should correlate with happiness in all cultures. Reich and Zautra (1981) postulated that personal causation or efficacy is a ubiquitous source of positive affect, and Csikszentmihalyi and Figurski (1982) found that voluntariness is a positive aspect of experience. The importance of social support to happiness (Campbell et al., 1976) suggests that this could be a ubiquitous need. An optimum level of arousal has also been proposed as a major source of happiness. Scitovsky (1976) maintained that the correct level of stimulation or novelty increases positive affect.

Goals and desires are usually thought of as more conscious than needs. Most individuals have had the experience of feeling happy when they achieve some important goal. However, a key question is whether goal fulfillment leads to longer-term differences in SWB between persons, rather than just short-term mood elevations. Some theorists (e.g., Chekola, 1975) argued that happiness depends on the continuing fulfillment of one's life plan, the total integrated set of a person's goals. Some goals may be in conflict with others. Thus, according to the life plan approach, happiness depends on two key related factors: harmonious integration of one's goals and fulfillment of these goals.

In a vein similar to the life plan approach, Palys and Little (1983) hypothesized that people have personal projects or concerns and that these projects can be integrated into a total project system. They measured these projects and found that dissatisfied people were committed to goals that held the prospect of long-term reward, but that had little short-term reinforcement or enjoyment. Their projects were difficult and long term. More satisfied individuals had projects that were more enjoyable, less difficult, and more important at that time.

According to telic approaches, there are several things that can interfere with SWB. First, individuals may desires goals that bring short-term happiness but have long-term consequences that are deleterious to happiness because they interfere with other goals. Second, people's goals and desires may be in conflict, and thus it is impossible to satisfy them fully. Because their needs or desires might be unconscious, it would be difficult to identify and integrate them if they were in conflict. Third, individuals could be bereft of happiness because they had no goals or desires. Finally, people may be unable to gain their goals because of poor conditions or skills, or because the goals are so lofty.

There are several shortcomings to the current telic approaches. They have rarely been formulated in a clear way and then tested. Many of these approaches are not falsifiable. Needs or goals are sometimes described in a circular way, depending on the observations the concept is to explain. Clear measures of needs and goals are needed, and longitudinal methodologies would help indicate whether achieving the goals actually heightens SWB. Gordon (1975) compared the importance of various types of resources and examines how the need for these may have developed in childhood. Theoretical work such as this is needed in which various types of goals or needs and their fulfillment are related to various types of SWB. Formulations such as Bentham's law of diminishing marginal utility can be tested empirically in relation to SWB. One limitation to the law of marginal utility is that it seems to apply to some things (e.g., money), but not to others (e.g., skills).

Pleasure and Pain

The idea that gaining goals or needs leads to happiness raises a theme that is found throughout the happiness literature: Pleasure and pain are intimately related. An individual only has goals or needs to the extent that something is missing in that person's life. Thus, most need and goal formulations presume that lack or deprivation is a necessary precursor of happiness. One assumption in these approaches is that the greater the deprivation (and hence unhappiness), the greater the joy upon achieving the goal. The idea that fulfilling needs leads to happiness is the opposite of the idea that having all needs permanently fulfilled will lead to the maximum happiness. According to the present formulation, if an individual's desires and goals are totally fulfilled, it may be impossible to achieve great happiness. Houston (1981) maintained that "our genetic make-up is such that we are probably happiest when we experience deprivation-based need and are able to satisfy that need" (p. 7). Similarly, according to Wilson (1960), "the recurrent needs are cyclical in nature and the most rewarding state of affairs is for the cycles to repeat themselves in a normal and orderly way" (p. 76). From this perspective, it is fortunate that biological desires are self-renewing with time and that a person who achieves goals will often set other goals. However, Wilson (1960) postulated that the maximum fulfillment at all times is most rewarding for sensory and acquired needs.

The idea that pleasure and pain (happiness and unhappiness) are somehow connected is an idea that has been frequently advanced (Tatarkiewicz, 1976). For example, the Italian writer Verri proposed that pleasure is always proceded by distress. There are additional reasons why happiness and unhappiness should be connected. As mentioned earlier, people who experience more intense negative emotions (Diener et al., in press). Another reason that pleasure and pain are connected has to do with psychological investment or involvement with the goal. If a person has an important goal and has worked hard to attain it, failure will produce substantial unhappiness and success will lead to much happiness. If a person has little interest in reaching a goal, failure to achieve it will not bring great unhappiness. In the words of Tatarkiewicz, "if the sources of pleasure are multiplied, so automatically are the sources of pain" (1976, p. 50). Thus, commitment, involvement, and effort seem to raise the intensity of affect that a person will feel.

Another theory that suggests pleasure and pain are intimately connected is the opponent process theory of Solomon (1980). According to this formulation, the loss of something good leads to unhappiness and the loss of something bad leads to happiness. In addition, specific predictions are made about the magnitude of affect. A person will habituate to a good or bad object, and thus it will bring less happiness or unhappiness with repeated exposure. However, the crucial component of the theory is that opposing affect when the object is lost will be greatest after habituation. For example, if an individual was habituated to an automobile and it brought little pleasure and if the automobile was stolen, that person would be more unhappy than he or she would be if the car was new. Note that this is an addiction type of model which states that with repeated exposure, good items lose their power to produce happiness, but after repeated exposure their loss will produce greater unhappiness. Initial studies on this theory of happiness have not been supportive (Sandvik & Diener, 1983).

Activity Theories

Whereas telic theories place the locus of happiness in certain-end states, activity theories maintain that happiness is a by-product of human activity. For example, the activity of climbing a mountain might bring greater happiness than reaching the summit. Aristotle was a major proponent of one of the earliest and most important activity theories. He maintained that happiness comes about through virtuous activity, that is, from activity that is performed well. According to Aristotle's theory, there are certain human abilities, and happiness arises when these are performed in an excellent manner. In contrast, activity theory in modern gerontology refers to activity in more global terms. For example, hobbies, social interaction, and exercise are all considered to be activities.

One frequent theme in activity theories is that self-awareness will decrease happiness, and there is some empirical evidence for this (Csikszentmihalyi & Figurski, 1982). This is consonant with the popular idea that concentrating on gaining happiness may be self-defeating. According to this approach, one should concentrate on important activities and goals, and happiness will come as an unintended by-product. These ideas have not yet been rigorously formulated or empirically tested, although they appear frequently in the literature.

Perhaps the most explicit formulation about activity and SWB is the theory of flow (Csikszentmihalyi, 1975). Activities are seen as pleasurable when the challenge is matched to the person's skill level. If an activity is too easy, boredom will develop; if it is too difficult, anxiety will result. When a person is involved in an activity that demands intense concentration and in which the person's skills and the challenge of the task are roughly equal, a pleasurable flow experience will result. Surgery and mountain climbing are offered as prototypes of this pleasurable experience. People's lives will be happier to the extent that they are involved in interesting and involving activities. Unlike goal theorists, activity theorists propose that happiness arises from behavior rather than from achieving endpoints. However, the two ideas are not necessarily incompatible and thus could possibly be integrated.

Top-Down Versus Bottom-Up Theories

The distinction between bottom-up and top-down approaches is popular in modern psychology, and parallel questions can be found throughout the scholarly history of happiness. For example, some philosophers maintained that happiness is simply the sum of many small pleasures (bottom-up theory). According to this view, when a person judges whether his or her life is happy, some mental calculation is used to sum the momentary pleasures and pains. A happy life in this view is merely an accumulation of happy moments. In philosophy this view is related to Lockean reductionistic or atomistic views (Kozma & Stones, 1980). In contrast, the top-down approach assumes that there is a global propensity to experience things in a positive way, and this propensity influences the momentary interactions an individual has with the world. In other words, a person enjoys pleasures because he or she is happy, not vice versa. In this more Kantian view, causation proceeds from the higher-order elements down through the lower or more elemental levels.

In the top-down approach to happiness, global features of personality are thought to influence the way a person reacts to events. For example, a person with a sanguine temperament might interpret a large number of events as positive. Philosophers have frequently placed the locus of happiness in attitudes, thus suggesting a top-down approach. For example, Democritus maintained "that a happy life does not depend on good fortune or indeed on any external contingencies, but also, and even to a greater extent, on a man's cast of mind.... The important thing is not what a man has, but how he reacts to what he has" (Tatarkiewicz, 1976, p. 29). Andrews and Withey (1974) reported data that supports a top-down approach. In predicting life satisfaction, they found that the type of domain satisfactions that were used as predictors did not matter and that weighting the domains did not produce much better predictions. These findings suggest that satisfaction with the domains may result from rather than cause global life satisfaction. In the bottom-up approach, a person should develop a sunny disposition and sanguine outlook as positive experiences accumulate in the person's life. For example, hedonists counsel that one can be happy if pleasures are carefully selected and accumulated (bottom-up theory).

Although both formulations may be partly true, the challenge is to uncover how top-down or internal factors and bottom-up molecular events interact. Because people react to events as subjectively perceived, some top-down processes must be involved. However, it also appears that certain events are pleasurable to most people, and this suggests that bottom-up principles may also be useful. An understanding is needed of how cognitions and personality factors may be altered by an accumulation of events. It is also necessary to study the process by which a person acquires a sanguine temperament and how resistant this temperament is to change. The interaction of large-scale life events and small daily pleasures in producing long- and short-term happiness requires further research. The top-down and bottom-up dichotomy should serve as a useful device for generating theoretical alternatives and as a heuristic for generating research ideas.

There are two debates in the area of SWB that relate to the bottom-up and top-down distinction. The first debate deals with happiness as a trait or a state. Those who maintain that it is a predisposition or trait suggest that happiness is not happy feelings per se but a propensity to react in a happy way. This top-down approach suggests that a happy person might currently be unhappy. The bottom-up or state approach suggests that a happy person is one with many happy moments. Chekola (1975) has described this as the collection view of happiness because happiness is seen as simply a large collection of happy moments. Happiness can be defined as either a trait or a state, and these will possibly follow different principles.

The second debate concerns the role of pleasant events in creating happiness (Lewinsohn & Amenson, 1978; Lewinsohn & MacPhillamy, 1974). Lewinsohn and his colleagues' contention that a lack of pleasant events leads to depression appears to be a bottom-up approach. However, critics maintain that depression leads to a failure to feel pleasure when engaged in normally pleasant events (Sweeney et al., 1982), and this is a top-down approach. Research is needed to determine whether (or under what conditions) a lack of pleasant events causes or results from depression.

Associationistic Theories

There are a number of models that seek to explain why some individuals have a temperament that is predisposed to happiness. Many of these theories are based on memory, conditioning, or cognitive principles that can be subsumed under the broad rubric of associationistic models. Cognitive approaches to happiness are in their infancy. One cognitive approach rests on the attributions people make about the events happening to them (Schwarz & Clore, 1983). It might be, for example, that good events bring the most happiness if they are attributed to internal, stable factors. Another possibility is that events that are perceived as good lead to happiness, regardless of the attributions made.

One general cognitive approach to happiness has to do with associative networks in memory. Bower (1981) has shown that people will recall memories that are affectively congruent with their current emotional state. Research on memory networks suggests that persons could develop a rich network of positive associations and a more limited and isolated network of negative ones. In such persons, more events or ideas would trigger happy ideas and affect. Thus, a person with such a predominantly positive network would be predisposed to react to more events in a positive way.

A related type of theory is based on a classically conditioned elicitation of affect. Research has shown that affective conditioning can be extremely resistant to extinction. Thus, happy persons might be those who have had very positive affective experiences associated with a large number of frequent everyday stimuli. Zajonc's (1980) contention that affective reactions occur independently of and more rapidly than cognitive evaluation of stimuli is compatible with a conditioning approach to happiness.

Conditioning and memory networks may function without explicit conscious intervention. However, there is some evidence that a person can give conscious direction to the affective associations in his or her life. Fordyce (1977a) offered evidence that a conscious attempt to reduce negative thoughts can increase happiness, and Kammann (1982) found that reciting positive statements in the morning leads to a happier day. Goodhart (in press) has found that positive thinking similar to that recommended by Norman Peale is correlated with SWB. Thus, explicit conscious attempts to avoid unhappy thoughts and to think of happy ones may to some extent increase happiness.

Certain individuals may have built up a strong network of positive associations and learned to react habitually in positive ways. These individuals are perhaps those characterized by philosophers as possessing a happy temperament. A person with a Pollyanna approach to life (Matlin & Stang, 1978) is perhaps the prototype of a person who has formed positive associations to the world. Several studies (Dember & Penwell, 1980; Matlin & Gawron, 1979) have found a relationship between happiness, a cognitive bias toward positive associations, and high Pollyanna personality scores.

An interactional approach could be developed that would integrate the influence of external events and the influence of personality. A person might have associative networks that cause a predisposition to happy reactions. However, although the response to incoming events is biased by these associations, current events could alter the associations over time. In other words, a person's associative networks might be more or less permeable to the influence of new associations.

Judgment Theories

A number of theories postulate that happiness results from a comparison between some standard and actual conditions. If actual conditions exceed the standard, happiness will result. In the case of satisfaction, such comparisons may be conscious.

However, in the case of affect, comparison with a standard may occur in a nonconscious way. Although judgment theories usually do not predict what events will be positive or negative, they do help to predict the magnitude of affect that events will produce.

One way to partition the judgment theories is based on the standard that is used. In social comparison theory, one uses other people as a standard. If a person is better off than others, that person will be satisfied or happy (Carp & Carp, 1982; Emmons et al., 1983; Michalos, 1980). In adaptation (Brickman, Coates, & Janoff-Bulman, 1978) and the range-frequency theory (Parducci, 1968, 1982), a person's past life is used to set the standard. If the individual's current life exceeds this standard, that person will probably be happy. The individual may also acquire a standard in other ways. For example, the individual might aspire to a certain level of attainment based on self-concept or based on what that person is told by his or her parents.

Although standards may come about in different ways according to each theory, in each case they are used as the basis for judging conditions. In social comparison theories, proximal others are usually weighted heavily because of their salience. However, Dermer, Cohen, Jacobsen, and Anderson (1979) demonstrated that even people who are remote in time can be used as a standard of comparison if they are made salient. Seidman and Rapkin (1983) reviewed evidence that suggests social comparison can influence mental health, and Wills (1981) showed that downward comparison with less fortunate persons can increase SWB, Kearl (1981–1982) found that believing others live in poor circumstances can enhance one's life satisfaction. Easterlin (1974) argued persuasively that the amount of income that will satisfy people depends on the income of others in their society. One shortcoming to extant social comparison theories is that they do not make clear when a person will need to make comparisons with others. As Freedman (1978) pointed out, for some things such as sex, social comparison may not be important to happiness because people have an internal standard based upon their own values or needs. However, Emmons et al. (1983) found that social comparison was the strongest predictor of satisfaction in most domains.

Adaptation to events means that when they first occur, events can produce either happiness or unhappiness, depending on whether they are good or bad. However, over time the events lose their power to evoke affect. The person adapts to good conditions so they no longer evoke happiness, and a similar adaptation process occurs for bad events. Adaptation theory is based on a standard derived from an individual's own experience. If current events are better than the standard, the individual will be happy. However, if the good events continue, adaptation will occur; the individual's standard will rise so that it eventually matches the newer events (Brickman & Campbell, 1971). Thus, according to the adaptation theory recent changes produce happiness and unhappiness because a person will eventually adapt to the overall level of events. Therefore, this theory predicts that changes in income and so forth are much more important to happiness than is the average level of the events. An individual's standard will eventually move up or down to any level or circumstance; it is only departures from this level that can produce affect.

Brickman et al. (1978) reported that lottery winners are no happier, and quadriplegics no less happy, than normal controls. They interpreted these findings by suggesting that people adapt to all events, no matter how fortunate or unfortunate. Wortman and Silver (1982) confirmed this conclusion with longitudinal data. They found that spinal cord-injury victims were extremely unhappy after their accidents. However, their affect quickly began moving back toward happiness, suggesting that adaptation was occurring rapidly even to this extreme misfortune. Cameron (1974) and Feinman (1978) also reported evidence indicating that other handicapped groups are as happy as controls. Detailed descriptive longitudinal data on adaptation are needed: How long does it take to adapt, to what conditions do people adapt, and do people completely adapt? What amount of time or accumulation of experiences is included in one's standard, and how are more recent events weighted? The psychological process underlying adaptation also warrants further consideration. It seems unlikely that people will completely adapt to all conditions. Positive factors such as health or income do correlate with SWB. It may be that adaptation reduces, but does not eliminate, the effect of circumstances. Although adaptation seems to be a powerful process, its limits or the parameters that influence it are not well understood.

Parducci (1968) developed a provocative theory of happiness based on laboratory models of human judgment. The range-frequency model predicts a precise standard (based on the person's experience) against which incoming events are judged. In laboratory settings this theory outperforms adaptation level approaches. The model has the most interesting implications for persons who have skewed distributions of life events. It predicts that the greatest happiness will occur for those who have a negatively skewed distribution of events. As explained earlier, the average level of goodness of the events happening to a person does not influence happiness because the person adapts to the events. However, the range-frequency model establishes the standard of comparison point approximately halfway between the midpoint of the range and the median of the events happening to that person. Events above this point will make the person happy. A person with a negatively skewed distribution will be happy a majority of the time because most events will fall above this comparison point. The absolute level of goodness of the events does not matter, but the shape of the distribution is crucial. A positively skewed distribution of events will produce unhappiness a majority of the time. Thus, persons with a few ecstatic moments in their lives may be doomed to unhappiness. As Parducci (1968) noted, "if the best can come only rarely, it is better not to include it in the range of experiences at all" (p. 90). This prediction contradicts the common sense idea that some very happy times can enrich one's life. One strength of the range–frequency theory is that its predictions are very specific and thus testable.

One popular form of judgment theory is aspiration level, which maintains that happiness will depend on the discrepancy in a person's life between actual conditions and aspirations (e.g., Carp & Carp, 1982). McGill (1967) and Wilson (1960) agreed that happiness depends on the ratio of fulfilled desires to total desires. According to this theory, high aspirations are as much a threat to happiness as are bad conditions. As the ancient Cyrenaics noted, no person can be rich whose desires for money can never be met. The level of aspirations presumably comes from an individual's previous experience, goals, and so forth. Easterlin (1974) outlined the dramatic differences in aspirations for income between people in various countries. Recall that Gibbs (1973) attributed the declining happiness of more fortunate blacks in the U.S. to the rising aspirations of this group. Although there is evidence that supports the idea that the discrepancy between actual conditions and the level a person aspires to correlates with happiness, this relationship in general does not appear to be strong (Emmons et al., 1983; Gerrard, Reznikoff, & Riklan, 1982; Kammann, 1982; Wilson, 1960).

One question related to all judgment theories is whether comparisons occur only within domains (e.g., income) or generalize across domains. Dermer et al. (1979) found that comparison did not generalize to all areas. In addition, they found that although making a negative standard salient led to increased satisfaction, it also led to more negative affect. Thus, the positivity of affect did not simply increase as satisfaction judgments rose.

Another question related to judgments theories deals with when each type of comparison takes precedence. For example, when will social comparison be most important, and when will adaptation or one's own prior conditions be more important? The work of Emmons et al. (1983) and Dermer et al. (1979) suggests that social comparison may be important to many satisfaction judgments. However, one's own prior experience may usually have more influence on affect. A final question concerning these theories deals with their limits. Critics have dubbed the social comparison approach to happiness with the appellation, "If everyone has a pain, then mine doesn't hurt." Clearly there must be limits to the influence that comparison to standards can have. Note that judgment theories do not indicate how events come to have a particular hedonic value prior to the judgment, that is, why some events are good and why some are better than others.

Future Directions

It is clear that much work is needed to develop more sophisticated theories of happiness. Not only should factors that affect trait versus state happiness be differentiated, but types of SWB such as joy versus satisfaction may also depend on different processes. Constructs should be more rigorously defined, and falsifiable propositions must be developed. A number of important questions are evident in this review of the theories. These questions can be answered by programmatic research in which there is a continuous interchange between data and theoretical propositions. The limiting conditions of each theoretical approach need to be explored. Extant theories make different predictions in a number of instances, and these represent opportunities for research. Thus far, few theories have received rigorous propositional development or probing empirical analyses. In addition, there has been no attempt to integrate the theories.

References

Adams, D. L. (1969). Analysis of a life satisfaction index. *Journal of Gerontology, 24*, 470–474.

Adams, D. L. (1971). Correlates of satisfaction among the elderly. *The Gerontologist, 11*, 64–68.

Allen-Kee, D. (1980). The relationship of psychological androgyny to self-esteem and life satisfaction in career-oriented and home-oriented women (Doctoral dissertation, University of Southern California, 1980). *Dissertation Abstracts International, 41*, 1479A.

Alston, J. P., Lowe, G. D., & Wrigley, A. (1974). Socio-economic correlates for four dimensions of self-perceived satisfaction, 1972. *Human Organization, 33*, 99–102.

Anderson, M. R. (1977). A study of the relationship between life satisfaction and self-concept, locus of control, satisfaction with primary relationships, and work satisfaction (Doctoral dissertation, Michigan State University, 1977). *Dissertation Abstracts International, 38*, 2638 9A. (University Microfilms No. 77-25,214).

Andrews, F. M., & Inglehart, R. F. (1979). The structure of well-being in nine western societies. *Social Indicators Research, 6*, 73–90.

Andrews, F. M., & Withey, S. B. (1974). Developing measures of perceived life quality: Results from several national surveys. *Social Indicators Research, 1*, 1–26.

Andrews, F. M., & Withey, S. B. (1976). *Social indicators of well-being: America's perception of life quality*. New York: Plenum Press.

Baker, E. K. (1977). Relationship of retirement and satisfaction with life events to locus-of-control (Doctoral dissertation, University of Wisconsin—Madison, 1976). *Dissertation Abstracts International, 37*, 4748B. (University Microfilms No. 76-28, 900)

Barnston, A. G. (1975). *The effect of weather on mood, productivity, and frequency of emotional crisis in a temperate continental climate in early autumn*. Unpublished master's thesis, University of Illinois at Urbana—Champaign.

Barry, H., Jr., & Bousfield, W. A. (1935). A quantitative determination of euphoria and its relation to sleep. *Journal of Abnormal and Social Psychology, 29*, 385–389.

Beiser, M. (1974). Components and correlates of mental well-being. *Journal of Health and Social Behavior, 15*, 320–327.

Bortner, R. W., & Hultsch, D. F. (1970). A multivariate analysis of correlates of life satisfaction in adulthood. *Journal of Gerontology, 25*, 41–47.

Bousfield, W. A. (1938). Further evidence of the relation of the euphoric attitude to sleep and exercise. *Psychological Record, 2*, 334–344.

Bousfield, W. A. (1942). Certain subjective correlates of sleep quality and their relation to the euphoric attitude. *Journal of Applied Psychology, 26*, 487–498.

Bower, G. H. (1981). Mood and memory. *American Psychologist, 36*, 129–148.

Bradburn, N. M. (1969). *The structure of psychological well-being*. Chicago: Aldine.

Bradburn, N. M., & Caplovitz, D. (1965). *Reports on happiness*. Chicago: Aldine.

Brandt, A. S. (1980). Relationship of locus of control, environmental constraint, length of time in the institution and twenty-one other variables to morale and life satisfaction in the institutionalized elderly (Doctoral dissertation, Texas Woman's University, 1979). *Dissertation Abstracts International, 40*, 5802B. (University Microfilms No. 80-12, 153).

Braun, P. M. W. (1977). Psychological well-being and location in the social structure (Doctoral dissertation, University of Southern California, 1976). *Dissertation Abstracts International, 38*, 2351A.

Brenner, B. (1975). Enjoyment as a preventive of depressive affect. *Journal of Community Psychology, 3*, 346–357.

Brickman, P., & Campbell, D. T. (1971). Hedonic relativism and planning the good society. In M. H. Appley (Ed.), *Adaptation level theory: A symposium* (pp. 287–302). New York: Academic Press.

Brickman, P., Coates, D., & Janoff-Bulman, R. (1978). Lottery winners and accident victims: Is happiness relative? *Journal of Personality and Social Psychology, 36*, 917–927.

Bryant, F. B., & Veroff, J. (1982). The structure of psychological well-being: A sociohistorical analysis. *Journal of Personality and Social Psychology, 43*, 653–673.

Bull, C. N., & Aucoin, J. B. (1975). Voluntary association participation and life satisfaction: A replication note. *Journal of Gerontology, 30*, 73–76.

Bultena, G. L., & Oyler, R. (1971). Effects of health on disengagement and morale. *Aging and Human Development, 2*, 142–148.

Cameron, P. (1974). Social stereotypes: Three faces of happiness. *Psychology Today, 8*, 63–64.

Cameron, P. (1975). Mood as an indicant of happiness: Age, sex, social class, and situational differences. *Journal of Gerontology, 30*, 216–224.

Cameron, P., Titus, D. G., Kostin, J., & Kostin, M. (1973). The life satisfaction of nonnormal persons. *Journal of Consulting and Clinical Psychology, 41*, 207–214.

Campbell, A. (1976). Subjective measures of well-being. *American Psychologist, 31*, 117–124.

Campbell, A. (1981). *The sense of well-being in America: Recent patterns and trends.* New York: McGraw-Hill.

Campbell, A., Converse, P. E., & Rodgers, W. L. (1976). *The quality of American life.* New York: Russell Sage Foundation.

Cantril, H. (1965). *The pattern of human concerns.* New Brunswick, NJ: Rutgers University Press.

Carp, F. M., & Carp, A. (1982). Test of a model of domain satisfactions and well-being: Equity considerations. *Research on Aging, 4*, 503–522.

Catalano, R., & Dooley, C. D. (1977). Economic predictors of depressed mood and stressful life events in a metropolitan community. *Journal of Health and Social Behavior, 18*, 292–307.

Chekola, M. G. (1975). The concept of happiness (Doctoral dissertation, University of Michigan, 1974). *Dissertation Abstracts International, 35*, 4609A. (University Microfilms No. 75–655).

Cherlin, A., & Reeder, L. G. (1975). The dimensions of psychological well-being: A critical review. *Sociological Methods and Research, 4*, 189–214.

Clemente, F., & Sauer, W. J. (1976a). Life satisfaction in the United States. *Social Forces, 54*, 621–631.

Clemente, F., & Sauer, W. J. (1976b). Racial differences in life satisfaction. *Journal of Black Studies, 7*, 3–10.

Coan, R. W. (1977). *Hero, artist, sage, or saint?* New York: Columbia University.

Cohn, R. M. (1979). Age and the satisfactions from work. *Journal of Gerontology, 34*, 264–272.

Conte, V. C., & Salamon, M. J. (1982). An objective approach to the measurement and use of life satisfaction with older persons. *Measurement and Evaluation in Guidance, 15*, 194–200.

Costa, P. T., & McCrae, R. R. (1980). Influence of extraversion and neuroticism on subjective well-being: Happy and unhappy people. *Journal of Personality and Social Psychology, 38*, 668–678.

Csikszentmihalyi, M. (1975). *Beyond boredom and anxiety.* San Francisco: Jossey-Bass.

Csikszentmihalyi, M., & Figurski, T. J. (1982). Self-awareness and aversive experience in everyday life. *Journal of Personality, 50*, 15–24.

Culberson, C. E. (1977). A holistic view of joy in relation to psychotherapy derived from Lowen, Maslow, and Assagioli (Doctoral dissertation, California School of Professional Psychology, 1977). *Dissertation Abstracts International, 38*, 2853B. (University Microfilms No. 77–27, 591)

Cumming, E., Dean, L. R., & Newell, D. S. (1958). What is "morale"? A case history of a validity problem. *Human Organization, 17*, 3–8.

Cutler, S. J. (1973). Voluntary association participation and life satisfaction: A cautionary research note. *Journal of Gerontology, 28*, 96–100.

Cutler, S. J. (1976). Membership in different types of voluntary associations and psychological well-being. *The Gerontologist, 16*, 335–339.

Cutler, N. E. (1979). Age variations in the dimensionality of life satisfaction. *Journal of Gerontology, 34*, 573–578.

Czaja, S. J. (1975). Age differences in life satisfaction as a function of discrepancy between real and ideal self-concepts. *Experimental Aging Research, 1*, 81–89.

DeGuire, K. S. (1974). Activity choice, psychological functioning, degree of satisfaction, and personality factors in educated, middle-aged women (Doctoral dissertation, Fordham University,

1974). *Dissertation Abstracts International, 35*, 2424B. (University Microfilms No. 74–25, 045).

Dember, W. N., & Penwell, L. (1980). Happiness, depression, and the Pollyanna principle. *Bulletin of the Psychonomic Society, 15*, 321–323.

Dermer, M., Cohen, S. J., Jacobsen, E., & Anderson, E. A. (1979). Evaluative judgments of aspects of life as a function of vicarious exposure to hedonic extremes. *Journal of Personality and Social Psychology, 37*, 247–260.

Dicken, P., & Lloyd, P. E. (1981). *Modern western society: A geographical perspective on work, home and well-being*. London: Harper & Row.

Diener, E., & Emmons, R. A. (in press). The independence of positive and negative affect. *Journal of Personality and Social Psychology*.

Diener, E., Emmons, R., Larsen, R., & Griffin, S. (1983). *The Satisfaction with Life scale*. Manuscript submitted for publication, University of Illinois at Urbana—Champaign.

Diener, E., & Griffin, S. (in press). Happiness and life satisfaction: Bibliography. *Psychological Documents*.

Diener, E., & Larsen, R. J. (in press). Temporal stability and cross-situational consistency of positive and negative affect. *Journal of Personality and Social Psychology*.

Diener, E., Larsen, R. J., & Emmons, R. A. (in press). Person × situation interactions: Choice of situations and congruence response models. *Journal of Personality and Social Psychology*.

Diener, E., Larsen, R. J., Levine, S., & Emmons, R. A. (in press). Frequency and intensity: The underlying dimensions of positive and negative affect. *Journal of Personality and Social Psychology*.

Dixon, L. K., & Johnson, R. C. (1980). *The roots of individuality: A survey of human behavior genetics*. Monterey, CA: Brooks/Cole.

Dobson, C., Powers, E. A., Keith, P. M., & Goudy, W. J. (1979). Anomia, self-esteem, and life satisfaction: Interrelationships among three scales of well-being. *Journal of Gerontology, 34*, 569–572.

Drumgoole, W. P. (1981). Self-concept and life satisfaction as perceived by young, middle-aged, and senior adults (Doctoral dissertation, East Texas State University, 1980). *Dissertation Abstracts International, 41*, 2939A. (University Microfilms No. 80–27, 666).

Dupuy, H. J. (1978). *The research edition of the general psychological well-being schedule*. Unpublished manuscript.

Easterlin, R. A. (1974). Does economic growth improve the human lot? Some empirical evidence. In P. A. David & M. W. Reder (Eds.), *Nations and households in economic growth* (pp. 89–125). New York: Academic Press.

Edwards, N. J., & Klemmack, D. L. (1973). Correlates of life satisfaction: A re-examination. *Journal of Gerontology, 28*, 497–502.

Eisenberg, D. M. (1981). Autonomy, health and life satisfaction among older persons in a life care community (Doctoral dissertation, Bryn Mawr College, 1980). *Dissertation Abstracts International, 41*, 3724A. (University Microfilms No. 81–03, 906).

Emmons, R. A., & Diener, E. (1983). *Influence of impulsivity and sociability on positive and negative affect*. Manuscript submitted for publication, University of Illinois at Champaign—Urbana.

Emmons, R. A., Larsen, R. J., Levine, S., & Diener, E. (1983, May). *Factors predicting satisfaction judgments*. Paper presented at the meeting of the Midwestern Psychological Association Convention, Chicago.

Estes, R. J., & Wilensky, H. L. (1978). Life cycle squeeze and the morale curve. *Social Problems, 25*, 277–292.

Falkman, P. W. (1973). Objective, subjective and continuity correlates of life satisfaction in an elderly population (Doctoral dissertation, Iowa State University, 1972). *Dissertation Abstracts International, 33*, 4556–7A. (University Microfilms No. 73–3880).

Feinman, S. (1978). The blind as "ordinary people." *Journal of Visual Impairment and Blindness, 72*, 231–238.

Fellows, E. W. (1956). A study of factors related to a feeling of happiness. *Journal of Educational Research, 50*, 231–234.

Felton, B., & Kahana, E. (1974). Adjustment and situationally bound locus of control among institutionalized aged. *Journal of Gerontology, 29*, 295–301.

Fordyce, M. W. (1977a). Development of a program to increase personal happiness. *Journal of Counseling Psychology, 24*, 511–521.

Fordyce, M. W. (1977b). *The Happiness Measures: A sixty second index of emotional well-being and mental health.* Unpublished manuscript, Edison Community College, Ft. Myers, Florida.

Fordyce, M. W. (1978). *Prospectus: The self-description inventory.* Unpublished manuscript, Edison Community College, Ft. Myers, Florida.

Fordyce, M. W. (1983). A program to increase happiness: Further studies. *Journal of Counseling Psychology, 30*, 483–498.

Forrester, N. G. (1980). Factors contributing to life satisfaction of divorced women (Doctoral dissertation, Arizona State University, 1980). *Dissertation Abstracts International, 41*, 1401A. (University Microfilms No. 80–21,663)

Freedman, J. (1978). *Happy people: What happiness is, who has it, and why.* New York: Harcourt Brace Jovanovich.

Freudiger, P. T. (1980). Life satisfaction among American women (Doctoral dissertation, North Texas State University, 1979). *Dissertation Abstracts International, 40*, 6438A. (University Microfilms No. 80–12,882).

Gallup, G. H. (1976–1977). Human needs and satisfactions: A global survey. *Public Opinion Quarterly, 40*, 459–467.

George, L. K. (1979). The happiness syndrome: Methodological and substantive issues in the study of social psychological well-being in adulthood. *The Gerontologist, 19*, 210–216.

George, L. K., & Bearon, L. B. (1980). *Quality of life in older persons: Meaning and measurement.* New York: Human Sciences Press.

Gerrard, C. K., Reznikoff, M., & Riklan, M. (1982). Level of aspiration, life satisfaction and locus of control in older adults. *Experimental Aging Research, 8*, 119–121.

Gershon, E. S., Bunney, W. E., Lecksman, J. F., Van Erwegh, M., & DeBauche, B. A. (1976). The inheritance of affective disorders: A review of data and hypotheses. *Behavior Genetics, 6*, 227–261.

Gibbs, B. A. M. (1973). Relative deprivation and selfreported happiness of blacks: 1946–1966 (Doctoral dissertation, The University of Texas, 1972). *Dissertation Abstracts International, 34*, 885A. (University Microfilms No. 73–18,429).

Ginandes, C. S. (1977). Life satisfaction and self-esteem values in men of four different socioeconomic groups (Doctoral dissertation, Boston University, 1977. *Dissertation Abstracts International, 38*, 1880B. (University Microfilms No. 77–21,590).

Glenn, N. D. (1975). The contribution of marriage to the psychological well-being of males and females. *Journal of Marriage and the Family, 37*, 594–600.

Glenn, N. D. (1981). The well-being of persons remarried after divorce. *Journal of Family Issues, 2*, 61–75.

Glenn, N. D., & McLanahan, S. (1981). The effects of offspring on the psychological well-being of older adults. *Journal of Marriage and the Family, 43*, 138–150.

Glenn, N. D., & Weaver, C. N. (1979). A note on family situation and global happiness. *Social Forces, 57*, 960–967.

Glenn, N. D., & Weaver, C. N. (1981a). The contribution of marital happiness to global happiness. *Journal of Marriage and the Family, 43*, 161–168.

Glenn, N. D., & Weaver, C. N. (1981b). Education's effects on psychological well-being. *Public Opinion Quarterly, 45*, 22–39.

Goodhart, D. (in press). Some psychological effects associated with positive and negative thinking about stressful event outcomes: Was Pollyanna right? *Journal of Personality and Social Psychology.*

Goodstein, J., Zautra, A., & Goodhart, D. (1982). A test of the utility of social indicators for behavioral health service planning. *Social Indicators Research, 10*, 273–295.

Gordon, R. M. (1975). The effects of interpersonal and economic resources upon values and the quality of life (Doctoral dissertation, Temple University, 1975). *Dissertation Abstracts International, 36,* 3122B. (University Microfilms No. 75–28, 220).

Gorman, B. S. (1972). A multivariate study of the relationships of cognitive control and cognitive style principles to reported daily mood experiences. (Doctoral dissertation, City University of New York, 1971). *Dissertation Abstracts International, 32,* 4211B. (University Microfilms, No. 72–5071).

Graney, M. J. (1975). Happiness and social participation in aging. *Journal of Gerontology, 30,* 701–706.

Gurin, G., Veroff, J., & Feld, S. (1960). *Americans view their mental health.* New York: Basic Books.

Guttmann, D. (1978). Life events and decision making by older adults. *The Gerontologist, 18,* 462–467.

Hadaway, C. K. (1978). Life satisfaction and religion: A re-analysis. *Social Forces, 57,* 636–643.

Harding, S. D. (1982). Psychological well-being in Great Britain: An evaluation of the Bradburn Affect Balance Scale. *Personality and Individual Differences, 3,* 167–175.

Harry, J. (1976). Evolving sources of happiness for men over the life cycle: A structural analysis. *Journal of Marriage and the Family, 38,* 289–296.

Hartmann, G. W. (1934). Personality traits associated with variations in happiness, *Journal of Abnormal and Social Psychology, 29,* 202–212.

Hasak, P. A. (1978). Relationships among decentration, personality, and life satisfaction in the elderly (Doctoral dissertation, University of Kentucky, 1977). *Dissertation Abstracts International, 39,* 2986B. (University Microfilms No. 78–24, 397).

Higgins, D. H. (1978). Self-concept and its relation to everyday stress in middle-aged women: A longitudinal study (Doctoral dissertation, Illinois Institute of Technology, 1977). *Dissertation Abstracts International, 38,* 4537B. (University Microfilms No. 78–00,865).

Houston, J. P. (1981). *The pursuit of happiness.* Glenview, IL: Scott, Foresman.

Hoyt, D. R., & Creech, J. C. (1983). The Life Satisfaction Index: Methodological and theoretical critique. *Journal of Gerontology, 38,* 111–116.

Hoyt, D. R., Kaiser, M. A., Peters, G. R., & Babchuk, N. (1980). Life satisfaction and activity theory: A multidimensional approach. *Journal of Gerontology, 35,* 935–941.

Jasper, H. H. (1930). The measurement of depressionelation and its relation to a measure of extraversion–introversion. *Journal of Abnormal and Social Psychology, 25,* 307–318.

Jones, H. M. (1953). *The pursuit of happiness.* Cambridge, MA: Harvard University Press.

Joshi, B. L. (1964). Personality correlates of happiness (Doctoral dissertation, University of California, Berkeley, 1964). *Dissertation Abstracts, 25,* 2083. (University Microfilms No. 64–9039).

Kammann, R. (1982, August). *Personal circumstances and life events as poor predictors of happiness.* Paper presented at the 90th Annual Convention of the American Psychological Association, Washington, DC.

Kammann, R. (1983). Objective circumstances, life satisfactions and sense of well-being: Consistencies across time and place. *New Zealand Psychologist, 12,* 14–22.

Kammann, R., & Campbell, K. (1982). Illusory correlation in popular beliefs about the causes of happiness. *New Zealand Psychologist, 11,* 52–62.

Kammann, R., Christie, D., Irwin, R., & Dixon, G. (1979). Properties of an inventory to measure happiness (and psychological health). *New Zealand Psychologist, 8,* 1–9.

Kammann, R., Farry, M., & Herbison, P. (1982). *The analysis and measurement of the sense of well-being.* Manuscript submitted for publication, University of Otago, New Zealand.

Kammann, R., & Flett, R. (1983). Affectometer 2: A scale to measure current level of general happiness. *Australian Journal of Psychology, 35,* 257–265.

Kearl, M. C. (1981–1982). An inquiry into the positive personal and social effects of old age stereotypes among the elderly. *International Journal of Aging and Human Development, 14,* 277–290.

Kimmel, D. C., Price, K. F., & Walker, J. W. (1978). Retirement choice and retirement satisfaction. *Journal of Gerontology, 33*, 575–585.

Klemmack, D. L., Carlson, J. R., & Edwards, J. N. (1974). Measures of well-being: An empirical and critical assessment. *Journal of Health and Social Behavior, 15*, 267–270.

Knapp, M. R. J. (1976). Predicting the dimensions of life satisfaction. *Journal of Gerontology, 31*, 595–604.

Knippa, W. B. (1979). The relationship of antecedent and personality variables to the life satisfaction of retired military officers (Doctoral dissertation, University of Texas at Austin, 1979). *Dissertation Abstracts International, 40*, 1360A. (University Microfilms No. 79–20,146).

Kozma, A., & Stones, M. J. (1978). Some research issues and findings in the study of psychological well-being in the aged. *Canadian Psychological Review, 19*, 241–249.

Kozma, A., & Stones, M. J. (1980). The measurement of happiness: Development of the Memorial University of Newfoundland Scale of Happiness (MUNSH). *Journal of Gerontology, 35*, 906–912.

Kozma, A., & Stones, M. J. (1982). *Predictors of happiness.* Unpublished manuscript, Memorial University of Newfoundland.

Kozma, A., & Stones, M. J. (1983). *Rater bias in the assessment of happiness.* Unpublished manuscript, Memorial University of Newfoundland.

Kuhlen, R. G. (1948). Age trends in adjustment during the adult years as reflected in happiness ratings. *American Psychologist, 3*, 307.

Kushman, J., & Lane, S. (1980). A multivariate analysis of factors affecting perceived life satisfaction and psychological well-being among the elderly. *Social Science Quarterly, 61*, 264–277.

Larsen, R. J. (1983). *Manual for the Affect Intensity Measure.* Unpublished manuscript, University of Illinois at Champaign—Urbana.

Larsen, R. J., Diener, E., & Emmons, R. A. (1983a). *An evaluation of subjective well-being measures.* Manuscript submitted for publication, University of Illinois at Champaign—Urbana.

Larsen, R. J., Diener, E., & Emmons, R. A. (1983b). *Affect intensity and reactions to daily life events.* Manuscript submitted for publication, University of Illinois at Champaign—Urbana.

Larsen, R. J., Emmons, R. A., & Diener, E. (1983, May). *Validity and meaning of measures of subjective well-being.* Paper presented at the Midwestern Psychological Association Convention, Chicago.

Larson, R. (1978). Thirty years of research on the subjective well-being of older Americans. *Journal of Gerontology, 33*, 109–125.

Lawler, E. E., & Suttle, J. L. (1972). A causal correlational test of the need hierarchy concept. *Organizational Behavior and Human Performance, 7*, 265–278.

Lawton, M. P. (1972). The dimensions of morale. In D. P. Kent, R. Kastenbaum, & S. Sherwood (Eds.), *Research, planning and action for the elderly* (pp. 144–165). New York: Behavioral Publications.

Lawton, M. P. (1975). The Philadelphia Geriatric Center Morale Scale: A revision. *Journal of Gerontology, 30*, 85–89.

Laxer, R. M. (1964). Relation of real self-rating to mood and blame, and their interaction in depression. *Journal of Consulting Psychology, 28*, 538–546.

Lemon, B. W., Bengston, V. L., & Peterson, J. A. (1972). An exploration of the activity theory of aging: Activity types and life satisfaction among in-movers to a retirement community. *Journal of Gerontology, 27*, 511–523.

Lewinsohn, P. M., & Amenson, C. S. (1978). Some relations between pleasant and unpleasant events and depression. *Journal of Abnormal Psychology, 87*, 644–654.

Lewinsohn, P. M., & MacPhillamy, D. J. (1974). The relationship between age and engagement in pleasant activities. *Journal of Gerontology, 29*, 290–294.

Liang, J., Kahana, E., & Doherty, E. (1980). Financial well-being among the aged: A further elaboration. *Journal of Gerontology, 35*, 409–420.

Lohmann, N. L. P. (1977). Comparison of life satisfaction, morale and adjustment scales on an elderly population (Doctoral dissertation, Brandeis University, 1977). *Dissertation Abstracts International, 38*, 418B. (University Microfilms No. 77–15,272).

London, M., Crandall, R., & Seals, G. W. (1977). The contribution of job and leisure satisfaction to quality of life. *Journal of Applied Psychology, 62*, 328–334.

Maddox, G. L. (1963). Activity and morale: A longitudinal study of selected elderly subjects. *Social Forces, 42*, 195–204.

Mancini, J. A., & Orthner, D. K. (1980). Situational influences on leisure satisfaction and morale in old age. *Journal of the American Geriatrics Society, 28*, 466–471.

Markides, K. S., & Martin, H. W. (1979). A causal model of life satisfaction among the elderly. *Journal of Gerontology, 34*, 86–93.

Mathes, E. W., & Kahn, A. (1975). Physical attractiveness, happiness, neuroticism and self-esteem. *Journal of Psychology, 90*, 27–30.

Matlin, M. W., & Gawron, V. J. (1979). Individual differences in Pollyannaism. *Journal of Personality Assessment, 43*, 411–412.

Matlin, M. W., & Stang, D. (1978). *The Pollyanna principle*. Cambridge, MA: Schenkman.

McGill, V. J. (1967). *The idea of happiness*. New York: Praeger.

McClure, R. F., & Loden, M. (1982). Religious activity, denomination membership and life satisfaction. *Psychology, A Quarterly Journal of Human Behavior, 19*, 12–17.

McKennell, A. (1974). Surveying subjective welfare: Strategies and methodological considerations. In B. Strumpel (Ed.), *Subjective elements of well-being* (pp. 45–72). Paris: Organization for Economic Development and Cooperation.

Medley, M. L. (1980). Life satisfaction across four stages of adult life. *International Journal of Aging and Human Development, 11*, 193–209.

Messer, M. (1968). Race differences in selected attitudinal dimensions of the elderly. *The Gerontologist, 8*, 245–249.

Michalos, A. C. (1980). Satisfaction and happiness. *Social Indicators Research, 8*, 385–422.

Miller, M. L. (1980). Adaptation and life satisfaction of the elderly (Doctoral dissertation, Boston College, 1980). *Dissertation Abstracts International, 41*, 7367B. (University Microfilms No. 80–16,611).

Mitchell, R. M. (1976). Paths to happiness: residence locality and interpersonal relationships (Doctoral dissertation, University of Notre Dame, 1976). *Dissertation Abstracts International, 37*, 3944A. (University Microfilms No. 76–27,291).

Morawetz, D. (1977). Income distribution and self-rated happiness: Some empirical evidence. *The Economic Journal, 87*, 511–522.

Morganti, J. B., Nehrke, M. F., & Hulicka, I. M. (1980). Resident and staff perceptions of latitude of choice in elderly institutionalized men. *Experimental Aging Research, 6*, 367–384.

Moriwaki, S. Y. (1974). The Affect Balance Scale: A validity study with aged samples. *Journal of Gerontology, 29*, 73–78.

Morris, A. F., & Husman, B. F. (1978). Life quality changes following and endurance conditioning program. *American Correctional Therapy Journal, 32*, 3–6.

Morris, J. N., & Sherwood, S. (1975). A retesting and modification of the Philadelphia Geriatric Center Morale Scale. *Journal of Gerontology, 30*, 77–84.

Natale, M., & Hantas, M. (1982). Effect of temporary mood states on selective memory about the self. *Journal of Personality and Social Psychology, 42*, 927–934.

Near, J. P., Rice, R. W., & Hunt, R. G. (1978). Work and extra-work correlates of life and job satisfaction. *Academy of Management Journal, 21*, 248–264.

Near, J. P., Rice, R. W., & Hunt, R. G. (1980). The relationship between work and nonwork domains: A review of empirical research. *Academy of Management Review, 5*, 415–429.

Neugarten, B. L., Havighurst, R. J., & Tobin, S. S. (1961). The measurement of life satisfaction, *Journal of Gerontology, 16*, 134–143.

Noberini, M. R. (1977). Adaptive behavior in middle-aged women: A follow-up study (Doctoral dissertation, University of Chicago, 1976). [*Dissertation Abstracts International, 38*, 881B. Maryland, 1979).] *Dissertation Abstracts International, 40*, 5211A. (University Microfilms No. 80–07,107).

Okun, M. A., Stock, W. A., Haring, M. J., & Witter, R. A. (in press-a). Health and subjective well-being: A meta-analysis. *Journal of Aging and Human Development.*

Okun, M. A., Stock, W. A., Haring, M. J., & Witter, R. A. (in press-b). A quantitative synthesis of the social activity/subjective well-being relationship. *Research on Aging.*

Olsen, J. K. (1980). The effect of change in activity in voluntary associations on life satisfaction among people 60 and over who have been active through time (Doctoral dissertation, University of Maryland, 1979). *Dissertation Abstracts International, 40,* 5211A. (University Microfilms No. 80–07,107).

O'Sullivan, W. M. (1980). A study of the relationship between life satisfaction of the aged and perceptions they hold concerning their own masculinity or femininity (Doctoral dissertation, New York University, 1980). *Dissertation Abstracts International, 41,* 6745B. (University Microfilms No. 80–17,520).

Paintal, H. K. (1978). A correlational study of the three tools for measuring successful aging. *Indian Journal of Clinical Psychology, 5,* 69–76.

Palmore, E. (1979). Predictors of successful aging. *The Gerontologist, 19,* 427–431.

Palmore, E., & Kivett, V. (1977). Change in life satisfaction: A longitudinal study of persons aged 46–70. *Journal of Gerontology, 32,* 311–316.

Palmore, E., & Luikart, C. (1972). Health and social factors related to life satisfaction. *Journal of Health and Social Behavior, 13,* 68–80.

Palys, T. S., & Little, B. R. (1983). Perceived life satisfaction and the organization of personal projects systems. *Journal of Personality and Social Psychology, 44,* 1221–1230.

Parducci, A. (1968). The relativism of absolute judgements. *Scientific American, 219,* 84–90.

Parducci, A. (1982, August). *Toward a relational theory of happiness.* Paper presented at the 90th Annual Convention of the American Psychological Association, Washington, DC.

Perry, G., & Warr, P. (1980). The measurement of mothers' work attitudes. *Journal of Occupational Psychology, 53,* 245–252.

Peterson, J. L. (1975). Personality effects of self-esteem, need motivation, and locus of control on the life satisfaction of older black adults (Doctoral dissertation, University of Michigan, 1974). *Dissertation Abstracts International, 35,* 5700B. (University Microfilms No. 75–10,256).

Phillips, D. L. (1967). Social participation and happiness. *American Journal of Sociology, 72,* 479–488.

Pierce, J. R. (1981). The relationship between continuing education and life satisfaction in older adults (Doctoral dissertation, Georgia State University, 1980). *Dissertation Abstracts International, 41,* 3909A. (University Microfilms No. 81–06, 835).

Pomerantz, S. C. (1978). Adolescent identity, self-esteem, and physical self-satisfaction as a function of age and sex: Do they predict satisfaction with one's social milieu? (Doctoral dissertation, Temple University, 1978). *Dissertation Abstracts International, 39,* 961B. (University Microfilms No. 78–12, 191).

Ray, R. O. (1979). Life satisfaction and activity involvement: Implications for leisure service. *Journal of Leisure Research, 11,* 112–119.

Reffruschini, J. O. (1978). Some multi-dimensional and value aspects of happiness (Doctoral dissertation, University of Arizona, 1978). *Dissertation Abstracts International, 39,* 2479B. (University Microfilms No. 78–20, 402).

Reich, J. W., & Zautra, A. (1981). Life events and personal causation: Some relationships with satisfaction and distress. *Journal of Personality and Social Psychology, 41,* 1002–1012.

Reich, J. W., & Zautra, A. (1983). Demands and desires in daily life: Some influences on well-being. *American Journal of Community Psychology, 11,* 41–58.

Reid, D. W., & Ziegler, M. (1977). A survey of the reinforcements and activities elderly citizens feel are important for their general happiness. *Essence, 2,* 5–24.

Reid, D. W., & Ziegler, M. (1980). Validity and stability of a new desired control measure pertaining to psychological adjustment of the elderly. *Journal of Gerontology, 35,* 395–402.

Rhodes, A. A. (1980). The correlates of life satisfaction in a sample of older Americans from a rural area (Doctoral dissertation, University of Arkansas, 1980). *Dissertation Abstracts International, 41,* 1958–9A. (University Microfilms No. 80–26, 072).

Rice, R. W., Near, J. P., & Hunt, R. G. (1979). Unique variance in job and life satisfaction associated with workrelated and extra-workplace variables. *Human Relations, 32,* 605–623.

Rice, R. W., Near, J. P., & Hunt, R. G. (1980). The job satisfaction/life satisfaction relationship: A review of empirical research. *Basic and Applied Social Psychology, 1*, 37–64.

Riddick, C. C. (1980). The life satisfaction of retired and employed older women: A re-examination of the disengagement theory (Doctoral dissertation, Pennsylvania State University, 1980). *Dissertation Abstracts International, 41*, 2327A. (University Microfilms No. 80–24, 483).

Roth, T., Kramer, M., & Roehrs, T. (1976). Mood before and after sleep. *The Psychiatric Journal of the University of Ottawa, 1*, 123–127.

Rux, J. M. (1977). Widows and widowers: Instrumental skills, socio-economic status, and life satisfaction (Doctoral dissertation, Pennsylvania State University, 1976). *Dissertation Abstracts International, 37*, 7352A. (University Microfilms No. 77–09, 724).

Sandvik, E., & Diener, E. (1983). *An evaluation of an opponent process theory of happiness.* Manuscript submitted for publication, University of Illinois at Champaign—Urbana.

Sauer, W. (1977). Morale of the urban aged: A regression analysis by race. *Journal of Gerontology, 32*, 600–608.

Schaffer, N. G. (1977). The influence of activity level, personality traits, and social-demographic variables on life satisfaction in elderly women (Doctoral dissertation, Catholic University of America, 1977). *Dissertation Abstracts International, 37*, 5845B. (University Microfilms No. 77–11,042).

Schneider, M. (1975). The quality of life in large American cities: Objective and subjective social indicators. *Social Indicators Research, 1*, 495–509.

Schwarz, N., & Clore, G. L. (1983). Mood, misattribution, and judgments of well-being: Informative and directive functions of affective states. *Journal of Personality and Social Psychology, 45*, 513–523.

Scitovsky, T. (1976). *The joyless economy.* Oxford: Oxford University Press.

Seidman, E., & Rapkin, B. (1983). Economics and psychosocial dysfunction: Toward a conceptual framework and prevention strategies. In R. D. Felner, L. A. Jason, J. N. Moritsugu, & S. S. Farber (Eds.), *Preventive psychology* (pp. 175–198). New York: Pergamon Press.

Sherman, L. K. G. (1980). The correlates of happiness in post-separation adjustment (Doctoral dissertation, University of Oregon, 1979). *Dissertation Abstracts International, 40*, 5022B. (University Microfilms No. 80–05,800).

Shin, D. C., & Johnson, D. M. (1978). Avowed happiness as an overall assessment of the quality of life. *Social Indicators Research, 5*, 475–492.

Sigelman, L. (1981). Is ignorance bliss? A reconsideration of the folk wisdom. *Human Relations, 34*, 965–974.

Silver, M. (1980). Money and happiness? Towards "eudaimonology." *Kyklos, 33*, 157–160.

Smith, H. C. (1961). *Personality adjustment.* New York: McGraw-Hill.

Smith, T. W. (1979). Happiness: Time trends, seasonal variations, intersurvey differences, and other mysteries. *Social Psychology Quarterly, 42*, 18–30.

Smith, K. J., & Lipman, A. (1972). Constraint and life satisfaction. *Journal of Gerontology, 27*, 77–82.

Solomon, R. L. (1980). The opponent-process theory of acquired motivation: The costs of pleasure and the benefits of pain. *American Psychologist, 35*, 691–712.

Solomowitz, N. (1979). Life styles, life satisfaction and ego development in late adulthood (Doctoral dissertation, University of Kentucky, 1979). *Dissertation Abstracts International, 40*, 2857B. (University Microfilms No. 79–27, 719).

Spreitzer, E., & Snyder, E. E. (1974). Correlates of life satisfaction among the aged. *Journal of Gerontology, 29*, 454–458.

Springer, N. N., & Roslow, S. A. (1935). A study in the estimation of feelings. *Journal of Applied Psychology, 19*, 379–384.

Stock, W., Okun, M., Stock, S., Haring, M., & Witter, R. A. (1982, August). *Reporting reliability: A case study of life satisfaction research.* Paper presented at the 90th Annual Convention of the American Psychological Association, Washington, DC.

Stock, W. A., Okun, M. A., Haring, M. J., & Witter, R. A. (1983). Age and subjective well-being: A metanalysis. In R. J. Light (Ed.), *Evaluation studies: Review annual* (Vol. 8, pp. 279–302). Beverly Hills, CA: Sage.

Suchman, E., Phillips, B., & Strieb, G. (1958). An analysis of the validity of health questionnaires. *Social Forces, 36*, 223–232.

Sudman, S., Greeley, A. M., & Pinto, L. J. (1967). The use of self-administered questionnaires. In S. Sudman (Ed.), *Reducing the cost of surveys* (pp. 46–57). Chicago: Aldine.

Sundre, D. L. (1978). *The relationship between happiness and internal–external locus of control.* Unpublished master's thesis, California State University, Chico.

Sweeney, P. D., Schaeffer, D. E., & Golin, S. (1982). Pleasant events, unpleasant events, and depression. *Journal of Personality and Social Psychology, 43*, 136–144.

Tatarkiewicz, W. (1976). *Analysis of happiness.* The Hague, Netherlands: Martinus Nijhoff.

Tellegen, A. (1979). *Differential Personality Questionnaire.* Unpublished manuscript, University of Minnesota.

Tolor, A. (1978). Personality correlates of the joy of life. *Journal of Clinical Psychology, 34*, 671–676.

Toseland, R., & Rasch, J. (1979–1980). Correlates of life satisfaction: An AID analysis. *International Journal of Aging and Human Development, 10*, 203–211.

Tredway, V. A. (1978). Mood and exercise in older adults (Doctoral dissertation, University of Southern California, 1978). *Dissertation Abstracts International, 39*, 2531B.

Underwood, B., & Framing, W. J. (1980). The mood survey: A personality measure of happy and sad moods. *Journal of Personality Assessment, 44*, 404–414.

Usui, W. M., Keil, T. J., & Phillips, D. C. (1983). Determinants of life satisfaction: A note on a race-interaction hypothesis. *Journal of Gerontology, 38*, 107–110.

VanCoevering, V. G. R. (1974). An exploratory study of middle-aged and older widows to investigate those variables that differentiate high and low life satisfaction (Doctoral dissertation, Wayne State University, 1973). *Dissertation Abstracts International, 34*, 3895A. (University Microfilms No. 73–31, 788).

Wahba, M. A., & Bridwell, L. G. (1976). Maslow reconsidered: A review of research on the need hierarchy theory. *Organizational Behavior and Human Performance, 15*, 212–240.

Warr, P. (1978). A study of psychological well-being. *British Journal of Psychology, 69*, 111–121.

Warr, P., Barter, J., & Brownbridge, G. (1983). On the independence of negative and positive affect. *Journal of Personality and Social Psychology, 44*, 644–651.

Washburne, J. N. (1941). Factors related to the social adjustment of college girls. *Journal of Social Psychology, 13*, 281–289.

Watson, G. (1930). Happiness among adult students of education. *The Journal of Educational Psychology, 21*, 79–109.

Weaver, C. N. (1978). Job satisfaction as a component of happiness among males and females. *Personnel Psychology, 31*, 831–840.

Weinstein, L. (1982). Positive contrast as due to happiness. *Bulletin of the Psychonomic Society, 19*, 97–98.

Wessman, A. E. (1957). A psychological inquiry into satisfactions and happiness (Doctoral dissertation, Princeton University, 1956). *Dissertation Abstracts International, 17*, 1384. (University Microfilms No. 00–20, 168).

Wessman, A. E., & Ricks, D. F. (1966). *Mood and personality.* New York: Holt, Rinehart & Winston.

Wills, T. A. (1981). Downward comparison principles in social psychology. *Psychological Bulletin, 90*, 245–271.

Wilson, W. R. (1960). An attempt to determine some correlates and dimensions of hedonic tone (Doctoral dissertation, Northwestern University, 1960). *Dissertation Abstracts, 22*, 2814. (University Microfilms No. 60–6588).

Wilson, W. (1967). Correlates of avowed happiness. *Psychological Bulletin, 67*, 294–306.

Wilson, R. S., & Matheny, A. P. (1983). Assessment of temperament in infant twins. *Developmental Psychology, 19*, 172–183.

Wiltsey, R. G. (1967). Some relationship between verbal reports of pleasant and unpleasant moods, sleep duration and sleep quality variables in college students (Doctoral dissertation, University of Rochester, 1967). *Dissertation Abstracts International, 28*, 346–7B. (University Microfilms No. 67–8982).

Wish, C. W. (1977). The relationship of sex role typing to life satisfaction in older persons (Doctoral dissertation, Ohio State University, 1976). *Dissertation Abstracts International, 37*, 5820-1B. (University Microfilms No. 77–10,627).

Wolk, S., & Telleen, S. (1976). Psychological and social correlates of life satisfaction as a function of residential constraint. *Journal of Gerontology, 31*, 89–98.

Wood, V., Wylie, M. L., & Sheafor, B. (1969). An analysis of a short self-report measure of life satisfaction: Correlation with rate judgments. *Journal of Gerontology, 24*, 465–469.

Wortman, C., & Silver, R. (1982, August). *Coping with undesirable life events.* Paper presented at the 90th Annual Convention of the American Psychological Association, Washington, DC.

Wright, J. D. (1978). Are working women really more satisfied? Evidence from several national surveys. *Journal of Marriage and the Family, 40*, 301–313.

Zajonc, R. B. (1980). Feeling and thinking: Preferences need no inferences. *American Psychologist, 35*, 151–175.

Zautra, A. J. (1983). Social resources and the quality of life. *American Journal of Community Psychology, 11*, 275–290.

Zautra, A., Hempel, A. (1983). *Subjective well-being and physical health: A review of literature and some suggestions for future research.* Manuscript submitted for publication, Arizona State University.

Zautra, A., & Reich, J. W. (1980). Positive life events and reports of well-being: Some useful distinctions. *American Journal of Community Psychology, 8*, 657–670.

Zautra, A. J., & Reich, J. W. (1983). Life events and perceptions of life quality: Developments in a two-factor approach. *Journal of Community Psychology, 11*, 121–132.

Zeglen, M. E. (1977). The impact of primary relationships on life satisfaction of the elderly (Doctoral dissertation, Washington State University, 1976). *Dissertation Abstracts International, 37*, 5372A. (University Microfilms No. 77–2892).

Zevon, M. A., & Tellegen, A. (1982). The structure of mood change: An idiographic/nomothetic analysis, *Journal of Personality and Social Psychology, 43*, 111–122.

In Pursuit of Happiness: Empirical Answers to Philosophical Questions

Pelin Kesebir and Ed Diener

Abstract In this article, we provide an overview of what various philosophers throughout the ages have claimed about the nature of happiness, and we discuss to what extent psychological science has been able to substantiate or refute their claims. We first address concerns raised by philosophers regarding the possibility, desirability, and justifiability of happiness and then turn to the perennial question of how to be happy. Integrating insights from great thinkers of the past with empirical findings from modern behavioral sciences, we review the conditions and causes of happiness. We conclude our discussion with some thoughts about the future of happiness studies.

It is not astonishing that the history of philosophy abounds with inquiries about the nature of happiness and the good life. The notion that what matters in life is not just to live but to live well is most likely as old as human existence. Down through the ages philosophers have speculated endlessly on the ways of rising above mere existence and achieving a desirable life. In this article, we examine the important issues philosophers and other great minds of history have raised regarding happiness, and we attempt to uncover the contributions of contemporary psychologists to the understanding of happiness.

We will begin our discussion with a brief history of the concept of happiness, which will be followed by a broader review of what philosophers have thought and what psychologists have discovered about the nature of happiness. Can people be happy? If they have both the ability and the desire to be happy, ought they pursue happiness for themselves and others? If they can, want, and ought to be happy, how should they go about realizing this goal? We will review answers to these and other similar questions, standing on the shoulders of great philosophers and psychologists.

E. Diener (✉)

Department of Psychology, University of Illinois, Urbana-Champaign, Champaign, IL 61820, USA

e-mail: ediener@uiuc.edu

E. Diener (ed.), *The Science of Well-Being: The Collected Works of Ed Diener*, Social Indicators Research Series 37, DOI 10.1007/978-90-481-2350-6_3,

A Short History of Happiness

In his review of Darrin M. McMahon's book, *Happiness: A History*, Jim Holt (2006) remarks, half in jest, that the history of the idea of happiness could be summarized in a series of bumper sticker equations: happiness=luck (Homeric era), happiness=virtue (classical era), happiness=heaven (medieval era), happiness= pleasure (Enlightenment era), and happiness=a warm puppy (contemporary era). Imagine just how undemanding our task would be if only the history of happiness would yield itself to such simple, orderly classification. Yet, reality is almost always more complex than bumper stickers would have us believe, and the history of the idea of happiness, spanning more than two millennia, is a particularly intricate one. Providing a comprehensive account of this history would be beyond the scope of this article. Rather, we wish to present a brief history of happiness in Western culture that will allow us to bridge the past and the present and put the findings of current happiness researchers into context.

As is the case with many affairs of knowledge, Ancient Greece was the place and time in which the topic of the good life received serious philosophical attention. Democritus ($\sim$ 460 BC–370 BC), who suggested that a happy life is not exclusively the product of a favorable fate or of external circumstances but rather of a man's cast of mind, is considered to be the first philosopher in the Western world to inquire into the nature of happiness (Tatarkiewicz, 1976). Democritus's subjectivist view seems not to have been endorsed by Socrates or by his student Plato, who conceptualized happiness in more objective and absolute terms, such as the "secure enjoyment of what is good and beautiful" (Plato, 1999, p. 80). On the other hand, Aristotle, in his influential work *Nicomachean Ethics*, in which happiness (*eudaemonia*) was the central issue, asserted that happiness was not out of one's hands but is realizable for anyone willing to lead a life in accordance with the most valued virtues (Aristotle, 1992).

Hellenistic history also saw schools of philosophy that propounded hedonism as the royal road to the good life. A prominent example of these schools of thought was the Cyrenaics, whose founder, Aristippus, argued that "No considerations should restrain one in the pursuit of pleasure, for everything other than pleasure is unimportant, and virtue is least important of all" (Tatarkiewicz, 1976, p. 317). Nevertheless, such a view appears to be uncharacteristically extreme even for the hedonists of Ancient Greece. In the ancient world, there was a broad consensus, first among the Greeks and then the Romans, that a good life devoid of reason and morality was simply not achievable. Even Epicurus, whose doctriness have at times been dismissed as self-indulgent hedonism, was possessed of the conviction that virtue and pleasure were interdependent and that it was simply impossible "to live pleasantly without living prudently, honorably, and justly" (Epicurus, 1994, p. 31). The Stoic philosopher Cicero was such a staunch advocate of the felicific powers of virtue that he believed a man in possession of virtue could be happy even while being tortured (McMahon, 2006).

Christian philosophers of the Middle Ages also considered a life of virtue as indispensable to the good life; nonetheless, virtue was no longer considered to be sufficient for happiness. Happiness was an ethereal, spiritual matter; it now lay in the hands of God, attainable only by means of devoted faith and the grace of God. Whereas earthly happiness was fallible—albeit not impossible—the Kingdom of Heaven promised complete and eternal happiness (Tatarkiewicz, 1976).

In the Age of Enlightenment, the idea of happiness grew more secular and less otherworldly. In parallel, there was an increased emphasis in Western cultures on pleasure as a path to, and even as a synonym for, happiness. These changes were best illustrated by the utilitarian philosophy of the early 19th century, which determined that happiness equaled utility was derived from maximum pleasure. Utilitarians, such as the English philosopher Jeremy Bentham, regarded the maximum surplus of pleasure over pain as the cardinal goal of human striving and advocated that the greatest happiness of the greatest number of people should be the basis of morals and legislation.

The idea that humans are entitled to pursue and attain happiness gained widespread acceptance in the modern era, as manifested by the preamble to the American Declaration of Independence and the crowded self-help aisles of bookstores. Classical and medieval conceptions of happiness as "virtue" or "perfection" have been largely ignored or rendered obsolete in recent centuries. In McMahon's apt words, humans in this day and age think of happiness "more as *feeling* good than *being* good" (2006, p. 65). Philosphical treatments of the issue of human well-being are rarer in this era than in centuries past, whereas both the behavioral and social sciences have begun to devote considerable attention to the topic (Haybron, 2007b).

What is this Thing Called Happiness?

Philosophers of happiness tend to agree, if on nothing else, on the difficulty of defining happiness. For science to progress, however, clearly defined and operationalized concepts are in dispensable. As a way to capture what lay people mean by "happiness," psychologists pioneering the scientific study of happiness proposed the term *subjective well-being* (SWB; Diener, 1984). SWB refers to people's evaluations of their lives and encompasses both cognitive judgments of satisfaction and affective appraisals of moods and emotions.

This conceptualization emphasizes the subjective nature of happiness and holds individual human beings to be the single best judges of their own happiness. Classical philosophers such as Socrates, who did not have faith in the intellectual prowess of the masses and distinguished between the "hoi polloi" and the "wise," would probably disapprove of regaling personal authority to ordinary people in matters of happiness (Haybron, 2007b). Concerns regarding the adequacy of measuring happiness through self-reports have also been expressed by contemporary philosophers and psychologists (e.g., Haybron, 2007a; Schwarz & Strack, 1999). Although there is room for improvement in SWB measures and multimethod assessments should certainly be implemented whenever possible, several studies attest to the reliability and validity of self-report happiness measures in informing research (e.g., Diener & Suh, 1997).

Modern psychologists perhaps cannot hope to define *happiness* to everyone's satisfaction; nonetheless, they have made a discovery of significance—namely, the separable components of subjective well-being that cohere in understandable ways. These components include life satisfaction (global judgments of one's life), satisfaction with important life domains (satisfaction with one's work, health, marriage, etc.), positive affect (prevalence of positive emotions and moods), and low levels of negative affect (prevalence of unpleasant emotions and moods). A careful examination reveals that these components have often been part of the philosophical discourse on happiness at one point or another in the last two and a half millennia. For instance, the enunciation of frequent positive affect and rare negative affect as being conductive to happiness is directly traceable to the hedonist tradition in philosophy. SWB's acknowledgment of subjective life satisfaction as a crucial ingredient of happiness, on the other hand, resonates most with contemporary philosopher Wayne Sumner's ideas, for whom "happiness (or unhappiness) is a response by a subject to her life conditions *as she sees them*" (1999, p. 156).

Ryff and Singer's (1996) concept of psychological well-being and Ryan and Deci's (2000) self-determination theory are two other prominent accounts of happiness and well-being put forth by psychologists. These theories have a less subjective and more prescriptive character in that they specify certain needs that must be fulfilled (such as autonomy, self-acceptance, and mastery) as a prerequisite of human well-being. In that sense, they are akin to the eudaemonist flourishing theories of the classical era, such as those of Aristotle (Tiberius, 2006).

It is important for the purposes of our discussion to emphasize that most of the empirical studies conducted in psychology regarding happiness, as well as most research mentioned in our article, conceive of happiness not in the eudaimonic sense—embodying a value judgment about whether a person is leading a commendable life—but rather in the sense of subjective well-being. Clearly, high subjective well-being and eudaimonic happiness are not necessarily interchangeable concepts, and it is easily imaginable that a person could feel subjectively happy without leading a virtuous life. However, we believe, and many contemporary philosophers (Haybron, 2005; Sumner, 1999) agree, that subjective well-being and eudaimonic well-being are sufficiently close. It is reasonable to use subjective well-being as a proxy for well-being, even if it is not a perfect match. Admittedly, current empirical psychological research cannot directly answer the ancient philosophical question of how to live well. As researchers of subjective well-being, our hope is that we answer this question indirectly by illuminating a *sine qua non* of the good life—namely, subjective well-being.

Can People Be Happy?

In attempting to answer this question, we believe that a distinction between *ideal happiness* and *actual happiness* (Tatarkiewicz, 1976) would be beneficial at the outset. Ideal happiness can be defined as happiness that is complete and lasting and that touches the whole of life. Such a happiness—perfect, pure, and perpetual—has extremely high standards and may indeed be beyond anyone's reach. However, it is still possible for people to experience predominantly positive emotions and be satisfied with their lives. Actual happiness, as it has been called, is what psychologists are interested in as an object of scientific inquiry. This attainable type of happiness in the focus of our article as well.

It has been argued that the conflict between pessimism and optimism in philosophy is practically as old as philosophy itself (Tatarkiewicz, 1976). On the one end of the spectrum, we find Leibniz (1646–1716), famous for his statement that we are living in the best of all possible worlds. On the other end of the spectrum, there is Hegesias, a figure from 3rd century BC Alexandria, also known as *Peisithanatos* (the death persuader) because he believed that happiness was unattainable, life was not worth living, and that the sage would choose death (Matson, 1998). Such pessimists saw human happiness as either impossible to attain or at least quite improbable, depicting the suffering and tragedy in the world as an inevitable source of unhappiness. It is also not to be forgotten that all philosophical stances inevitably reflect the soul of the times and places they have originated in. Many a distrustful claim regarding the posibility of happiness was advanced in a social context of much lower quality of life and more common unhappiness in comparison with modern times (Veenhoven, 2005).

Scientific psychology can attempt to shed some light on the issue of whether happiness is possible by addressing two pertinent questions: Do people report being happy, and is happiness an adaptive, evolutionarily feasible phenomenon? Evidence from worldwide surveys suggests that the answer to the first question is affirmative. In an article suitably titled "Most People Are Happy," Diener and Diener (1996) reviewed the available evidence and concluded that an overwhelming majority of individuals fall in the positive range of the happiness scale, including people with apparent disadvantages, such as quadriplegics or those in the lowest income groups. A recent opinion poll corroborates this finding by revealing that 84% of Americans see themselves as either "very happy" or "pretty happy" (Pew Research Center, 2006). Likewise, 86% of the 43 nations included in Diener and Diener's study had average happiness levels above the midpoint of the happiness scale.

Though it is rare for people to be constantly elated or ecstatic, most people report being happy most of the time. All this evidence is discordant with a view of life as a "vale of tears" and of modern society as a "sink of unhappiness." Humans appear to have a predisposition to mild levels of happiness, which brings us to our second query: What are the adaptive functions of happiness?

It has been long recognized that negative emotions (e.g., fear, anger, and anxiety) make an individual focus on the immediate threat or problem, thereby contributing to evolutionary fitness. It is only recently, however, that we have begun to understand the adaptive advantages engendered by positive feelings. Barbara Frederickson's "broaden-and-build theory" (1998) proposes that positive feelings allow individuals to broaden their thought–action repertories and build intellectual, psychological, social, and physical resources over time. In other words, positive affect and general well-being produce a state from which individuals can confidently explore the environment and approach new goals, thus allowing them to build important personal resources. It follows that happiness is not just an epiphenomenon, it is also adaptive from an evolutionary point of view and brings about various benefits, as we will explore in greater detail later in our discussion.

The psychological discoveries of the past few decades seem to refute the pessimistic idea that happiness is an impossible human ambition or a fool's dream. Let us now examine the arguments about the improbability of happiness. In the humanities, one of the most frequently encountered ideas concerning happiness is that although people are not doomed to an unhappy existence, the search for happiness will necessarily be self-defeating, and that the harder people strive for happiness, the further they will retreat from it. Schopenhauer, for instance, observed that wherever joy makes its appearance, "it as a rule comes uninvited and unannounced, by itself and *sans façon*" (Schopenhauer, 2001, p. 409). Several philosophers agreed that happiness will only lead to a wild-goose chase when pursued directly as a goal of existence and that it has to be found along the way as the byproduct of other activities. John Stuart Mill eloquently stated that only those are happy who "have their minds fixed on some object other than their own happiness; on the happiness of others, on the improvement of mankind, even on some art or pursuit, followed not as a means, but as itself an ideal end" (Mill, 1944, p. 100).

One psychological study, conducted by Schooler, Ariely, and Loewenstein (2003), suggests that the conscious pursuit of happiness and the continuous assessment of one's happiness may indeed prove deleterious to one's well-being. In this study, participants listened to Stravinsky's *Rites of Spring* under one of three conditions. In the first condition, the participants simply listened to the music; in the second, they were asked to make themselves as happy as possible while listening to the recording; and in the last conditions, they were instructed to adjust a movable measurement scale to point to their real-time happiness. As it turned out, those in the first condition who simply listened to the recording—without trying to be as happy as possible or without constantly monitoring their level of happiness—enjoyed it most. This finding dovetails with studies showing that happy moods are associated with low degrees of self-focused attention (Green, Sedikides, Saltzberg, Wood, & Forzano, 2003).

Yet at the same time, we find support for the effectiveness of interventions to increase happiness (Fordyce, 1977; Lyubomirsky, Sheldon, & Schkade, 2005). This means that whereas being self-conscious and abessive about one's happiness may backfire, there are still certain activities individuals can consciously choose to partake or lifestyle changes that they can deliberately make that will increase their happiness, such as meditation and counting one's blessings.

In *Anna Karenina*, Tolstoy observes that "there are no conditions to which a person cannot grow accustomed" (2004, p. 706). Adam Smith, in a similar vein, talks of "the never-failing certainty with which all men, sooner or later, accommodate themselves to whatever becomes their permanent situation" (2002, p. 172). Since the early studies showing that lottery winners were not happier than controls and that even paralyzed accident victims revert approximately to their initial levels of happiness (e.g., Brickman, Coates, & Janoff-Bulman, 1987), the hedonic treadmill theory—the idea that our emotional systems adjust to almost anything that happens in our lives, good or bad—has been embraced by psychologists as a guiding principle in happiness research. In affiliation with the hedonic treadmill model, the set-point theory posits that major life events, such as marriage, the death of a child, or unemployment, affect a person's happiness only temporarily, after which the person's happiness level regresses to a default determined by genotype (Lykken & Tellegen, 1996). The implication of these assertions is that no matter how hard we try to be happier, adaptation on the one hand and our temperament on the other will ensure that our venture will remain just a futile rat race with an illusory goal.

Our conviction is that the time is ripe for a revision of hedonic adaptation theories. Accumulating evidence reveals that, even though adaptation undeniably occurs to some extent and personal aspirations do rise and adjust, people do not adapt quickly and/or completely to everything (Diener, Lucas, & Scollon, 2006). Lucas, Clark, Georgellis, and Diener (2003, 2004), for example, have observed in a 15-year longitudinal study that individuals who experienced unemployment or widowhood did not, on average, fully recover and return to their earlier life satisfaction levels. Other studies have shown that people hardly, if ever, adapt to certain elements in their lives such as noise, long commutes, or interpersonal conflict (Haidt, 2006), whereas other events such as plastic surgery may have long-lasting positive effects on one's psychological well-being (Rankin, Borah, Perry, & Wey, 1998).

Do People Want to Be Happy?

From antiquity to the present, the notion that happiness is a fundamental human drive has almost had an axiomatic quality in philosophy. Alexander Pope called happiness "our being's end and aim," and the same view finds one of its most elegant expressions in Pascal's words:

> All men seek happiness. There are no exceptions. However different the means they may employ, they all strive towards this goal. The reason why some go to war and some do not is the same desire in both, but interpreted in two different ways. The will never takes the least step except to that end. This is the motive of every act of every man, including those who go and hang themselves (1995, p. 45).

Whether or not happiness embodies the *summum bonum*—the highest good—is not a question that can be answered by the methods available to science. What psychologists can and did do, however, is ask people how much they desire happiness. Surveys conducted with college students in 41 nations showed that on a 7-point scale—where 7 indicated *extraordinarily important and valuable*—respondents rated happiness a 6.39 on average (Diener, Sapyta, & Suh, 1998). Similarly, King and Napa (1998) reported that Americans see happiness as more relevant to the judgment of a good life than are wealth or moral goodness, and they even think that happy people are more likely to go to heaven.

It is also worth pointing out that the desirability of happiness does not rule out the value of other human strivings. We agree with Tatarkiewicz that "it would be ig-headed and dangerous to think of happiness as the only good" (1976, p. 126). It is immensely difficult to imagine a desirable life that is devoid of happiness. As much as happiness is necessary to the good life, however, it is not sufficient. When we deem happiness a worthwhile object of study, it is because we trust that pursuing happiness is one form of the good life, but not the only one.

Should People Be Happy?

One recent development in happiness studies has been the discovery that, on both the individual and societal levels, happiness precedes and causes a plethora of positive outcomes, instead of merely being the product of these positive outcomes (Lyubomirsky, King, & Diener, 2005). More specifically, happiness leads to better health, better work performance, better social relationships, and to more ethical behavior. In this section, we will discuss these findings, while at the same time comparing and contrasting them with the views of the great minds of the past.

Health

French writer Marcel Proust observes in *Remembrance of Things Past* that happiness is salutary to the body, whereas it is unhappiness that develops the forces of the mind. Although he seems to have gotten the part about unhappiness cultivating the mind wrong, as we will elaborate on shortly, current research strongly supports his insight that happiness leads to better physical health. One of the most impressive studies revealing this link was conducted by Danner, Snowdon, and Friesen (2001), who demonstrated that positive affective content in handwritten autobiographies of Catholic sisters, composed when they were at the mean age of 22, strongly predicted their longevity six decades later. Experimental data similarly testify to the salutary effects of happiness on the body: In a study in which researchers infected participants with a cold virus, those who reported high levels of happiness were found to be less vulnerable to the common cold (Cohen, Doyle, Turner, Alper, & Skoner, 2003).

Achievement

Confirming Fredrickson's broaden-and-build theory of positive emotions, happiness emerges from available data as the resource leading to the development and better use of intellectual skills and resources. The fairly common characterization of happiness as a catalyst for dumbing people down must be connected to an understanding of happiness as giddy, empty-headed hedonism. Decades of research reveals, however, that happiness primarily emanates not from the ceaseless pursuit of pleasure, but from striving for and making progress towards goals derived from one's most-prized values. Feelings of meaning, purpose, and fulfillment thus typically trump pleasure as predictors of happiness.

Proust's sadder-but-wiser maxim is contradicted by research indicating that those who are dispositionally happy or artificially put in a happy mood outperform others in various tasks such as accurate decision making, clerical error checking, anagram solving, or original and flexible thinking (Diener & Seligman, 2004). There seems to be only one sense in which people experiencing elevated moods can be considered "stupid" and that is their increased inclination to rely on heuristics (Lyubomirsky, King, & Diener, 2005).

Happiness is also linked to higher achievement in professional life. Accordingly, happy individuals are more likely to graduate from college, secure a job, receive favorable evaluations from their supervisors, and earn higher incomes, and they are less likely to lose their job and are quicker to be reemployed if they are laid off (Diener, Nickerson, Lucas, & Sandvik, 2002; Diener & Seligman, 2004).

Social Relationships and Prosocial Behavior

Most noteworthy among the arguments raised against the justifiability of happiness has been the view equating happiness with self-centeredness and insensitivity to the problems darkening the world. George Eliot (1996), for instance, talks about how happiness is considered "a well-fleshed indifference to sorrow outside it" (p. 796), and another English novelist, Sir Hugh Walpole, notes that "to confess to happiness implies a smug complacency and callousness to the general misfortunes of the world" (as cited in Tatarkiewicz, 1976, p. 348). Study after study, however, fails to substantiate the portrayal of happiness as an egotistic and apathetic state; instead, they disclose the opposite pattern. Happiness appears to bring out the best in humans, making them more social, more cooperative, and even more ethical. Illustrating this, people with chronically high or experimentally increased positive affect evaluate persons they have recently met in more positive affect evaluate persons they have recently met in more positive terms, become more interested in social interaction, and also become more prone to self-disclosure (Diener & Seligman, 2004). Those who report higher life satisfaction exhibit more generalized trust in others (Brehm & Rahn, 1997), and when asked how justifiable they find some hypothetical ethical scenarios (such as buying something they knew to be stolen or avoiding a fare on public transport), participants with higher happiness levels respond in more ethical ways (James & Chymis, 2004). Furthermore, as Tov and Diener (2007) point out in their review, the virtuous relationship between happiness and socially desirable outcomes also holds true on a national level. Happier countries tend to score higher on generalized trust, volunteerism, and democratic attitudes.

How to Be Happy?

John Locke observed that men take "various and contrary ways" to reach happiness, albeit "all aim at being happy" (1894, p. 190). The annals of philosophy are equally filled with the various and contrary ways of achieving happiness. For almost every page written on the merits of a certain quality in inducing happiness, there exists another page condemning that quality and lauding the opposite one. Yet, unavoidably, some advice is sounder than the rest, and some methods of achieving happiness are more effective than others. Scientific methods fortunately permit us to distinguish the contenders from the pretenders.

As sociologists and quality-of-life researchers expressed interest in the subject of happiness earlier than psychologists did, the first investigations about the concomitants and causes of happiness primarily involved demographic factors (e.g., age, gender, race) and life-status variables (e.g., marital status, health). This research tradition led to the somewhat astounding discovery that objective life circumstances play a fairly minor role in explaining happiness. Scholars have estimated that demographic factors account for 8–15% of the variance in happiness (Diener, Suh, Lucas, & Smith, 1999).

The inadequacy of external circumstances in predicting happiness led psychologists to focus on other correlates of happiness. In this section, we will contemplate some of the conditions and sources of happiness as they are discussed by the distinguished minds of the past and as revealed by modern research.

Wealth

Aristotle believed that wealth was a necessary ingredient of happiness (1991). Stoics, in contrast, believed that material possessions and wealth were in no way required for happiness. Inhabiting the middle ground were the Epicureans, who maintained that although we should have sufficient money to shelter us from harm and pain, money ceases to offer greater levels of happiness beyond a certain threshold. "Nothing satisfies the man who is not satisfied with a little" was Epicurus's conviction (De Botton, 2000, p. 62). Research reveals a significant positive correlation between wealth and happiness. At the same time, Epicurus and his followers seem to have touched upon a keen insight about happiness with their belief in the diminishing effect of income on happiness. Frey and Stutzer (2002) established that although increased income contributes significantly to happiness at low levels of development across nations, once the threshold of around US $10,000 annual per capita income has been passed, there is not a strong correlation between wealth and life satisfaction. In a similar vein, Diener, Horowitz, and Emmons (1985) documented that very wealthy people, chosen from the *Forbes* list of the wealthiest Americans, were only modestly happier than a control group who lived in the same geographical area. Research, all in all, suggests that an adequate amount of money is a necessary condition of happiness, albeit not a sufficient one.

Friends and Social Relationships

Arthur Schopenhauer, displaying his signature misanthropy, advocated that loneliness was a superior condition to human company. He can perhaps find consolation in the fact that this idea of his would hardly attract any company. Philosophers through the ages have repeatedly pointed out, approvingly, the value and importance of friendship. Aristotle was of the conviction that "no one would choose to live without friends, even if he had all the other goods" (2000, p. 143), and Epicurus believed that "of all the things that wisdom provides to help one live one's entire life in happiness, the greatest by far is the possession of friendship" (De Botton, 2000, p. 57). Empirical studies strongly corroborate these views. Diener and Seligman (2002) found in their study of very happy people that every single one of them had excellent social relationships. Quantity and, more importantly, quality of friendships correlate positively with happiness, and perceived loneliness is robustly linked to depression. In light of this and other parallel findings, Reis and Gable (2003) have suggested that good social relationships may be the single most important source of happiness. It must be true that "it is man, who is essential to man's happiness" (Tatarkiewicz, 1976, p. 130), and as much as some may believe that hell is other people, so, apparently, is heaven.

Religion

As mentioned earlier, medieval Christian scholars believed that happiness lay in God and that religious devotion was the only means of achieving it. For instance, the 6th century philosopher Boethius reasoned that if true happiness is the perfect good, it must reside in the most supreme deity (Boethius, 1999). Atheists, on the other hand, argued that God was an illusion, and some nonbelievers claimed that genuine happiness was only possible for those who realized this. One of them, Karl Marx, famously believed that religion is the opiate of the masses and perceived "the overcoming of religion as the illusory happiness of the people" as a necessity for real happiness (McMahon, 2006, p. 391). Research is powerless and therefore irrelevant when it comes to answering the question of whether God is real or an illusion; nonetheless, multiple studies reveal that religion does make people happier. More specifically, participation in religious services, strength of religious affiliation, relationship with God, and prayer all seem to contribute to happiness (Ferriss, 2002; Poloma & Pendleton, 1990). Still, it is important to point out that the positive association between happiness and religious beliefs and practices is not a universal one, with religious people in certain countries (e.g., Lithuania, Slovakia) reporting lower levels of life satisfaction.

Personality

Investigators of happiness unambiguously agree that dispositional differences in responding to people and events have an important effect on individuals' happiness levels. Lykken and Tellegen (1996) reported that such stable temperamental tendencies resulting from genetic inheritance account for as much as 50% of variability in happiness.

Thirty years ago, Tatarkiewicz brilliantly foreshadowed the empirical findings of personality scientists when he wrote about personality having a dual influence on happiness: "Firstly because it predisposes one to feel joy or sorrow, and secondly because it shapes a man's life in such a way as to cause him joy or sorrow" (1976, p. 194). Research indeed shows that certain personality traits (e.g., extraversion) render individuals more likely to experience positive affect, whereas other personality traits (e.g., neuroticism) predispose individuals to negative affect (Rusting & Larsen, 1997). At the same time, confirming the second part of Tatarkiewicz's claim, extraversion predicts the frequency of positive objective life events, and neuroticism predicts the frequency of negative objective events (Magnus, Diener, Fujita, & Pavot, 1993). Other than extraversion and neuroticism, personality traits such as self-esteem, optimism, trust, agreeableness, repressive defensiveness, desire for control, and hardiness have been found to be strong predictors of happiness (DeNeve & Cooper, 1998; Lucas, Diener, & Suh, 1996).

Where Do We Go from Here?

In this article, we have presented a chronicle of the idea of happiness from antiquity to modern times and contemplated the questions of the possibility, desirability, and justifiability of happiness as discussed by philosophers and investigated by psychologists. This was followed by an overview of the conditions and sources of happiness. The reader can gather from our analysis alone that there still remain many unanswered and even unexamined questions about the nature of happiness.

Some of the issues in happiness research that await illumination are of an empirical nature; in other words, they are directly answerable by science. Hence, we believe that, as complex as they may be, their resolution is ultimately only a matter of time. Adaptation, specifically, its exact effect on happiness and its limits, is one such issue, as is the nature of the interaction between temperament and environment in determining happiness levels. Similarly, the correlates and causes of the distinct components of happiness (i.e., positive affect, negative affect, and life satisfaction) constitute an important yet understudied topic. The field would also vastly benefit from learning more about the correlates of different conceptualizations of happiness, such as Ryff and Singer's concept of psychological well-being and Ryan and Deci's self-determination model. Another topic we deem to be extremely important and timely is the relationship between religious belief and happiness. The recent controversy surrounding the publication of several books that view religious belief as "an irrational embrace of myth" (Harris, 2005, p. 26; see also Dawkins, 2006) and argue that even moderate religion is pernicious to humanity further underscores the need for rigorous research on the costs and benefits of religion.

On the other hand, other questions of great concern to our field call for value judgments and are thus more philosophical and less empirical in nature. One of these questions is whether happiness should be the aim of formal education. We, as scholars of happiness, clearly believe in the value of enlightening people about where happiness can in fact be found. Whether the ultimate objective of education should be to make people happy, however, is not a question that can be answered directly, but it is one that can instead be approached through the accumulation of relevant data and through vigorous philosophical discussions about the implications of these data.

A similar value question concerns whether the aim of national policymaking should be the happiness of citizens. Numerous philosophers from Aristotle to Jeremy Bentham believed that it should be so, and several social reformers agreed with such philosophers. William Beveridge, who established Britain's welfare state after the Second World War, observed, "The objective of government in peace and in war is not the glory of rulers or races, but the happiness of the common man." Recently, some psychologists have proposed that, in addition to the prevailing economic and social indicators of the day, governments should use a national index of happiness to guide them in policymaking (Diener & Seligman, 2004). Putting aside the debate regarding the ultimate aim of governments, we believe that such an index would be a valuable complement to the current approaches used to gauge human welfare (Kesebir & Diener, 2008).

On the Shoulders of Giants

Philosopher Nicholas White believed, "Philosophers' concrete advice about how to become happy isn't any better (in fact, it's probably worse) than that of the average person. They generally don't know enough of the relevant facts, and they don't have the right temperament" (White, 2006, p. 15). Our discussion suggests that, though some thinkers' insights about the nature of happiness were penetrating and profound, the arguments of numerous other philosophers simply could not be substantiated by available data. These great minds provided the most important questions regarding happiness, yet their answers disagreed with each other more often than not. It was by looking at the questions posed by philosophers and by using the methods of science that we have been able to provide some initial answers to crucial questions that have vexed thinkers for millennia. If we have seen farther than our betters, it was by standing on the shoulders of the great philosophers and on the platform of science. It is our hope that the fields of philosophy and psychology will continue to mutually inspire and enrich each other, so that future psychologists and philosophers will be able to see even farther.

References

Aristotle. (1991). *On rhetoric: A theory of civic discourse* (G. A. Kennedy, Trans.). New York: Oxford University Press.
Aristotle. (1992). *Eudaemian ethics* (2nd ed., M. Woods, Trans.). Oxford, United Kingdom: Clarendon Press.

Aristotle. (2000). *Nicomachean ethics* (R. Crisp, Ed.). Cambridge, England: Cambridge University Press.

Boethius. (1999). *The consolation of philosophy* (P. G. Walsh, Trans.). Oxford, United Kingdom: Clarendon Press.

Brehm, J., & Rahn, W. (1997). Individual-level evidence for the causes and consequences of social capital. *American Journal of Political Science, 41*, 999–1024.

Brickman, P., Coates, D., & Janoff-Bulman, R. (1978). Lottery winners and accident victims: Is happiness relative? *Journal of Personality and Social Psychology, 36*, 917–927.

Cohen, S., Doyle, W. J., Turner, R. B., Alper, C. M., & Skoner, D. P. (2003). Emotional style and susceptibility to the common cold. *Psychosomatic Medicine, 65*, 652–657.

Danner, D., Snowdon, D., & Friesen, W. (2001). Positive emotions in early life and longevity: Findings from the nun study. *Journal of Personality and Social Psychology, 80*, 814.

Dawkins, R. (2006). *The god delusion.* Boston: Houghton Mifflin.

De Botton, A. (2000). *The consolations of philosophy.* New York: Vintage Books.

DeNeve, K. M., & Cooper, H. (1998). The happy personality: A metaanalysis of 137 personality traits and subjective well-being. *Psychological Bulletin, 124*, 197–229.

Diener, E. (1984). Subjective well-being. *Psychological Bulletin, 95*, 542–575.

Diener, E., & Diener, C. (1996). Most people are happy. *Psychological Science, 7*, 181–185.

Diener, E., Horowitz, J., & Emmons, R. A. (1985). Happiness of the very wealthy. *Social Indicators Research, 16*, 263–274.

Diener, E., Lucas, R. E., & Scollon, C. N. (2006). Beyond the hedonic treadmill: Revisions to the adaptation theory of well-being. *American Psychologist, 61*, 305–314.

Diener, E., Nickerson, C., Lucas, R. E., & Sandvik, E. (2002). Dispositional affect and job outcomes. *Social Indicators Research, 59*, 229–259.

Diener, E., Sapyta, J. J., & Suh, E. M. (1998). Subjective well-being is essential to well-being. *Psychological Inquiry, 9*, 33–37.

Diener, E., & Seligman, M. E. P. (2002). Very happy people. *Psychological Science, 13*, 81–84.

Diener, E., & Seligman, M. E. P. (2004). Beyond money: Toward an economy of well-being. *Psychological Science in the Public Interest, 5*, 1–31.

Diener, E., & Suh, E. (1997). Measuring quality of life: Economic, social, and subjective indicators. *Social Indicators Research, 40*, 189–216.

Diener, E., Suh, E. M., Lucas, R. E., & Smith, H. L. (1999). Subjective well-being: Three decades of progress. *Psychological Bulletin, 125*, 276–302.

Eliot, G. (1996). *Daniel Deronda.* London: Penguin Classics.

Epicurus. (1994). *The Epicurus reader: Selected writings and testimonia* (L. P. Gerson & B. Inwood, Eds. & Trans.). Indianapolis, IN: Hackett Publishing.

Ferriss, A. L. (2002). Religion and the quality of life. *Journal of Happiness Studies, 3*, 199–215.

Fordyce, M. W. (1977). Development of a program to increase happiness. *Journal of Counseling Psychology, 24*, 511–521.

Frey, B. S., & Stutzer, A. (2002). *Happiness and economics: How the economy and institutions affect human well-being.* Princeton, NJ: Princeton University Press.

Green, J. D., Sedikides, C., Saltzberg, J. A., Wood, J. V., & Forzano, L.-A. B. (2003). Happy mood decreases self-focused attention. *British Journal of Social Psychology, 28*, 147–157.

Haidt, J. (2006). *The happiness hypothesis: Finding modern truth in ancient wisdom.* New York: Basic Books.

Harris, S. (2005). *The end of faith: Religion, terror, and the future of reason.* New York: W.W. Norton.

Haybron, D. (2005). On being happy or unhappy. *Philosophy and Phenomenological Research, 71*, 287–317.

Haybron, D. (2007a). Life satisfaction, ethical reflection, and the science of happiness. *Journal of Happiness Studies, 8*, 99–138.

Haybron, D. (2007b). Philosophy and the science of subjective well-being. In M. Eid & R. J. Larsen (Eds.), *The science of subjective well-being* (pp. 17–43). New York: Guilford Press.

Holt, J. (2006, February 12). Oh, joy [Review of the book *Happiness: A history*]. *The New York Times*, p. 20.

James, H. S., & Chymis, A. (2004). *Are happy people ethical people? Evidence from North America and Europe* (Working Paper No. AEWP 2004-8). Columbia, MO: University of Missouri, Department of Agricultural Economics.

Kesebir, P., & Diener, E. (2008). In defense of happiness: Why policymakers should care about subjective well-being. In L. Bruni, M. Pugno, & F. Comim (Eds.), *Capabilities and happiness.* New York: Oxford University Press.

King, L. A., & Napa, C. K. (1998). What makes a life good? *Journal of Personality and Social Psychology, 75,* 156–165.

Locke, J. (1894). *An essay concerning human understanding.* London: George Routledge and Sons.

Lucas, R. E., Clark, A. E., Georgellis, Y., & Diener, E. (2003). Reexamining adaptation and the set point model of happiness: Reactions to changes in marital status. *Journal of Personality and Social Psychology, 84,* 527–539.

Lucas, R. E., Clark, A. E., Georgellis, Y., & Diener, E. (2004). Unemployment alters the set point for life satisfaction. *Psychological Science, 15,* 8–13.

Lucas, R. E., Diener, E., & Suh, E. (1996). Discriminant validity of well-being measures. *Journal of Personality and Social Psychology, 71,* 616–628.

Lykken, D., & Tellegen, A. (1996). Happiness is a stochastic phenomenon. *Psychological Science, 7,* 186–189.

Lyubomirsky, S., King, L., & Diener, E. (2005). The benefits of frequent positive affect: Does happiness lead to success? *Psychological Bulletin, 131,* 803–855.

Lyubomirsky, S., Sheldon, K. M., & Schkade, D. (2005). Pursuing happiness: The architecture of sustainable change. *Review of General Psychology, 9,* 111–131.

Magnus, K., Diener, E., Fujita, F., & Pavot, W. (1993). Extraversion and neuroticism as predictors of objective life events: A longitudinal study. *Journal of Personality and Social Psychology, 65,* 1046–1053.

Matson, W. I. (1998). Hegesias; the death-persuader; or, the gloominess of hedonism. *Philosophy, 73,* 553–557.

McMahon, D. M. (2006). *Happiness: A history.* New York: Atlantic Monthly Press.

Mill, J. S. (1944). *Autobiography of John Stuart Mill.* New York: Columbia University Press.

Pascal, B. (1995). *Pensées* (A. J. Krailsheimer, Trans.). London, England: Penguin Books. (Original work published 1669)

Pew Research Center. (2006). *Are we happy yet?* Retrieved November 10, 2006, from http://pewresearch.org/assets/social/pdf/AreWe-HappyYet.pdf

Plato. (1999). *The symposium* (W. Hamilton, Trans.). London: Penguin Classics.

Poloma, M. M., & Pendleton, B. F. (1990). Religious domains and general well-being. *Social Indicators Research, 22,* 255–276.

Rankin, M., Borah, G. L., Perry, A. W., & Wey, P. D. (1998). Quality-of-life outcomes after cosmetic surgery. *Plastic and Reconstructive Surgery, 102,* 2139–2145.

Reis, H. T., & Gable, S. L. (2003). Toward a positive psychology of relationships. In C. L. Keyes & J. Haidt (Eds.), *Flourishing: The positive person and the good life* (pp. 129–159). Washington, DC: American Psychological Association.

Rusting, C. L., & Larsen, R. J. (1997). Extraversion, neuroticism, and susceptibility to positive and negative affect: A test of two theoretical models. *Personality and Individual Differences, 22,* 607–612.

Ryan, R. M., & Deci, E. L. (2000). Self-determination theory and the facilitation of intrinsic motivation, social development and well-being. *American Psychologist, 55,* 68–78.

Ryff, C. D., & Singer, B. (1996). Psychological well-being: Meaning, measurement, and implications for psychotherapy research. *Psychotherapy and Psychosomatics, 65,* 14–23.

Schooler, J. W., Ariely, D., & Loewenstein, G. (2003). The pursuit and assessment of happiness may be self-defeating. In I. Brocas & J. D. Carrillo (Eds.), *The psychology of economic decisions: Vol. 1. Rationality and well-being* (pp. 41–70). New York: Oxford University Press.

Schopenhauer, A. (2001). *Parerga and paralipomena* (E. F. J. Payne, Trans.). New York: Oxford University Press.

Schwarz, N., & Strack, F. (1999). Reports of subjective well-being: Judgmental processes and their methodological implications. In D. Kahneman, E. Diener, & N. Schwarz (Eds.), *Well-being: The foundations of hedonic psychology* (pp. 61–84). New York: Russell Sage Foundation.

Smith, A. (2002). *The theory of moral sentiments* (K. Haakonssen, Ed.). Cambridge, England: Cambridge University Press. (Original work published 1759)

Sumner, L. W. (1999). *Welfare, happiness, and ethics.* Oxford, United Kingdom: Clarendon Press.

Tatarkiewicz, W. (1976). *Analysis of happiness.* Warsaw: Polish Scientific Publishers.

Tiberius, V. (2006). Well-being: Psychological research for philosophers. *Philosophy Compass, 1,* 493–505.

Tolstoy, L. (2004). *Anna Karenina* (R. Pevear & L. Volokhonsky, Trans.). New York: Penguin Books. (Original work published 1877)

Tov, W., & Diener, E. (2007). The well-being of nations: Linking together trust, cooperation, and democracy. In B. A. Sullivan, M. Snyder, & J. L. Sullivan (Eds.), *Cooperation: A powerful force in human relations.* Malden, MA: Blackwell.

Veenhoven, R. (2005). Is life getting better? How long and happy people live in modern society. *European Psychologist, 10,* 330–343.

White, N. (2006). *A brief history of happiness.* Malden, MA: Blackwell Publishing.

Personality and Subjective Well-Being

Richard E. Lucas and Ed Diener

Abstract Personality has been found to be more strongly associated with subjective well-being in many instances than are life circumstances. In part, this might be due to the fact that temperament and other individual differences can influence people's feelings and evaluations of their lives, but also because people's emotions are an inherent part of personality. This chapter discusses the heritability of "happiness," that portion of subjective well-being that is due to genetic differences between individuals. The stability of subjective well-being over time is substantial, and this is likely due in part to the stability of personality. Specific personality traits are related to various types of well-being. For example, extroversion appears to be more strongly related to positive emotions, while neuroticism is more related to negative feelings. Although personality is an important correlate of subjective well-being, situations and life circumstances can in some cases have a considerable influence as well. Furthermore, personality can to some degree change over time, and with it, levels of subjective well-being can change.

Subjective well-being (SWB) reflects the extent to which people think and feel that their life is going well. This construct—which is often referred to more colloquially as happiness—plays somewhat of an unusual role within personality psychology. On the one hand, neither the previous two editions of this handbook (Pervin, 1990; Pervin & John, 1999) nor Hogan, Johnson, and Briggs's (1997) *Handbook of Personality Psychology* included chapters on the topic (though these handbooks did address the topic of emotion). This absence suggests that well-being research has not played a central role in personality theory. Yet on the other hand, the strong influence of personality is seen as one of the most replicable and most surprising findings to emerge from the last four decades of research on SWB. In fact, Gilovich and Eihach (2001) suggested that the relatively weak influence of situational factors and the relatively strong influence of personality factors in an important, counter intuitive finding that came as a considerable surprise to social psychologists. If the links between personality and SWB are so strong and so

R.E. Lucas (✉)
Department of Psychology, Michigan State University, East Lansing, MI 48824, USA
e-mail: lucasri@msu.edu

E. Diener (ed.), *The Science of Well-Being: The Collected Works of Ed Diener*, Social Indicators Research Series 37, DOI 10.1007/978-90-481-2350-6_4,
© Springer Science+Business Media B.V. 2009

surprising, why hasn't SWB research played a more important role in personality theory? Furthermore, why are personality effects in the SWB domain viewed as being so surprising in the first place?

We believe that part of the answer to these questions comes when we consider the dual nature of the construct. SWB can be thought of both as an outcome for which individuals strive and as part of a functional process that helps individuals to achieve other goals. In reference to the first point. William James suggested that "how to keep, how to gain, how to recover happiness is . . . for most men at all times the secret motive for all they do" (1902, p. 76). We would argue that the only thing that James got wrong in this statement is the suggestion that this motive is secret. Most people agree that being happy is the ultimate goal toward which they strive. For instance, one study reported that being happy was raced to be more important than having good health, a high income, or high levels of attractiveness; and it was rated as being more important than experiencing love or meaning in life (Diener & Oishï, 2004). Thus, happiness is seen as an ultimate goal that guides individual choices and that can be achieved if the external circumstances in a person's life coincide with his or her desires (for a different view/emphasis, see Ryff & Keyes, 1995; Ryff, 2008).

When people concepruize happiness in this way—as an outcome that can be achieved if things go well—they naturally think about it as something that can change. Not surprisingly, initial work in the area focused on identifying the external life cumstances that reliably correlate with SWB (Wilson, 1967). It was thought that these correlations could reveal basic human needs, and that by understanding these needs, psychologists could identify pathways to greater well-being. These efforts have continued over the years, and some progress has been made in identifying interventions that can lead to lasting changes in happiness (Lyubomirsky, Sheldon, & Schkade, 2005; Seligman, Steen, Park, & Peterson, 2005). In fact, psychologists and economists have increasingly advocated for the implementation of large-scale surveys of well-being so that population levels can be tracked over time (Diener, 2000; Diener & Seligman, 2004; Kahneman, Krueger, Schkade, Schwarz, & Stone, 2003). Again, the principle that underlies this suggestion is that by identifying macro-level characteristics that reliably affect well-being, policy decisions could be optimized to increase well-being for all.

If happiness is conceptualized as an outcome that reflects the conditions in a person's life, it may seen counterintuitive and even somewhat distressing when research suggests that happiness is stable over time and unresponsive to changes in life circumstances. It is this outcome-focused aspect of well-being research and theory that makes strong personality effects seem so surprising. Yet when SWB is thought of not as an outcome but as an integral part of an ongoing process, the strong effects of personality and the relatively weak effects of situations should come as no surprise. For at the heart of well-being judgments lie affective reactions (Lucas & Diener, 2008), and these emotions and moods likely play a functional role in people's lives (Fredrickson, 1998; Gross, 1999; Lyubomirsky, King, & Diener, 2005). Negative affect does not simply relay the news that something in one's life is not going well. Instead it provides the motivation and perhaps even the tools that allow for corrections. Similarly, pleasant feelings are not simply a reward for a job well done; these feelings are functional. Thus, negative emotions should not cease when a person's life circumstances become ideal, nor should pleasure endure forever when all important goals are achieved. In fact, the pleasure that one experiences after the achievement of a goal may actually promote the desire to seek new goals (Carver, 2003; Fredrickson, 1998). If there are individual differences in these underlying affective processes, then SWB will also exhibit the characteristics of a personality trait. Thus, well-being should be play an important role in personality research.

In the current chapter, we first discuss general issues regarding the nature of SWB. We then address concerns about the measurement of well-being. Finally, we review the evidence linking personality and well-being constructs. We believe that confusion about the dualistic nature of well-being has sometimes led to the misinterpretation of existing research, particularly when it comes to questions about the impact of external circumstances and the possibility for change. Although we believe that personality processes matter, research suggests that happiness can change and that life circumstances can have important consequences.

Defining SWB

Although researchers sometimes discuss happiness and well-being as if they reflect a unitary construct, there is no single judgment that captures the entirety of SWB. Instead, SWB researchers divide the domain into narrower classes of constructs that tap into distinct ways in which one's life could be evaluated (see Schimmack, 2008, for a more detailed review). For instance, SWB researchers often distinguish cognitive judgments of well-being from affective experience (Diener, 1984). The cognitive components assess an individual's reflective judgment that his or her life or the circumstances of that life are going well. To assess this component, researchers often administer measures of life satisfaction or domain satisfaction—measures that ask people to consider and consciously evaluate the conditions in their lives.

This type of reflective judgment can be contrasted with the emotions and moods that individuals actually experience as they live their lives. Experience sampling studies (i.e., those studies that assess experience repeatedly over time) show that there are very few moments that are affectively neutral: People report some affective feeling almost all the time (Diener, Sandvik, & Pavor, 1991). Furthermore, one of the most basic features of these feelings is that people can tell whether they are pleasant or unpleasant (Kahneman, 1999). Thus, a life could be considered to be a good one if there were more pleasant experiences than unpleasant ones over an extended period of time. Thus, *reflective judgments* and *affective experiences* provide two distinct ways in which a person's life could be evaluated.

In addition, affective experiences themselves can be further divided into narrower categories. The study of these more precise affect variables often reveals unique information about the quality of a person's life and the processes that underlie the evaluation of that life. For instance, although it is tempting to conceptualize affective experience simply as the ratio of positive to negative, much information is lost when such an index is constructed. Two individuals who have equal amounts of positive and negative experiences may have very different lives, depending on the intensity of their experiences. In addition, because positive and negative feelings are not polar opposites, it may be inappropriate to combine them in a single index. As early as 1969, Bradburn recognized that pleasant and unpleasant affect were empirically separable. Following up on this work, Watson, Tellegen, and their colleagues suggested that positive and negative affect are distinct and orthogonal factors (Watson, Clark, & Tellegen, 1988; Watson & Tellegen, 1985; Zevon & Tellegen, 1982). Furthermore, these distinct factors often correlate with unique sets of predictors (e.g., Carver, Sutton, & Scheier, 2000; Costa & McCare, 1980; Elliott & Thrash, 2002; Tellegen, 1985). To be sure, the independence view is not without its critics (see Schimmack, 2008, for a review), but SWB researchers often recommend assessing positive and negative affect separately.

Although it is easy to understand the conceptual distinctions among the various facets of well-being, it is still important to ask how the various components interrelate, both at a theoretical and empirical level. First, it is clear that the various components are, in fact, separable. For instance, multi-method studies show that when different methods of assessment are used to measure distinct well-being components, different measures of the same construct tend to correlate more strongly than do different constructs assessed by similar methods (Lucas, Diener, & Suh, 1996). This means that at a measurement level, the various components are distinct.

However, at a theoretical level it is necessary to explain the associations among the various constructs and to develop theories about the factors that will influence each. For instance, one major debate that has implications for personality theory concerns the top-down versus bottom-up issue (Diener, 1984; Heller, Watson, & Ilies, 2004; Schimmack, 2008). According to bottom-up models, individuals construct global well-being judgments by evaluating the various characteristics in their lives. People might examine the various domains in their lives, calculate satisfaction scores for each domain, and then aggregate across domains to arrive at an overall judgment of life satisfaction. In this model (which is consonant with the SWB-as-outcome view described above), life circumstances affect intermediate judgments of domain satisfaction along with day-to-day emotional experience, and these intermediate judgements and experiences combine to affect global judgments of well-being.

Although bottom-up models are intuitively appealing, the strong forms of these models do not appear to be correct. For one thing, the amount of information that one must aggregate to calculate a global judgment of happiness is probably too large to allow for quick and efficient ratings. Reaction time studies suggest that once people are asked to evaluate relatively long periods of time (i.e., longer than a few hours), they do not search their memory for relevant information. Instead, they rely on existing beliefs about their happiness to make a global judgment (Robinson & Clore, 2002). We must caution that this finding does not necessarily mean that these quick judgments are not valid; it simply suggests that people do not conduct an exhaustive search of information about satisfaction with lower-level domains before coming up with a global judgment. This fact, combined with research showing that the associations among domain satisfaction ratings are too high to be explained by a simple bottom-up model (Schimmack, 2008), shows that well-being judgments are not constructed in a purely bottom-up manner. Instead, top-down processes likely play a role.

Top-down models posit that personality processes influence the general affective tone that a person experiences, and this general tendency colors all aspects of that person's life. A happy person will not only experience frequent positive emotions and infrequent negative emotions, but he or she will view the various aspects of life as being more positive than they really are. Thus, the moderate association between domain and life satisfaction could be explained by the tendency for happy people to be satisfied with all aspects of their lives, rather than by a causal effect of domains on global judgments. According to this top-down model, life circumstances have weak effects on happiness because personality-based processes affect how one views the world (see, e.g., Brief, Butcher, George, & Link, 1993; Feist, Bodner, Jacobs, Miles, & Tan, 1995; Judge & Watanabe, 1993; Saris, 2001; Schyns, 2001).

The final structural consideration concerns the links between the affective and cognitive components. As the evidence from discriminant validity studies shows, life satisfaction judgments do not simply reflect the sum of one's affective experiences over time (Lucas et al., 1996). Instead, these cognitive judgments and affective experiences provide different information about the quality of one's life as a whole. It appears that affective experience may provide one source of information that individuals can use to judge the overall quality of their lives. However, they may also consider additional factors, including the objective conditions in their lives or their satisfaction with narrower domains (Schimmack, 2008).

Furthermore, the role that these affective experiences play in the construction of global judgments may vary across individuals. For instance, we showed that positive and negative affect predicted life satisfaction to different degrees in different cultures (Suh, Diener, Oishi, & Triandis, 1998). Among participants from individualist cultures, affective experience was strongly correlated with life satisfaction, whereas among participants from collectivist cultures, the associations were somewhat weaker. Because people living in individualist cultures tend to view the self as an autonomous, self-sufficient entity (Markus & Kitayama, 1991), feelings and emotions weigh heavily as determinants of behavior. Collectivist cultures, on the other hand, stress harmony with family and friends rather than stressing one's autonomy from these people. Feelings about the self (including emotional reactions) weigh less heavily in these cultures. Thus, people appear to rely on their emotions when making satisfaction judgments, but the exact role that these experiences play may vary depending on the value that individuals place on these experiences (see Kim-Prieto, E. Diener, Tamir, Scollon, & M. Diener, 2005, for a more detailed discussion of the processes that link the various components of SWB).

In summary, SWB can be defined as an individual's subjective belief or feeling that his or her life is going well. There is no single judgment that can capture the diverse ways that life can be evaluated. Instead, a variety of cognitive and affective components are needed to provide a relatively complete picture of one's life as a whole. It is important to stress that each component may be affected by different predictors and may result from distinct but overlapping processes (Kim-Prieto et al., 2005). Thus, researchers who study SWB must carefully consider which components are most useful for their purposes—not all components will behave in similar ways. An important goal for ongoing and future research will be to identify and explain the links between these diverse ways of evaluating a person's life.

Measuring SWB

Because SWB researchers place value on an individual's own opinion about his or her life, it is sometimes assumed that self-reports of well-being provide the "gold standard" measure of the construct. But this is simply not the case. Although it is true that self-reports are used quite frequently within the field, there are also reasons to be skeptical of these measures. For instance, people may not want to reveal their true level of happiness, and method factors such as scale use or acquiescence bias could overwhelm the true variance that is captured by self-report techniques. Furthermore, if certain cognitive theories are correct, people may not have the cognitive capacity to report accurately on their experiences over time (Robinson & Clore, 2002; Schwarz & Strack, 1999). Thus, the validity of self-reports must not be taken for granted simply because they have strong face validity as measures of subjective feelings. Researchers must make sure that responses to these measures make sense in a larger nomological network that includes non-self-report measures and criteria.

Research examining the psychometric properties of SWB measures has shown that self-report scales tend to be reliable and valid. For instance, multiple-item measures of life satisfaction, domain satisfaction, and positive and negative affect scales all show high reliability, regardless of whether reliability is assessed using interitem correlations or short-term test-retest correlations (Diener, Suh, Lucas, & Smith, 1999). More importantly, there is increasing evidence for the validity of these measures. Different measures of the same well-being construct tend to correlate more strongly with one another than with measures of related but theoretically distinct constructs (Lucas et al., 1996). In addition, these measures also coverage with non-self-report methods of assessment. For instance, Lucas et al. showed that self-reports of life satisfaction, positive affect, and negative affect correlated between 0.35 and 0.52 with informant reports of the same constructs. Similarly, Sandvik, Diener, and Seidlitz (1993) showed that expert ratings of participants' happiness correlated approximately 0.50 with self-reports. Even indirect measures, such as the number of positive versus negative life events that an individual could remember and list, tend to correlate with self-report measures of happiness (Sandvik et al., 1993). Finally, well-being measures are correlated with physiological indicators, including asymmetrical hemispheric activation in the prefrontal cortex (Davidson, 2004). This evidence suggests that unwanted method variance does not overwhelm the valid variance that is captured by self-report methods of assessment.

Research also shows that self-report measures are responsive to life events and sensitive to different life circumstances. Although we review this evidence in more detail when we discuss the factors that influence well-being, it is worth noting here that well-being measures change when significant life events occur (Headey & Wearing, 1989; Lucas, 2005, 2006; Lucas, Clark, Georgellis, & Diener, 2003, 2004; Magnus, 1991; Suh, Diener, & Fujita, 1996). Furthermore individuals living in disadvantaged circumstances tend to report lower well-being than do those living in more ideal settings. For instance, Biswas-Diener and Diener (2001) found that individuals living in the slums of Calcutta reported life satisfaction scores that were considerably lower than individuals living in more affluent circumstances. Similarly, individuals with severe spinal cord injuries or other lasting disabilities tend to report well-being scores that are much lower than those of individuals without such injuries (Brickman, Coates, & Janoff-Buiman, 1978; Dijkers, 1997; Lucas, 2007).

In fact, even among individuals with spinal cord injuries, well-being measures are able to distinguish between those who have additional complications and those who do not. For instance, Putzke, Richards, Hicken, and DeVivo (2002) used the Satisfaction With Life Scale (SWLS: Diener, Emmons, Larsen, & Griffin, 1985) to examine life satisfaction in a cohort of 940 adults with traumatic onset spinal cord injury. The entire sample of participants reported relatively low levels of life satisfaction ($M = 17.3$, $SD = 7.7$) when compared to adult norms, which tend to average between 23 and 27 in most samples (Pavot & Diener, 1993). But more importantly, a number of additional characteristics were significantly related to SWLS scores. For example, spinal-cord injured patients with no additional medical complications (e.g., bladder management, ventilator use, autonomic dysreflexia, and deep vein thrombosis) were significantly more satisfied than individuals with either one or more than one complication. Similarly, individuals who had required no additional hospitalizations following injury were significantly more satisfied than individuals who had undergone one or more than one subsequent hospitalization (effect sizes were in the small to moderate range). Thus, life circumstances seem to matter, and the effects of these circumstances are reflected in SWB measures.

It is also the case that SWB measures predict relevant behaviors and outcomes. For instance, Koivumaa-Honkanen and colleagues have examined the predictive validity of self-report life satisfaction and happiness measures in a sample of over 29,000 Finnish adults (mostly twins) who were followed for up to 20 years. Their analyses show that life satisfaction prospectively predicts outcomes that include suicide (Koivumaa-Honkanen, Honkanen, Koskenvuo, & Kaprio, 2003; Koivumaa-Honkanen, Honkanen, Vinamaki, Heikkilä, Kaprio, & Koskenvuo, 2001) and the onset of depression (Koivumaa-Honkanen, Kaprio, Honkanen, Vinamaki, & Koskenvuo, 2004). Even measures of domain satisfaction predict outcomes that might be expected to occur among those who are unsatisfied with a particular area of their lives. For instance, research shows that job satisfaction measures predict absenreeism and the likelihood of changing jobs (Clark, Georgellis, & Sanfey, 1998; Frijters, 2000; Pelled & Xin, 1999). In other words, those who are not dissatisfied with their jobs tend to stay away from those jobs and tend to leave those jobs. These results show that people who say they are unsatisfied do things that psychologists would expect unsatisfied people to do.

Of course, this evidence does not mean that SWB measures are beyond reproach. Researchers have raised serious challenges to the validity, and these challenges must be acknowledged and addressed by any psychologist who wishes to use these measures. For instance, Schwarz, Strack, and their colleagues have argued that a variety of irrelevant contextual factors (including minor changes in instructions, setting, question wording, question order, or response options) can have a strong influence on well-being judgments and therefore that these reports should not be trusted. For instance, in a study that is often cited as evidence for the malleability of well-being reports, Strack, Martin, and Schwarz (1988) showed that simply changing the order of two questions could dramatically influence the correlation between them. In their study, when questions about satisfaction with a specific domain (e.g., relationship satisfaction) preceded a question about general life satisfaction, then the correlation between the two measures was strong. When the general life satisfaction question was asked first, however, then the two measures correlated quite weakly. This pattern of associations suggests that asking about specific life domains makes information about these domains salient when an individual is later asked to judge his or her life as a whole. It also implies that life satisfaction judgments are constructed "on the fly" and are susceptible to irrelevant contextual effects.

Schwarz and Strack have amassed an impressive body of research that provides insight into the processes that underlie self-reported judgments of well-being (see Schwarz, 1999, for a review of more general processes). Based on their review of the literature, they concluded that one might interprer this body of evidence to mean that "there is little to be learned from self-reports of global well-being" and that "what is being assessed, and how, seems too context-dependent to provide reliable information about a population's well-being" (Schwarz & Strack, 1999, p. 80). However, we believe that such statements are much too strong and are not supported by the large body of evidence showing that SWB measures are stable and valid. Experimental studies in controlled laboratory settings reveal important information about the processes that may underlie complex psychological phenomena. But it is important to remember that demonstrating that such processes exist does not reveal the extent to which these processes affect real-world judgments. Additional research is needed to determine the extent to which irrelevant contextual factors actually influence SWB measures, although existing research suggests that these influences are not strong.

For instance, Schimmack and Oishi (2005) conducted a meta-analysis of studies that had manipulated the order of life satisfaction and domain satisfaction ratings (along with five new replication studies of their own), and they showed that the item-order effect that Strack, Martin, and Schwarz (1988) identified is, on average, quite small. In addition, Schimmack and Oishi, along with Schimmack, Diener, and Oishi (2002), showed that people tend to use chronically accessible information rather than transient sources of information when constructing well-being judgments. Furthermore, contextual factors such as current mood have only a very small influence on well-being judgments that theoretically should be stable (Eid & Diener, 2004). Together, this evidence suggests that although people may be influenced by transient and irrelevant contextual information, these effects are not large.

In summary, evidence to date suggests that self-report measures of SWB are reliable and valid, sensitive to external circumstances, and responsive to change. They correlate with additional self-report measures in addition to non-self-report measures and criteria. Finally, they prospectively predict theoretically relevant behaviors and outcomes, which shows that they can be useful both in research and in practice. It is true that there may be times when contextual factors influence these judgments, but we are aware of no research that suggests that such contextual effects have a large impact on the validity of the measures. Thus, researchers can be confident that SWB can be assessed well with standard self-report measures. That being said, we also believe that self-report does not provide a gold standard, and thus alternative techniques should be used when possible. Experience sampling techniques (Scollon, Kim-Prieto, & Diener, 2003) or other self-report procedures that do not require memory for, and aggregation across, numerous events can help. In addition, non-self-report measures, including informant reports, psychophysiological measures, textual analysis, and other novel techniques, can provide important information about the extent to which a person's life is going well.

Evidence for the Importance of Personality

After decades of research on SWB researchers have often arrived at what to some seems like a startling conclusion: The most important factor in determining a person's SWB appears to be the personality with which he or she is born. Evidence for this conclusion comes from at least four lines of research. First, studies of objective life circumstances (including such factors as a person's income, age, education level, doctor-rated health, and social relationships) show that associations with such factors tend to be quite small. Second, SWB is moderately heritable, which means that some inborn factors are at work. Third, SWB is stable over time, sometimes even in the face of changing life circumstances. And finally, when effect sizes are compared directly, correlations with personality traits tend to be much larger than correlations with external circumstances. This evidence has been interpreted to mean that happiness cannot change and that individuals are stuck with a biologically determined level of happiness that is only weakly linked to the circumstances that they experience in life. In the following sections, we review evidence from these four different lines of research. Although we believe that personality plays an important role in SWB, a careful examination of the existing evidence suggests that life circumstances also matter and that there is room for change.

Associations with External Life Circumstances

People's behavior is often guided by their beliefs about the types of things that will make them happy (Gilbert, 2006). People may choose a high-paying job, an expensive house, or a short commute over other alternatives because they believe that these life circumstances will improve or maintain their happiness. Thus, one goal for psychological research is to identify the factors that actually do correlate with happiness. Through such research, people's intuitions could be tested, and practical guidance could be offered. Unfortunately, the most common conclusion from such inquiries is that very few objective life circumstances exhibit strong associations with any SWB variable. In one of the first attempts to quantify the links between SWB and a broad set of predictors, Andrews and Withey (1976) concluded that about 10% of the variance in well-being could be accounted for by demographic characteristics. In later reviews, Diener (1984) and Argyle (1999) suggested a slightly higher estimate of 15%. Below we review some of the findings from this literature, focusing not just on effect sizes but also on the practical implications of these effects.

Perhaps the most surprising finding in this line of research concerns the link between income and happiness. Many studies have been conducted, and a number of consistent findings have emerged (Diener & Biswas-Diener, 2002). Most important for the current discussion, research shows that at an individual level, correlations tend to be positive but very small. For instance, Lucas and Dyrenforth (2006) reviewed evidence from two meta-analyses (Haring, Stock, & Okun, 1984; Pinquart & Sörensen 2000), a more recent narrative review of cross-national results (Diener & Biswas-Diener, 2002), and many waves of an annual nationally representative survey (General Social Survey; Davis, Smith, & Marsden, 2003). This review showed that the correlation between income and happiness tends to fall between 0.17 and 0.21. The typical conclusion that one draws from these data is that people overestimate the importance of money, and that once people have their basic needs met, income does not matter.

Although we do not dispute the size of the correlations that have been found in previous research, we caution that such correlations need to be interpreted carefully. For instance, a 0.20 correlation would mean that each additional standard deviation of income would only "buy" one-fifth of a standard deviation in happiness. However, income standard deviations tend to be quite small relative to the range of the distribution. Thus, when people's intuition suggests that money will make them happier, they may by concerned with moving closer to the endpoint of the distribution rather than just moving one or two standard deviations away from their current position. Even with a relatively weak 0.20 correlation, the intuition that money matters could still be correct.

To illustrate, we examined data from the most recent wave of the German Socio-Economic Panel (GSOEP) study, a long-running, nationally representative panel study that is in its 22nd year (Lucas & Schimmack, 2007). We first transformed household income scores from Euros into U.S. dollars and then computed the correlation between income and life satisfaction. Consistent with previous research, the correlation was a small 0.18. However, this small correlation can result from very large differences between the various income groups (Fig. 1. For instance, those in the richest group report life satisfaction scores that are more than one-half of one standard deviation above the mean level of satisfaction and almost three-quarters of one standard deviation above the satisfaction of those living at the poverty level.

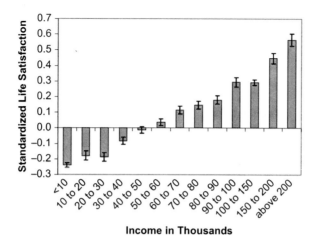

Fig. 1 Standardized life satisfaction plotted against income (in thousands of U.S. dollars) in the 2004 wave of the GSOEP

We do not consider these to be small effects, even though income can only explain a very small amount of the variance in life satisfaction measures among the full sample.

Additional interpretational concerns arise when inappropriate measures of the predictor variables are used. This problem can be illustrated by examining the association between health and well-being. Correlations with health tend to be small to moderate in size. Okun, Stock, Haring, and Wirtet (1984) conducted a meta-analysis of over 200 effect sizes, and they found correlations around 0.30. Similarly, Brief and colleagues (1993) found that subjective reports of health tended to correlate between 0.30 and 0.40 with life satisfaction. Effects of this size might suggest that health plays a reasonably important role in SWB. However, both groups of researchers have suggested that when more objective measures of health are obtained, the correlation drops close to zero. For instance, Okun and George (1984) found that physician ratings of health were not correlated with well-being, and Brief et al. found that the number of doctor visits only correlated about 0.10 with life satisfaction.

Although some have suggested that this type of discrepancy provides evidence that self-reports of health are not valid (e.g., Diener et al., 1999; Kahneman & Riis, 2005), there is some indication that the opposite might be true. Self-reports may in fact be more valid (at least in terms of content validity) than other objective measures. For instance, self-reports of health predict mortality over and above more objective measures (e.g., Ganz, Lee, & Siau, 1991; Mossey & Shapiro, 1982; Rumsfeld et al., 1999), and studies that have investigated the discrepancies between self- and doctor-rated health have found evidence that it may be the doctors' judgments that are wrong (e.g., Nelson et al., 1983). Finally, as was noted in the section on validity, there is considerable evidence that objective measures of specific health conditions, such as spinal cord injuries and severe disability, are associated with large and lasting differences in SWB.

The examples described above show that associations that appear to be very small can actually be quite large when alternative effect size indexes are examined or when appropriate measures of predictor variables are used. Unfortunately, the opposite can also be true. Effects that have been considered to be very large may not be so large when examined closely. Recently, we argued that this is the case with variables related to the existence of social relationships (Lucas & Dyrenforth, 2005, 2006). When predictors of SWB are compared, variables such as the existence of strong social relationships are presented as if they were the strongest correlates to emerge from the literature (e.g., Argyle, 2001). However, reviews of this literature often focus on satisfaction with relationships or the extent to which people value relationships, rather than on the existence of relationships themselves. If these more objective measures are evaluated, the correlations are similar to, and perhaps even smaller than, the association with income.

For example, Lucas and Dyrenforth (2006) reviewed the literature on the associations between SWB and the number of friends that people have, whether individuals have a close friend to whom they can talk, the amount of time that people spend with friends, and the amount of time that people spend with family members. Existing meta-analyses (e.g., Okun et al., 1984; Pinquart & Sörensen, 2000) along with new analyses of data from nationally representative surveys showed that correlations with these variables tended to be around 0.15 and very rarely exceeded 0.20. Even marital status, which has often been held up as one of the most important demographic predictors, only correlates 0.14 with measures of SWB (Haring-Hidore, Stock, Okun, & Witter, 1985). Thus, at least when relatively objective measures are assessed, these associations are smaller than the effect of income or health.

We acknowledge that the same concerns about the interpretation of effect sizes that we raised for income and health may also apply to correlations with social relationship variables. A very small correlation may be meaningful, and simple count- and frequency-based measures of social relationships may not adequately capture the quality of these relationships. Furthermore, social relationships, including marriage, predict a wide variety of outcomes that include risk for mental illness, poor physical health, and even death (e.g., Berkman & Syme, 1979; House, Landis, & Umberson, 1988; House, Robbins, & Merzner, 1982). Thus, the robustness of these effects across domains may be important, even if the individual effects are quite small. However, because it is difficult to say whether an individual effect size is practically important, researchers must be careful to compare apples to apples when drawing conclusions about the relative importance of different life circumstances.

The three domains reviewed above provide just a small sample of effects from the large body of literature linking SWB to demographic characteristics and other external life circumstances. Considerable amounts of research have also investigated factors such as age, gender, education, employment status, ethnicity, and religion. A more detailed review is beyond the scope of this chapter, though we refer the reader to other sources, including Argyle (1999, 2001) and one of our previous reviews (Diener et al., 1999) for more detailed coverage. Our goal here is to point out that although effect sizes have often been found to be quite small, these effects must be interpreted carefully. The types of characteristics reviewed in this section do not account for much variance in SWB scores, but this lack of variance does not necessarily mean that they are unimportant. Individuals who become unemployed, acquire a disability, or lose contact with a close friend may, in fact, experience lasting changes as a consequence of these losses. Thus, SWB may be more strongly influenced by life circumstances than has generally been assumed.

Heritability of SWB

The second piece of evidence for personality effects comes from behavioral genetic studies that examine the heritability of the various SWB components. In the typical design, identical and fraternal twins complete happiness measures and then the cross-twin correlations are compared. Simple additive genetic effects are implied when the cross-twin correlation for identical twins is approximately twice as large as the cross-twin correlation for fraternal twins. Nonadditive genetic effects are implied when the ratio of identical to fraternal twin correlations is higher than two (though more sophisticated designs are often required to isolate these effects). Extensions of the basic twin design can be used to examine additional questions about the heritability of happiness. For instance, the inclusion of twins who were raised in different households allows researchers to isolate shared-environment effects more precisely and to rule out alternative explanations of the results. In addition, by acquiring multiple waves of data over time, researchers can examine the genetic effects on stability and change.

A number of studies have been conducted to examine the heritability of various well-being measures, and most arrive at similar conclusions about the broad heritability of SWB. For instance, in perhaps the first such study, Tellegen and colleagues (1988) examined twins who were reared together and those who were reared apart to estimate the contribution of genes and environment to various scales from the Multidimensional Personality Questionnaire. The estimated heritabilities of the well-being facet and global positive emotionality factor were 0.48 and 0.40, respectively. The heritabilities of the stress reaction facet and negative emotionality factor were 0.53 and 0.55, respectively. These estimates suggest that about half of the variance in these well-being measures could be accounted for by shared genes. Importantly, this study also suggested that growing up in the same household played very little role in the similarity of twins. The only significant shared environment effect was for the global positive emotionality trait, where this component accounted for 22% of the variance.

One criticism that could be raised about this study is that the assessed measures were not developed as measures of subjective well-being. Instead, they were developed to assess stable personality characteristics that have an affective core. Thus, they may not reflect "happiness" as it is typically studied by SWB researchers. However, more recent studies have replicated this basic effect using a variety of measures. For instance, Roysamb, Harris, Magnus, Vitterso, and Tambs (2002; also see Roysamb, Tambs, Reichborn-Kjennerud, Neale, & Harris, 2003) examined the heritability of a four-item global well-being measure that assessed satisfaction, happiness, nervousness, and activity level. Like Tellegen and colleagues (1988), they found that about 50% of the variance could be accounted for by a genetic component, and the shared-environment component contributed very little. Similarly, Stubbe, Posthuma, Boomsma, and De Geus (2005) reported that 38% of the variability in the SWLS (Diener et al., 1985) was heritable.

These studies consistently show that regardless of the measure that is used, broad heritability estimates for well-being constructs tend to fall between 0.40 and 0.50. However, this does not mean that behavioral genetic research is without controversy. Perhaps the most controversial issue relates to questions regarding the heritability of the stable component of happiness. According to one prominent model of SWB, people have a setpoint level of happiness that is stable over time (Brickman & Camphell, 1971). Events and life circumstances can move people away from this setpoint, but eventually people adapt and return to baseline. Thus, at any given moment, a person's happiness score might reflect the combined effects of the stable baseline and the temporary influence of life events. If so, the heritability of happiness might be higher if the stable baseline could be isolated from these temporary deviations.

In 1996, Lykken and Tellegen attempted to accomplish this goal using data from identical and fraternal twins who completed happiness measures on two occasions separated by approximately 10 years. Lykken and Tellegen found that the stability of well-being was about 0.50, meaning that approximately 50% of the variance at either of the two occasions was stable trait variance. But more importantly, they found that the cross-time, cross-twin correlation was 0.40 in the identical twins. Because this cross-twin, cross-time correlation is 80% as large as the stability coefficient, Lykken and Tellegen estimated that 80% of the stable component of well-being is heritable. The authors suggested that this extremely high heritability means that "trying to be happier [may be] as futile as trying to be taller" (p. 189).

There are three reasons why this conclusion may be too extreme. First, as Rutter (1997) noted, estimates of heritability "provide no unambiguous implications for theory, policy, or practice" (p. 391). In other words, even if Lykken and Tellegen's (1996) estimate of heritability is correct, this does not necessarily mean that happiness cannot be changed. Until the mechanisms by which these genetic effects work are discovered, questions about the possibility for change remain even when the heritability is known to be strong.

Second, the high heritability only refers to the part of happiness that is stable over time, and this makes up only about half of the variance at any given wave in Lykken and Tellegen's (1996) study. Furthermore, these stability estimates appear to be at the upper bound for what is typically found in longitudinal studies of SWB. As we review in the section on stability below, most studies find 10-year stabilities that are somewhat lower than that found by Lykken and Tellegen. Thus, even if the stable component was 100% heritable and completely unchangeable, there would still be considerable room for change.

Finally, Lykken and Tellegen's (1996) conclusion is based on a single study with a relatively small sample of twins. Although a more recent study has replicated these findings in a much larger sample (Nes, Roysamb, Tambs, Harris, & Reichborn-Kjennerud, 2006), a second study has nor. Johnson, McGue, and Krueger (2005) presented cross-twin, cross-time correlations that suggest that 38% of the stable variance in well-being is heritable (though they did not set out to address this question and did not set out to address this question and did not explicitly analyze their data in this way). The major difference between these two samples was the age of the participants. The Johnson and colleagues study included older adults, whereas the Nes and colleagues study and the original Lykken and colleagues study included a sample of participants in their 20s. Thus, with only three studies available, the replicability of this more controversial effect (along with the role that age plays in this effect) cannot be evaluated.

Stability of SWB

It is tempting to interpret heritability statistics as an index of changeability. But as noted above, there is no direct and necessary correspondence between the heritability of a characteristic and the extent to which it can change. If the process linking genes to well-being is indirect, then even characteristics with very strong heritabilities could be changed if the underlying processes were identified and effective interventions were designed. Furthermore, because even stable biological characteristics can be changed under the right circumstances (e.g., Davidson et al., 2003), even a direct link from genes to physiology to SWB does not guarantee that change cannot occur. Therefore, for researchers interested in the stability of SWB over time, it is important to address this question directly. How stable is happiness, and is there evidence that lasting changes can occur under the right circumstances?

For decades, psychologists have recognized that there is considerable stability in people's affective and cognitive evaluations of their lives. This stability is reflected both in the consistency of individuals' affective reactions to distinct situations and in the maintenance of their relative level of global happiness over time. For instance, in his early studies on the consistency of personality, Epstein (1979) showed that affect during any one day correlates relatively weakly with affect on any other day. However, once affect is aggregared over multiple days, strong correlations emerge. Similarly, momentary affect was assessed across multiple situations using the experience sampling method (Diener & Larsen, 1984). Like Epstein, it was found that moment-to-moment correlations were quite weak. However, once affect ratings were aggregated within similar types of situations, average levels of affect were highly consistent over time and across situations. For instance, average positive affect at work correlated 0.70 with average positive affect experienced during recreation. Similarly, average negative affect at work correlated 0.74 with average negative affect during recreation. Thus, there are stable individual differences in the level of positive and negative affect that emerge even across diverse situations.

Of course, cross-situational consistency does not guarantee long-term stability, and therefore to determine whether happiness can change, it is necessary to conduct longitudinal studies over very long periods of time. Results of such studies show that the various SWB components exhibit moderate long-term stability. For instance, Schimmack and Oishi (2005) conducted a meta-analysis of existing studies that had examined the stability of life satisfaction measures. Not surprisingly, they found that stability decreased with increasing intervals. However, even after relatively long periods of time had elapsed, life satisfaction measures were moderately stable. For instance, the predicted 2−, 5−, and 10 year stabilities were approximately 0.60, 0.50, and 0.35, respectively.

More recently, Fujita and Diener (2005) and Lucas and Donnellan (2007) used data from large-scale panel studies to estimate the stability of a single-item life satisfaction measure. Fujita and Diener showed that even over a period of 17 years, the stability of life satisfaction was approximately 0.25. Lucas and Donnellan used the same data and an additional panel study to isolate stable trait variance from slowly changing autoregressive variance and unstable state variance. They calculated that between 34 and 38% of the variance in single-item life satisfaction measures is trait variance that is perfectly stable over time. Thus, these estimates predict that long-term stabilities should asymptote around 0.35.

Fewer studies have been conducted examining the long-term stability of affect measures, but the research that exists lead to comparable conclusions to those from studies of life satisfaction. For instance, Watson and Walker (1996) examined the 3-year stability of affect ratings and found correlations that ranged from 0.36 to 0.46. Lucas and colleagues (1996) found slightly higher estimates, with 3-year stabilities of 0.56 and 0.61 for positive and negative affect, respectively. They also showed that these stabilities only dropped slightly (to 0.42 and 0.45) when self-reports were used to predict informant reports 3 years later (Magnus, 1991, reported similar results for self and informant reports of life satisfaction). Thus, like life satisfaction, positive and negative affect are moderately stable over time.

It is important to note, however, that these stabilities tend to be lower than the stability of other personality traits. For instance, Schimmack and Oishi's 2005) meta-analysis and Lucas and Donnellan's (2007) analysis of the GSOEP data suggest that the 20-year stability for life satisfaction should be around 0.30–0.35. Roberts and DelVecchio (2000) conducted similar analyses using personality traits, and they estimated that the 20-year stability for personality traits would be around 0.41. However, because Roberts and DelVecchio only reported the predicted 20-year stability for the least stable group of adults in their meta-analysis (20-year-olds), this value probably underestimates the long-term stability of personality traits among a broader sample of participants. For example, Roberts and DelVecchio found that the average stability coefficient for 18- to 20-year-olds was 0.54, whereas the average stability coefficient for 50- to 59-year-olds was 0.74. Thus, these comparisons show that SWB variables, while moderately stable over long periods of time, rend to be less stable than other established personality traits (also see Vaidya, Gray, Haig, & Watson, 2002).

Examination of stability coefficients provides one important piece of information about the extent to which personality can change. However, there are alternative techniques for investigating change that go beyond simply assessing rank-order stability. For instance, stability coefficients alone cannot distinguish stochastic change (where a variety of factors causes random changes that accumulate over time) from systematic change resulting from major life events (Fraley & Roberts, 2005). To assess the reasons for change, more sophisticated designs are required.

Recently, we have turned to the analysis of large-scale, long-running, nationally representative panel studies to determine whether major life events have lasting effects on SWB. These studies allow us to examine long-term levels of SWB both before and after events occur. This means that preexisting differences between those who experienced a particular life event and those who did not can be separated from true longitudinal change. Three important conclusions can be drawn from these studies (for a review see Diener, Lucas, & Scollon, 2006).

First, life events can have important effects on long-term levels of SWB. Divorce (Lucas, 2005), unemployment (Lucas et al., 2003), and the onset of a long-term disability (Lucas, 2007) are all associated with lasting changes in life satisfaction, and the effects can sometimes be quite large. For instance, the onset of a lasting disability was associated with more than a half a standard deviation drop in life satisfaction. The effects of severe disabilities were even larger, with effect sizes over a full standard deviation.

Second, there is not single answer to the question of whether people adapt to major life events. Very little adaptation occurred following the onset of disability, even over very long periods of time (Lucas, 2006). For events such as unemployment and divorce, on the other hand, some amount of adaptation occurred, but this adaptation was incomplete (Lucas, 2005; Lucas et al., 2004). Finally, for events such as marriage and widowhood, a great deal of adaptation occurred, with average levels of happiness returning to pre-event levels (Lucas et al., 2003).

Finally, there are considerable individual differences in the amount of change that occurs following life events. Because pre-event levels of SWB are known in these studies, it is possible to examine both average change as well as variability around this average level. Analyses show that the amount of variability is often quite large. For instance, Lucas and colleagues (2003) showed that on average, people adapt to marriage. Within approximately 2 or 3 years after marriage, participants who got married were no happier than they were before they got married. However, the amount of variability in the change scores was almost as great as the variability that existed in pre-event baseline levels. Thus, many people reported lasting positive change in happiness following the marriage, but there were also many people who reported lasting negative changes. Importantly, results showed that those people who had very positive initial reactions to marriage were also still far from baseline many years later. Thus, the fact that happiness levels are not greater after marriage than they were before marriage does not mean that adaptation is inevitable. Instead, the results from this study of marriage show that the same event may affect individuals in different ways, and these differential reactions may hide the amount of true change that occurs.

Associations with Personality Traits

The final piece of evidence we review concerns the empirical links between personality and SWB. In 1967, Warner Wilson published one of the first reviews of the literature on the correlates of what he called "avowed happiness." Although this review was based on a fairly small body of evidence, Wilson's conclusions foreshadowed modern research quite well. Although some external circumstances were judged to be important, many of the most reliable findings concerned individuals' characteristic outlook on life. For instance, his summary suggests that the happy person is "extraverred, optimistic, worry free" and has high self-esteem and modest aspirations (p. 294). The research conducted since Wilson published this review confirms that personality characteristics often exhibit moderate to strong correlations with well-being variables.

The personality characteristics that have been most frequently studied in relation to SWB are extraversion and neuroticism (Diener & Lucas, 1999). As early as the 1930s, researchers had linked characteristics such as social interest and the tendency to worry to reports of subjective well-being (e.g., Jasper, 1930; see Wilson, 1967, for a review). Research on these characteristics continued in the years that followed, but the modern focus on these two traits is often traced to a landmark study by Costa and McCrae (1980). These researchers argued that the broad trait of extraversion influenced feelings of positive affect, the trait of neuroticism influenced negative affect, and together these two components of emotional well-being influenced overall feelings of life satisfaction. In support of this hypothesis, Costa and McCrae found that extraversion was correlated with feelings of positive affect, and neuroticism was correlated with negative affect. Although the correlations in their study were actually quite weak (e.g., as around 0.20), the fact that they were stable over time led Costa and McCrae to suggest that stable individual differences were important for well-being. The basic pattern of results that Costa and McCrae identified has been replicated often (Emmons & Diener, 1985; Headey & Wearing, 1989; Magnus, Diener, Fujita, & Pavor, 1993) and has been found using non-self-report measures of personality and subjective well-being (Lucas & Fujita, 2000).

Yet in a comprehensive meta-analysis of the literature on personality and SWB, DeNeve and Cooper (1998) found that the associations between these two personality traits and SWB were not particularly strong. For instance, the correlation between extraversion and SWB was only 0.17, and the correlation for neuroticism was only 0.22. These correlations were significantly different from zero, but surprisingly weak. In addition, they were approximately the same size as the correlations that emerged from meta-analysis of demographic predictors of well-being. Thus, DeNeve and Cooper's review suggested that once meta-analytic techniques were used, the correlations that had been emphasized in narrative reviews were not so large after all.

Although the scope of DeNeve and Cooper's (1998) meta-analysis is impressive, there are also reasons to interpret these results cautiously. As with all meta-analyses, decisions must be made about which studies to include and which predictors and outcomes are similar enough to be treated as equivalent. If trait measures that do not really tap the dimension in question are included in the analysis, then the average correlation with well-being may be diluted. Similarly, if correlations with different forms of SWB are aggregated even when chose different components are only weakly correlated with one another, then the meta-analytic averages may not accurately reflect the associations with the individual components themselves.

There is some evidence that these factors contributed to the surprisingly weak correlations found in DeNeve and Cooper's (1998) meta-analysis. For instance, it was suggested that the correlation between extraversion and positive affect would be higher if only established extraversion scales were assessed (Lucas & Fujita, 2000). Furthermore, it was argued that existing theory would predict that the association between extraversion and positive affect should be stronger than the correlation with the other components of SWB. Thus, this link should be examined separately. An updated meta-analysis was conducted that focused only on established extraversion scales and the positive affect component of SWB and a meta-analytic average correlation of 0.37 was found . . . considerably higher than the estimate found by DeNeve and Cooper.

This finding has been confirmed in a larger meta-analysis that focused specifically on the associations between SWB and the personality trait measures from three widely used personality inventories: the NEO Personality Inventory—Revised (NEO-PI-R; Costa & McCrae, 1992), the Eysenck Personality Inventory (EPI, H. J. Eysenck & S. B. G. Eysenck, 1968), and the Eysenck Personality Questionnaire (EPQ; S. B. J. Eysenck & H. J. Eysenck, 1975). Shultz, Schmidt, and Steel's (2008) analysis shows that when results from only established scales are used, correlations are much higher than those found by DeNeve and Cooper (1998). For instance, the correlations between extraversion and positive affect were 0.44 for the NEO, 0.35 for the EPQ, and 0.25 for the EPI (Lucas & Fujita, 2000, also found that the EPI exhibited weaker correlations, probably because of the inclusion of an impulsivity component). The correlations between neuroticism and negative affect were 0.54 for the NEO, 0.53 for the EPQ, and 0.46 for the EPI. These results confirm the importance of extraversion and neuroticism as predictors of SWB.

Both DeNeve and Cooper's (1998) and Shultz, Schmidt, and Steel's (2006) meta-analyses also show that extraversion and neuroticism are not the only traits that matter. For instance, Shultz et al. showed that correlations between agreeableness and SWB constructs were consistently significantly different from zero and ranged from 0.12 for positive affect to 0.30 for happiness. Similarly, correlations with conscientiousness ranged from −0.21 for negative affect to 0.40 for overall quality of life. DeNeve and Cooper (1998) found that repressiveness–defensiveness, trust, hardiness, and some forms of locus of control and self-esteem also exhibited relatively high correlations (though many of these correlations were derived from a very small number of studies). Finally, personality traits such as optimism and self-esteem reflect general positive views about the self and the world, and they too have been shown to correlate with well-being (e.g., Lucas et al., 1996; Schimmack & Diener, 2003).

Explanations for these associations generally take one of two forms. McCrae & Costa (1991) suggested that *instrumental theories* posit an indirect link from personality to SWB through choice of situations or the experience of life events. For example, extraverts may enjoy and participate in social activities, which may in turn affect the amounts of positive affect that they experience. These instrumental theories can be contrasted with *temperament theories*, which posit a direct link from the trait to the outcome in question. According to temperament theories, the association does not flow through life choices, life events, or life experiences.

The most widely studied temperament theories link extraversion and neuroticism to affect through two basic motivational systems that have been proposed and investigated by Gray (1970, 1981, 1991; see also Elliot & Thrash, 2002; Tellegen, 1985). According to Gray, much of the variability in personality can be explained by three fundamental systems; the behavioral activation system (BAS), which regulates reactions to signals of conditioned reward and nonpunishment; the behavioral inhibition system (BIS), which regulates reactions to signals of conditioned punishment and nonreward; and the fight–flight system (FFS), which regulates reactions to signals of unconditioned punishment and nonreward. Extraverts are though to be higher in BAS strength, and thus, they should be more sensitive to signals of reward. This reward sensitivity should be expressed in the form of enhanced information processing and increased positive emotions when exposed to positive stimuli. Similarly, the neuroticism dimension is thought to reflect individual differences in BIS strength. Thus, neurotics should be more sensitive than stable people to signals of punishment.

Tests of these hypotheses have proceeded either by ruling out instrumental explanations of the associations (e.g., by determining whether social activity mediates the association between extraversion and positive affect; e.g., Lucas, Le, & Dyrenforth, 2008) or by examining possible direct links between the constructs. For instance, Larsen and Kerelaar (1991) showed that extraverts are more sensitive than introverts to laboratory-based positive mood induction procedures and that neurotics are more sensitive than stable individuals to negative mood induction procedures (though, see Lucas & Baird, 2004, for meta-analytic evidence suggesting that the extraversion effect is not reliable). Other researchers have used paradigms that assess attention to and memory for positive and negative events (e.g., Derryberry & Reed, 1994; Rusting, 1998). Finally, researchers have linked these individual differences and affective reactions through specific psychophysiological processes (e.g., Canli, 2004; Depué & Collins, 1999; Depue & Morrone-Strupinsky, 2005). Theoretical progress on the links between these traits and well-being outcomes have advanced rapidly in recent years.

It is also important to note that personality traits are not the only personality constructs that have been studied in relation to SWB. Other stable individual differences have also been shown to be associated with well-being. For instance, Wilson's (1967) suggestion that aspirations affect well-being has been supported by more recent research. A number of studies show that the goals held by individuals are reliably associated with happiness constructs. For instance, Emmons (1986) showed that distinct characteristics of people's goals correlate with the various SWB components in different ways. Positive affect was associated with past fulfillment of goals and the degree of effort that the goal required, whereas negative affect was associated with lower perceived probability of success and high conflict between goals. Other personality researchers have examined stable individual differences in cognitive factors (e.g., Robinson & Compton, 2008) or emotion regulation strategies (e.g., John & Gross, 2004) that may play a role in SWB. A goal for future research will be to understand the processes that underlie the various characteristics that are related to well-being and to determine which are most important in driving this highly valued outcome.

Summary

The research reviewed in this chapter shows that when studying SWB, personality matters. Happiness, like most personality characteristics, is moderately heritable and moderately stable over time. In addition, happiness has been linked to specific personality traits and processes. In fact, the correlations between SWB and personality characteristics such as extraversion and neuroticism are stronger than correlations with any demographic predictor or major life circumstance that has been studied so far. Thus, a theory of well-being that fails to incorporate personality characteristics would be incomplete, and much of what we know about well-being comes from taking a personality perspective on the construct.

That being said, some caution is warranted when interpreting the evidence that has been presented in support of personality effects. For instance, it is important not to interpret strong heritabilities as evidence that happiness cannot change. Until researchers understand the processes that underlie stable individual differences in SWB, questions about the possibility for change remain unanswered. In addition, our review suggests that researchers should be careful not to dismiss effects that may appear to be quite small at first, but that have important implications for individual experience. Income may only account for about 5% of the variance in happiness, but this relatively small effect can hide the fact that the wealthy are considerably happier than individuals who live at the poverty level and below. Finally, although the stability of SWB over long periods of time is impressive, it appears that at most about 35% of the variance reflects a stable trait component that does not change over time (though the percentage of reliable variance is probably higher). In addition, the study of major life events shows that significant changes in life circumstances can have large and lasting effects on happiness. Thus, well-being is responsive to life events and changing life circumstances—which leaves hope that it can be improved.

Researchers and practitioners hoping to use SWB in applied settings are sometimes dismayed by the effects described in this chapter. But it is important to realize that even if there is a reasonable amount of stability and strong personality effects, attempts to improve overall levels of SWB can still be a worthwhile goal. As an analogue, we can consider physical health. If it was possible to construct a purely objective index of overall physical health, it is likely that this index would be moderately to strongly stable over time, moderately heritable, and at least some what related to personality traits. Yet these facts alone would probably not persuade medical researchers to give up their quest to improve levels of health. Instead, research on the stability and personality correlates of this construct would be incorporated into broad theories that explain the processes that underlie these stable individual differences in physical health. This should also be true of research on SWB. Much of what we know about the construct comes from studies that investigate the personality predictors of the trait. This research can be used to develop broad theories that explain both stability and change in happiness over time.

References

Andrews, R. M., & Withey, S. B. (1976). *Social indicators of well-being*. New York: Plenum Press.
Argyle, M. (1999). Causes and correlates of happiness. In D. Kahneman, E. Diener, & N. Schwarz (Eds.), *Well-being: The foundations of hedonic psychology* (pp. 353–373). New York: Sage Foundation.
Argyle, M. (2001). *The psychology of happiness* (2nd ed.). New York: Routledge.
Berkman, L. F., & Syme, S. L. (1979). Social networks, host resistance, and mortality: A nine year follow-up study of Alameda county residents. *American Journal of Epidemiology, 109*(2), 186–204.
Biswas-Diener, R., & Diener, E. (2001). Making the best of a bad situation: Satisfaction in the slums of Calcutta. *Social Indicators Research, 55*, 329–352.
Brickman, P., & Campbell, D. T. (1971). Hedonic relativism and planning the good society. In M. H. Appley (Ed.), *Adaptation level theory: A symposium* (pp. 287–302). New York: Academic Press.
Brickman, P., Coates, D., & Janoff-Buiman, R. (1978). Lottery winners and accident victims: Is happiness relative: *Journal of Personality and Social Psychology, 36*, 917–927.
Brief, A. P., Butcher, A. H., George, J. M., & Link, K. E. (1993). Integrating bottom-up and top-down theories of subjective well-being: The case of health. *Journal of Personality and Social Psychology, 64*(4), 646–653.
Canli, T. (2004). Functional brain mapping of extraversion and neuroticism: Learning from individual differences in emotion processing. *Journal of Personality, 72*, 1105–1132.
Carver, C. S. (2003). Pleasure as a sign you can attend to something else: Placing positive feelings within a general model of affect. *Cognition and Emotion, 17*(2), 241–261.
Carver, C. S., Sutton, S. K., & Scheier, M. F. (2000). Action, emotion, and personality: Emerging conceptual integration. *Personality and Social Psychology Bulletin, 26*, 741–751.
Clark, A., Georgellis, Y., & Sanfey, P. (1998). Job satisfaction, wage changes and quits: Evidence from Germany. *Research in Labor Economics, 17*, 95–121.
Costa, P. T., Jr., & McCrae, R. R. (1980). Influence of extraversion and neuroticism on subjective well-being. Happy and unhappy people. *Journal of Personality and Social Psychology, 38*, 668–678.
Costa, P. T., Jr., & McCrae, R. R. (1992). *Revised NEO Personality Inventory (NEO PI-R) and NEO Five-Factor Inventory (NEO-FFI): Professional manual*. Odessa, FL: Psychological Assessment Resources.
Davidson, R. J. (2004). Well-being and affective style: Neural substrates and biobehavioural correlates. *Philophical Transactions of the Royal Society of London B, 359*, 1395–1411.
Davidson, R. J., Kabar-Zinn, J., Schumacher, J., Rosenkranz, M., Muller, D., Santorelli, S. F., et al. (2003). Alterations in brain and immune function produced by mindfulness mediration. *Psychosomatic Medicine, 65*(4), 564–570.

Davis, J. A., Smith, T. W., & Marsden, P. V. (2003). *General social surveys, 1972–2002*. Ann Arbor, MI: Inter-University Consortium for Political and Social Research. Available at www.webapp.ictisr.umich.edulGSSI.

DeNeve, K. M., & Cooper, H. (1998). The happy personality: A meta-analysis of 137 personality traits and subjective well-being. *Psychological Bulletin, 124*, 197–229.

Depué, R. A., & Collins, P. F. (1999). Neurobiology of the structure of personality: Dopamine, facilitation of incentive motivation, and extraversion. *Behavioral and Brain Sciences, 22*, 491–569.

Depue, R. A., & Morrone-Strupinsky, J. V. (2005). A neurobehavioral model of affiliative bonding: Implications for conceptualizing a human trait of affiliation. *Behavioral and Brain Sciences, 28*, 313–395.

Derryberry, D., & Reed, M. A. (1994). Temperament and attention: Orienting toward and away from positive and negative signals. *Journal of Personality and Social Psychology, 66*, 1128–1139.

Diener, E. (1984). Subjective well-being. *Psychological Bulletin, 95*, 542–575.

Diener, E. (2000). Subjective well-being: The science of happiness and a proposal for a national index. *American Psychologist, 55*(1), 34–43.

Diener, E., & Biswas-Diener, R. (2002). Will money increase subjective well-being? A literature review and guide to needed research. *Social Indicators Research, 57*, 119–169.

Diener, E., Emmons, R. A., Larsen, R. J., & Griffin, S. (1985). The Satisfaction with Life Scale. *Journal of Personality Assessment, 49*(1), 71–75.

Diener, E., & Larsen, R. J. (1984). Temporal stability and cross-situational consistency of affective, behavioral, and cognitive responses, *Journal of Personality and Social Psychology, 47*, 871–883.

Diener, E., & Lucas, R. E. (1999). Personality and subjective well-being. In D. Kahneman, E. Diener, & N. Schwarz (Eds.), *Well-being: The foundations of bedonic psychology* (pp. 213–229). New York: Sage Foundation.

Diener, E., Lucas, R. E., & Scollon, C. (2006). Beyond the hedonic treadmill: Revising the adaptation theory of well-being. *American Psychologist, 61*, 305–314.

Diener, E., & Oishï, S. (2004). Are Scandinavians happier than Asians? Issues in comparing nations on subjective well-being. In F. Columbus (Ed.), *Asiant economic and political issues* (Vol. 10, pp. 1–25). Hauppauge, NY: Nova Science.

Diener, E., Sandvik, E., & Pavor, W. (1991). Happiness is the frequency, not the intensity, of positive versus negative affect. In F. Strack, M. Argyle, & N. Schwarz (Eds.), *Subjective well-being: An interdisciplinary perspective* (pp. 119–139). Elmsford, NY: Pergamon Press.

Diener, E., & Seligman, M. E. P. (2004). Beyond money: Toward an economy of well-being. *Psychological Science in the Public Interest, 5*, 1–31.

Diener, E., Suh, E. M., Lucas, R. E., & Smith, H. L. (1999). Subjective well-being: Three decades of progress. *Psychological Bulletin, 125*, 276–302.

Dijkers, M. (1997). Quality of life after spinal cord injury: A meta analysis of the effects of disablement components. *Spinal Cord, 35*, 829–840.

Eid, M., & Diener, E. (2004). Global judgments of subjective well-being: Situational variability and long-term stability. *Social Indicators Research, 65*, 245–277.

Elliot, A. J., & Thrash, T. M. (2002). Approach–avoidance motivation in personality: Approach and avoidance temperaments and goals. *Journal of Personality and Social Psychology, 82*, 804–818.

Emmons, R. A. (1986). Personal strivings: An approach to personality and subjective well-being. *Journal of Personality and Social Psychology, 51*(5), 1058–1068.

Emmons, R. A., & Diener, E. (1985). Personality correlates of subjective well-being. *Personality and Social Psychology Bulletin, 11*(1), 89–97.

Epstein, S. (1979). The stability of behavior I. On predicting most of the people much of the time. *Journal of Personality and Social Psychology, 37*, 1097–1126.

Eysenck, H. J., & Eysenck, S. B. G. (1968). *Manual of the Eysenck Personality Inventory*. San Diego, CA: Education and Industrial Testing Service.

Eysenck, S. B. J., & Eysenck, H. J. (1975). *Manual of the Eysenck Personality Questionnaire*. London: Hodder & Stoughton.

Feist, G. J., Bodner, T. E., Jacobs, J. F., Miles, M., & Tan, V. (1995). Integrating top-down and bottom-up structural models of subjective well-being: A longitudinal investigation. *Journal of Personality and Social Psychology, 68*(1), 138–150.

Fraley, R. C., & Roberts, B. W. (2005). Patterns of continuity: A dynamic model for conceptualizing the stability of individual differences in psychological constructs across the life course. *Psychological Review, 112*(1), 60–74.

Fredrickson, B. L. (1998). What good are positive emorions? *Review of General Psychology: New Directions in Research on Emotion, 2*(3), 300–319.

Frijters, P. (2000). Do individuals try to maximise general satisfaction? *Journal of Economic Psychology, 21*, 281–304.

Fujita, F., & Diener, F. (2005). Life satisfaction set point: Stability and change. *Journal of Personality and Social Psychology, 88*, 158–164.

Ganz, P. A., Lee, J. J., & Siau, J. (1991). Quality of life assessment: An independent prognostic variable for survival in lung cancer. *Cancer, 67*, 3131–3135.

Gilbert, D. (2006). *Stumbling on happiness*. New York: Knopf.

Gilovich, T., & Eihach, R. (2001). The fundamental attribution error where it really counts. *Psychological Inquiry, 12*(1), 23–26.

Gray, J. A. (1970). The psychophysiological basis of introversion–extraversion. *Behaviour Research and Therapy, 8*, 249–266.

Gray, J. A. (1981). A critique of Eysenck's theory of personality. In H. J. Eysenck (Ed.), *A model for personality* (pp. 246–276). New York: Springer-Verlag.

Gray, J. A. (1991). Neural systems, emotion, and personality. In J. Madden (Ed.), *Neurobiology of learning, emotion, and affect* (pp. 273–306). New York: Raven Press.

Gross, J. J. (1999). Emotion and emotion regulation. In L. A. Pervin & O. P. John (Eds.), *Handbook of personality: Theory and research* (2nd ed., pp. 525–552). New York: Guilford Press.

Haring, M., Stock, W. A., & Okun, M. A. (1984). A research synthesis of gender and social class as correlates of subjective well-being. *Human Relations, 37*, 645–657.

Haring-Hidore, M., Stock, W. A., Okun, M. A., & Witter, R. A. (1985). Marital status and subjective well-being: A research synthesis. *Journal of Marriage and the Family, 47*(4), 947–953.

Headey, B., & Wearing, A. (1989). Personality, life events, and subjective well-being: Toward a dynamic equilibrium model. *Journal of Personality and Social Psychology, 37*, 731–739.

Heller, D., Watson, D., & Ilies, R. (2004). The role of person versus situation in life satisfaction: A critical examination. *Psychological Bulletin, 130*, 574–600.

Hogan, R., Johnson, J. A., & Briggs, S. R. (Eds.). (1997). *Handbook of personality psychology*. San Diego, CA: Academic Press.

House, J. S., Landis, K. R., & Umberson, D. (1988). Social relationships and health. *Science, 241*(4865), 540–545.

House, J. S., Robbins, C., & Merzner, H. L. (1982). The association of social relationships and activities with normality: Prospective evidence from the Tecunseh Community Health Study. *American Journal of Epidemiology, 116*(1), 123–140.

James, W. (1902). *Varieties of religious experience: A study in human nature*. New York: Longmans Green.

Jasper, H. H. (1930). The measurement of depression–elation and its relation to a measure of extraversion–introversion. *Journal of Abnormal and Social Psychology, 25*, 307–318.

John, O. P., & Gross, J. J. (2004). Healthy and unhealthy emotion regulation: Personality processes, individual differences, and life span development. *Journal of Personality, 72*(6), 1301–1334.

Johnson, W., McGue, M., & Krueger, R. F. (2005). Personality stability in late adulthood: A behavioral genetic analysis. *Journal of Personality, 73*(2), 523–551.

Judge, T. A., & Watanabe, S. (1993). Another look at the job satisfaction–life satisfaction relationship. *Journal of Applied Psychology, 78*(6), 939–948.

Kahneman, D. (1999). Objective happiness. In D. Kahneman, E. Diener, & N. Schwarz (Eds.), *Well-being: The foundations of hedonic psychology* (pp. 3–25). New York: Sage Foundation.

Kahneman, D., Krueger, A. B., Schkade, D., Schwarz, N., & Stone, A. (2003). Toward national well-being accounts. *American Economic Review, 94*, 429–434.

Kahneman, D., & Riis, J. (2005). Living and thinking about it: Two perspectives on life. In P. A. Huppert, N. Baylis, & B. Keverne (Eds.), *The science of well-being* (pp. 285–304). New York: Oxford University Press.

Kim-Prieto, C., Diener, E., Tamir, M., Scollon, C. N., & Diener, M. (2005). Integrating the diverse definitions of happiness: A time-sequential framework of subjective well-being. *Journal of Happiness Studies, 6*(3), 261–300.

Koivumaa-Honkanen, H., Honkanen, R., Koskenvuo, M., Kaprio, J., & Alcohol Research. (2003). Self-reported happiness in life and suicide in ensuring 20 years. *Social Psychiatry and Psychiatric Epidemiology, 38*(5), 244–248.

Koivumaa-Honkanen, H., Honkanen, R., Vinamaki, H., Heikkilä, K., Kaprio, J., & Koskenvuo, M. (2001). Life satisfaction and suicide: A 20-year follow-up study. *American Journal of Psychiatry, 158*(3), 433–439.

Koivumaa-Honkanen, H. Kaprio, J., Honkanen, R., Vinamaki, H., & Koskenvuo, M. (2004). Life satisfaction and depression in a 15-year follow-up of healthy adults. *Social Psychiatry and Psychiatric Epidennology, 39*(12), 994–999.

Larsen, R. J., & Kerelaar, T. (1991). Personality and susceptibility to positive and negative emotional states. *Journal of Personality and Social Psychology, 61*, 132–140.

Lucas, R. E. (2005). Time does not heal all wounds: A longitudinal study of reaction and adaptation to divorce. *Psychological Science, 16*, 945–950.

Lucas, R. E. (2007). Long-term disability has lasting effects on subjective well-being: Evidence from two nationally representative panel studies. *Journal of Personality and Social Psychology, 92*, 717–730.

Lucas, R. E., & Baird, B. M. (2004). Extraversion and emotional reactivity. *Journal of Personality and Social Psychology, 86*, 473–485.

Lucas, R. E., Clark, A. E., Georgellis, Y., & Diener, E. (2003). Reexamining adaptation and the set point model of happiness: Reactions to changes in marital status. *Journal of Personality and Social Psychology, 84*, 527–539.

Lucas, R. E., Clark, A. E., Georgellis, Y., & Diener, E. (2004). Unemployment alters the set point for life satisfaction. *Psychological Science, 15*, 8–13.

Lucas, R. E., & Diener, E. (2008). Subjective well-being. In M. Lewis & J. M. Haviland (Eds.), *Handbook of emotions* (3rd ed., pp. 471–484). New York: Guilford Press.

Lucas, R. E., Diener, E., & Suh, E. (1996). Discriminant validity of well-being measures. *Journal of Personality and Social Psychology, 71*(3), 616–628.

Lucas, R. E., & Donnellan, M. B. (2007). Can happiness change?: Using the STARTS model to estimate the stability of subjective well-being. *Journal of Research in Personality, 41*, 1091–1098.

Lucas, R. E., & Dyrenforth, P. S. (2005). The myth of marital bliss? *Psychological Inquiry, 16*(2–3), 111–115.

Lucas, R. E., & Dyrenforth, P. S. (2006). Does the existence of social relationships matter for subjective well-being? In K. D. Vobs & E. J. Finkel (Eds.), *Self and relationships: Connecting intrapersonal and interpersonal processes* (pp. 254–273). New York: Guilford Press.

Lucas, R. E., & Fujita, F. (2000). Factors influencing the relation between extraversion and pleasant affect. *Journal of Personality and Social Psychology, 79*, 1039–1056.

Lucas, R. E., Le, K., & Dyrenforth, P. S. (2008). Explaining the extraversion/positive affect relation: Sociability cannot account for extraverts greater happiness. *Journal of Personality, 76*, 385–414.

Lucas, R. E., & Schimmack, U. (2007). *Money matters*. Manuscript in preparation, Michigan State University.

Lykken, D., & Tellegen, A. (1996). Happiness is a stochastic phenomenon. *Psychological Science, 7*, 186–189.

Lyubomirsky, S., King, L., & Diener, R. (2005). The benefits of frequent positive affect: Does happiness lead to success? *Psychological Bulletin, 131*, 803–855.

Lyubomirsky, S., Sheldon, K. M., & Schkade, D. (2005). Pursuing happiness: The architecture of sustainable change. *Review of General Psychology, 9*, 111-131.

Magnus, K. B. (1991). *A longitudinal analysis of personality, life events, and subjective well-being.* Unpublished manuscript. University of illinois.

Magnus, K. B., Diener, F., Fujita, F., & Pavor, W. (1993). Extraversion and neuroticism as predictors of objective life events: A longitudinal analysis. *Journal of Personality and Social Psychology, 65*, 316–330.

Markus, H. R., & Kitayama, S. (1991). Culture and the self: Implications for cognition, emotion, and motivation. *Psychological Review, 98*, 224–253.

McCrae, R. R., & Costa, P. T. Jr. (1991). Adding *Liebe and Arbeit*: The full five-factor model and well-being. *Personality and Social Psychology Bulletin, 17*, 227–232.

Mossey, J. M., & Shapiro, E. (1982). Self-rated health: A predictor of mortality among the elderly. *American Journal of Public Health, 72*, 800–808.

Nelson, E., Conger, B., Douglass, R., Gephart, D., Kirk, J., Page, R., et al. (1983). Functional health status levels of primary care patients. *Journal of the American Medical Association, 249*, 3331–3338.

Nes, R. B., Roysamb, E., Tambs, K., Harris, J. R., & Reichborn-Kjennerud, T. (2006). Subjective well-being: Genetic and environmental contributions to stability and change. *Psychological Medicine, 36*(7), 1033–1042.

Okun, M. A., & George, L. K. (1984). Physician and self-ratings of health, neuroticism and subjective well-being among men and women. *Personality and Individual Differences, 5*, 533–539.

Okun, M. A., Stock, W. A., Haring, M. J., & Wirtet, R. A. (1984). Health and subjective well-being: A meta-analysis. *International Journal of Aging and Human Development, 19*, 111–132.

Pavot, W., & Diener, E. (1993). Review of the Satisfaction with Life Scale. *Psychological Assessment, 5*(2), 164–172.

Pelled, L. H., & Xin, K. R. (1999). Down and out: An investigation of the relationship between mood and employee withdrawal behavior. *Journal of Management, 25*, 875–895.

Pervin, L. A. (Ed.). (1990). *Handbook of personality: Theory and research.* New York: Guilford Press.

Pervin, L. A., & John, O. P. (Eds.), (1999). *Handbook of personality: Theory and research* (2nd ed.). New York: Guilford Press.

Pinquart, M., & Sörensen, S. (2000). Influences of socioeconomic status, social network, and competence on subjective well-being in later life: A meta-analysis. *Psychology and Aging, 15*(2), 187–224.

Putzke, J. D., Richards, J. S., Hicken, B. L., & DeVivo, M. J. (2002). Predictors of life satisfaction: A spinal cord injury cohort study. *Archives of Physical Medicine and Rehabilitation, 83*, 555–561.

Roberts, B. W., & Del Vecchio, W. F. (2000). The rank-order consistency of personality traits from childhood to old age: A quantitative review of longitudinal studies. *Psychological Bulletin, 126*, 3–25.

Robinson, M. D., & Clore, G. L. (2002). Belief and feeling: Evidence for an accessibility model of emotional self-report. *Psychological Bulletin, 128*(6), 934–960.

Robinson, M. D., & Compton, R. J. (2008). The happy mind in action: The cognitive basis of subjective well-being. In M. Eid & R. J. Larsen (Eds.), *The science of subjective well-being* (pp. 220–238). New York: Guilford Press.

Roysamb, E., Harris, J. R., Magnus, P., Vitterso, J., & Tambs, K. (2002). Subjective well-being: Sex-specific effects of genetic and environmental factors. *Personality and Individual Differences, 32*(2), 211–223.

Roysamb, E., Tambs, K., Reichborn-Kjennerud, T., Neale, M. C., & Harris, J. R. (2003). Happiness and health: Environmental and genetic contributions to the relationship between subjective well-being perceived health, and somatic illness. *Journal of Personality and Social Psychology, 85*(6), 1136–1146.

Rumsfeld, J. S., McWhinney, S., McCarrhy, M., J., Shroyer, A. L., W., VillaNueva, C. B., O'Brien, M., et al. (1999). Health-related quality of life as a predictor of mortality following coronary artery bypass graft surgery. *Journal of the American Medical Association, 281*, 1298–1303.

Rusting, C. L. (1998). Personality, mood, and cognitive processing of emotional information: Three conceptual frameworks. *Psychological Bulletin, 124,* 165–196.

Rutter, M. L. (1997). Nature-nurture integration. The example of antisocial behavior. *American Psychologist, 52,* 390–398.

Ryff, C. D. (2008). Challenges and opportunities at the interface of aging, personality, and well-being. In O. John, R. Robins, & L. Pervin (Eds.), *Handbook of personality* (3rd ed., pp. 399–418). New York: Guilford.

Ryff, C. D., & Keyes, C. L. M. (1995). The structure of psychological well-being revisited. *Journal of Personality and Social Psychology, 69,* 719–727.

Sandvik, E., Diener, E., & Seidlitz, L. (1993). Subjective well-being: The convergence and stability of self-report and non-self report measures. *Journal of Personality, 61*(3), 317–342.

Saris, W. F. (2001). The relationship between income and satisfaction: The effect of measurement error and suppressor variables. *Social Indicators Research, 53*(2), 117–136.

Schimmack, U. (2008). The structure of subjective well-being. In M. Eid & R. J. Larsen (Eds.), *The science of subjective well-being* (pp. 97–123). New York: Guilford Press.

Schimmack, U., & Diener, E. (2003). Predictive validity of explicit and implicit: self-esteem for subjective well-being. *Journal of Research in Personality, 37*(2), 100–106.

Schimmack, U., Diener, E., & Oishi, S. (2002). Life-satisfaction is a momentary judgment and a stable personality characteristic: The use of chronically accessible and stable sources. *Journal of Personality, 70*(3), 345–384.

Schimmack, U., & Oishi, S. (2005). The influence of chronically and temporarily accessible information on life satisfaction judgments. *Journal of Personality and Social Psychology, 89*(3), 395–406.

Schwarz, N. (1999). Self-reports. How the questions shape the answers. *American Psychologist, 54*(2), 93–105.

Schwarz, N., & Strack, F. (1999). Reports of subjective well-being: Judgmental processes and their methodological implications. In D. Kahneman, E. Diener, & N. Schwarz (Eds.), *Well-being: The foundations of hedonic psychology* (pp. 61–84). New York: Sage Foundation.

Schyns, P. (2001). Income and satisfaction in Russia. *Journal of Happiness Studies, 2*(2), 173–204.

Scollon, C., Kim-Prieto, C., & Diener, E. (2003). Experience sampling: Promises and pitfalls, strengths and weaknesses. *Journal of Happiness Studies, 4,* 5–34.

Seligman, M. E. P., Steen, T. A., Park, N., & Peterson, C. (2005). Positive psychology progress: Empirical validation of interventions. *American Psychologist, 60,* 410–421.

Steel, P., Schnnidt, J., & Shultz, J. (2008). Refining the relationship between personality and subjective well-being. *Psychological Bulletin, 134,* 138–161.

Strack, E., Martin, L. L., & Schwarz, N. (1988). Priming and communication: Social determinants of information use in judgments of life satisfaction. *European Journal of Social Psychology, 18,* 429–442.

Stubbe, J. H., Posthuma, D., Boomsma, D. L., & De Geus, E. J. C. (2005). Heritability of life satisfaction in adults: A twin-family study. *Psychological Medicine, 35*(11), 1581–1588.

Suh, E., Diener, E., & Fujita, F. (1996). Events and subjective well-being: Only recent events matter. *Journal of Personality and Social Psychology, 70*(5), 1091–1102.

Suh, E. M., Diener, E., Oishi, S., & Triandis, H. (1998). The shifting basis of life satisfaction judgments across cultures. *Journal of Personality and Social Psychology, 70,* 1091–1102.

Tellegen, A. (1985). Structures of mood and personality and their relevance to assessing anxiety, with an emphasis on self-report. In A. H. Tuma & J. D. Maser (Eds.), *Anxiety and the anxiety disorders* (pp. 681–706). Hillsdale, NJ: Erlbaum.

Tellegen, A., Lykken, D. T., Bouchard, T. J., Wilcox, K. J., Segal, N. L., & Rich, S. (1988). Personality similarity in twins reared a part and together. *Journal of Personality and Social Psychology, 54*(6), 1031–1039.

Vaidya, J. G., Gray, E. K., Haig, J., & Watson, D. (2002). On the temporal stability of personality: Evidence for differential stability and the role of life experiences. *Journal of Personality and Social Psychology, 83,* 1469–1484.

Watson, D., Clark, L. A., & Tellegen, A. (1988). Development and validation of brief measures of positive and negative affect. The PANAS scales. *Journal of Personality and Social Psychology, 54*, 1063–1070.

Watson, D., & Tellegen, A. (1985). Toward a consensual structure of mood. *Psychological Bulletin, 98*(2), 219–235.

Watson, D., & Walker, L. M. (1996). The long-term stability and predictive validity of trait measures of affect. *Journal of Personality and Social Psychology, 70*, 567–577.

Wilson, W. (1967). Correlates of avowed happiness. *Psychological Bulletin, 67*, 294–306.

Zevon, M. A., & Tellegen, A. (1982). The structure of mood change. An idiographic/nomotheric analysis. *Journal of Personality and Social Psychology, 43*(1), 111–122.

Beyond the Hedonic Treadmill: *Revising the Adaptation Theory of Well-Being*

Ed Diener, Richard E. Lucas and Christie Napa Scollon

Abstract According to the hedonic treadmill model, good and bad events temporarily affect happiness, but people quickly adapt back to hedonic neutrality. The theory, which has gained widespread acceptance in recent years, implies that individual and societal efforts to increase happiness are doomed to failure. The recent empirical work outlined here indicates that 5 important revisions to the treadmill model are needed. First, individuals' set points are not hedonically neutral. Second, people have different set points, which are partly dependent on their temperaments. Third, a single person may have multiple happiness set points: Different components of well-being such as pleasant emotions, unpleasant emotions, and life satisfaction can move in different directions. Fourth, and perhaps most important, well-being set points can change under some conditions. Finally, individuals differ in their adaptation to events, with some individuals changing their set point and others not changing in reaction to some external event. These revisions offer hope for psychologists and policymakers who aim to decrease human misery and increase happiness.

Imagine a world in which the poorest diseased beggar with no family or friends is as happy as the healthy billionaire who has a surfeit of close and supportive relationships. Or imagine that individuals living in a cruel dictatorship where crime, slavery, and inequality are rampant are as satisfied with their lives as people living in a stable democracy where crime is minimal. Finally, imagine that no matter how much effort and care someone put into being happy, the long-term effects were no different than if he or she lived a profligate and dissolute life. Implausible? These surprising visions are based on a widely accepted model of subjective well-being. Brickman and Campbell (1971) described a *hedonic treadmill*, in which processes similar to sensory adaptation occur when people experience emotional reactions to life events. Just as people's noses quickly adapt to many scents and smells thereafter disappear from awareness, Brickman and Campbell suggested that one's emotion

E. Diener (✉)
Department of Psychology, University of Illinois, Champaign, IL 61820 USA
e-mail: ediener@uiuc.edu

E. Diener (ed.), *The Science of Well-Being: The Collected Works of Ed Diener*, Social Indicators Research Series 37, DOI 10.1007/978-90-481-2350-6_5,
© Springer Science+Business Media B.V. 2009

system adjusts to one's current life circumstances and that all reactions are relative to one's prior experience. Myers described adaptation as a key to understanding happiness. In his popular book *The Pursuit of Happiness*, David Myers (1992) wrote, "The point cannot be overstated: *Every* desirable experience—passionate love, a spiritual high, the pleasure of a new possession, the exhilaration of success—is transitory" (p. 53).

In the original treadmill theory, Brickman and Campbell (1971) proposed that people briefly react to good and bad events, but in a short time they return to neutrality. Thus, happiness and unhappiness are merely short-lived reactions to changes in people's circumstances. People continue to pursue happiness because they incorrectly believe that greater happiness lies just around the corner in the next goal accomplished, the next social relationship obtained, or the next problem solved. Because new goals continually capture one's attention, one constantly strives to be happy without realizing that in the long run such efforts are futile.

The hedonic treadmill theory is built on an automatic habituation model in which psychological systems react to deviations from one's current adaptation level (Helson, 1948, 1964). Automatic habituation processes are adaptive because they allow constant stimuli to fade into the background. Thus, resources remain available to deal with novel stimuli, which are most likely to require immediate attention (Fredrick & Loewenstein, 1999). The happiness system is thus hypothesized to reflect changes in circumstances rather than the overall desirability of the circumstances themselves. This idea was formalized by Carver and Scheier (1990), who maintained that emotions depend on the rate of change of important circumstances.

In 1978, Brickman, Coates, and Janoff-Bulman offered initial empirical support for the treadmill model. In studies that have become classics in the field, Brickman et al. concluded that lottery winners were not happier than nonwinners and that people with paraplegia were not substantially less happy than those who can walk. Although the empirical support for hedonic adaptation was, in fact, mixed, the studies captured the attention of psychologists. The idea of hedonic adaptation was appealing because it offered an explanation for the observation that people appear to be relatively stable in happiness despite changes in fortune. In addition, the treadmill theory explained the observation that people with substantial resources are sometimes no happier than those with few resources and that people with severe problems are sometimes quite happy. Thus, the research of Brickman and colleagues became central to the way many scientists understand happiness.

We and many other psychologists readily accepted the theory of adaptation because evidence frequently supported the idea. External conditions are often weak correlates of reports of happiness. For instance, all demographic variables taken together predict less than 20% of the variance in happiness (Campbell, Converse, & Rodgers, 1976). Diener, Sandvik, Seidlitz, and Diener (1993) found that income and happiness in the United States correlate only 0.13, and Diener, Wolsic, and Fujita (1995) similarly found that objective physical attractiveness correlated at very low levels with reports of well-being. Perhaps even more surprising, Okun and George (1984) found that objective health on average correlated only 0.08 with happiness, and Feinman (1978) found that people who were blind did not differ in happiness from those who were able to see.

In addition, longitudinal studies that tracked changes in happiness over time provided more direct evidence that adaptation can occur. For instance, Silver (1982) found that individuals with spinal cord injuries reported strong negative emotions one week after their crippling accident. However, two months later, happiness was their strongest emotion. Similarly, Suh, Diener, and Fujita (1996) found that good and bad life events affected happiness only if they occurred in the past two months. More distant past events did not predict happiness (although many of the events they studied were relatively mundane). Furthermore, in a number of studies, researchers have traced reactions to the death of a spouse, and these studies show that emotional reactions eventually rebound after this major life event (e.g., Bonanno et al., 2002; Bonanno, Wortman, & Nesse, 2004; Lucas, Clark, Georgellis, & Diener, 2003). Thus, parts of the hedonic treadmill model have received robust empirical support (see Fredrick & Loewenstein, 1999, for a review).

Our Research on Adaptation

Over the last decade, we and others have tested predictions derived from the treadmill theory, and our findings suggest that the model requires important modifications. Although the revisions leave certain core features of the adaptation model intact, our research reveals that the idea is in need of an update. After reviewing these revisions, we describe the important implications that they have for psychology.

Revision 1: Nonneutral Set Points

The original treadmill theory suggested that people return to a neutral set point after an emotionally significant event. However, decades of research show that this part of the hedonic treadmill theory is wrong. Instead, most people are happy most of the time (E. Diener & C. Diener, 1996). For instance, Diener and Diener reviewed studies using a variety of methods of assessment, and they concluded that approximately three quarters of the samples they investigated reported affect balance scores (positive moods and emotions – negative moods and emotions) above neutral. Similarly, Biswas-Diener, Vittersø, and Diener (2005) found that even in such diverse populations as the Amish, African Maasai, and Greenlandic Inughuit, most people are above neutral in well-being. In the most recent World Values Survey (a large-scale survey in which the nations with the largest populations are sampled using probability methods; European Values Study Group & World Values Survey Association, 2005), 80% of respondents said that they were very or quite happy. Thus, if people adapt and return to a baseline, it is a positive rather than neutral one.

A general tendency to experience positive emotions may provide the motivation to explore one's environment and to approach new goals (Fredrickson, 1998).

Lyubomirsky, King, & Diener (2005) showed that positive moods facilitate a variety of approach behaviors and positive outcomes. Thus, the ubiquity of a positive emotional set point, in concert with the less frequent experience of unpleasant emotions, likely results from the adaptive nature of frequent positive emotions.

Revision 2: Individual Set Points

The empirical research that has been conducted since the publication of Brickman and Campbell (1971) reveals that if people do have set points, they vary considerably across individuals. These individual differences are due, at least in part, to inborn, personality-based influences (Diener & Lucas, 1999). Support for this view comes from at least three different lines of research. First, research consistently shows that one's level of well-being is reasonably stable over time (e.g., Eid & Diener, 2004). Second, behavioral genetic studies show that well-being is moderately heritable. For instance, Tellegen et al. (1988) found that identical twins reared apart were much more similar in their levels of well-being than were dizygotic twins who were reared apart. Finally, research shows that personality factors are strong correlates of well-being variables. Whereas any single demographic factor typically correlates less than 0.20 (usually much less) with well-being reports, both self- and non-self-report measures of personality tend to correlate much more strongly with well-being (see Diener & Lucas, 1999, for a review). Thus, personality factors may predispose individuals to experience different levels of well-being.

Revision 3: Multiple Set Points

The idea of a happiness set point implies that well-being is a single entity with a single baseline. However, work by Lucas, Diener, and Suh (1996) indicates that the global category of happiness is composed of separable well-being variables. It is important to note that these variables sometimes move in different directions over time. Thus, the idea of a unitary set point is not tenable, because positive and negative emotions might both decline in tandem or life satisfaction might move upward while positive emotions decrease.

In Fig. 1, we present age trends in positive affect, negative affect, and life satisfaction from the first wave of the Victoria Quality of Life Panel Study (see Headey & Wearing, 1989, 1992; Scollon, 2004) and from the 1990 World Value Survey (Inglehart & Klingemann, 2000). Both studies are based on probability samples, the former from the state of Victoria in Australia and the latter from 42 nations around the world. As can be seen in this figure, there were significant age effects for all five variables (all $ps < 0.001$). However, these effects varied for the different well-being variables. For instance, at the same point in the life span that positive affect was declining (representing a decrease in overall well-being), negative affect also declined (representing an increase in overall well-being). During this same period, both work

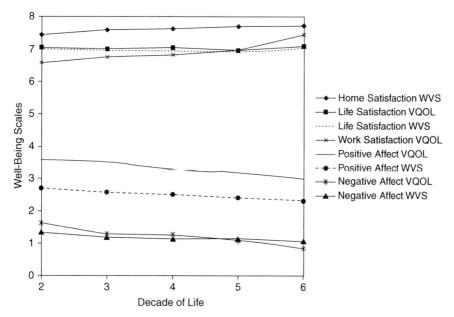

Fig. 1 Age trends in subjective well-being
Note: WVS = 1990 World Value Survey; VQOL = first wave of the Victoria Quality of Life Panel
Study.

and home satisfaction increased. These data indicate that (a) there is not a constant
global happiness set point that remains stable over the course of the entire life span
and (b) "happiness" is not a unitary concept with a single set point to which people
adapt. Instead, these findings suggest that different forms of well-being can move in
different directions (also see Easterlin, 2005).

We also used the longitudinal component of the Victoria Quality of Life Panel
Study to examine change in well-being within persons over time. Specifically, we
modeled change in work satisfaction and marital satisfaction over an eight-year
period using growth curve modeling. Significant individual differences in change
emerged on both variables, indicating that different people changed at different rates
and in different directions (Scollon & Diener, 2006). It is important to note that
the correlation between changes in the two variables was substantially less than 1
($r = 0.48$), even at the latent level. This shows that the two variables do not always
change in unison. Not all individuals who increased in work satisfaction increased
in marital satisfaction. At best, only one quarter of the variance in change could be
accounted for by the corresponding amounts of change in another variable. Thus, not
only do the various well-being components change in different ways over the course
of the life span, but changes in one domain do not fully correspond to changes in
other domains.

As a final test of the separability of well-being components, we examined the stability of positive and negative affect over time in the Victoria Quality of Life Panel

Table 1 Stability of subjective well-being measures in the Victoria Quality of Life Panel Study and the German Socio-Economic Panel Study

Time period between measurements	Positive affect[a]	Negative affect[a]	Life satisfaction[a]	Life satisfaction[b]
2 years	0.37	0.44	0.61	0.51
4 years	0.32	0.40	0.50	0.45
6 years	0.32	0.42	0.44	0.41
8 years	0.23	0.48	0.43	0.37

[a] Data are from the Victoria Quality of Life Panel Study.
[b] Data are from the German Socio-Economic Panel Study.

Study. We found that, consistent with the idea that there is no single set point, the various components exhibited differential stability. Specifically, long-term levels of negative affect were substantially more stable than were long-term levels of positive affect. In addition, the stability of positive affect and life satisfaction declined with longer time periods, whereas the stability of negative affect did not (see Table 1). These findings suggest that stable individual baselines might be more characteristic of negative affect than positive affect. However, over a period of a few years, life satisfaction was most stable.

Revision 4: Happiness Can Change

Perhaps the most controversial aspect of Brickman and Campbell's (1971) hedonic treadmill model is the idea that people cannot do much to change their long-term levels of happiness and life satisfaction. If the hedonic treadmill model is correct, adaptation is inevitable, and no change in life circumstance should ever lead to lasting changes in happiness. Although the work cited at the beginning of this article was suggestive of such an effect, until recently very little evidence has been available to provide longitudinal tests of this hypothesis. Thus, questions have remained about the extent to which important life events can permanently alter individuals' happiness set points.

One type of evidence demonstrating that life circumstances matter comes from well-being differences across nations. If there are strong national differences in well-being and these differences can be predicted from objective characteristics of those nations, then this would suggest that the stable external circumstances that vary across nations have a lasting impact on happiness. The first column of Table 2 presents affect balance scores (reported between 1981 and 1984) for several nations that differed markedly in affluence and human rights. The right column of Table 2 shows that these nations also differed in life satisfaction. Because the objective conditions in these countries remained consistent for many years, the cross-national differences in happiness suggest that people do not always completely adapt to conditions. Perhaps more important, these mean-level differences can be predicted from objective characteristics of the nations. For instance, E. Diener, M. Diener, and C. Diener (1995) found that the wealth and the human rights of nations were strong

Table 2 The happiness of selected nations

Nation	Affect balance (PA – NA), 1981–1984	Life satisfaction, 1999–2001
Canada	2.33	7.85
United States	2.23	7.66
China	1.46	6.53
West Germany	1.45	7.42
Mexico	1.38	8.14
India	0.72	5.14
Turkey	0.62	5.61
Russia	0.33	4.65

Note. Mean scores are taken from the World Value Survey, the Broadburn Affect Balance Scale, where affect balance can vary from 5 to −5, with 0 as the neutral point. The national differences in both positive affect (PA) and negative affect (NA) in the full sample are highly significant, $p < 0.001$. Life satisfaction scores, with a range of 1–10, were taken from the European Values Study Group and World Values Survey Association (2005) Data Wave 1999–2001.

predictors of average national well-being. Similarly, researchers at *The Economist* found that 85% of the variance in national levels of well-being could be explained by nine objective characteristics, including gross domestic product per person, life expectancy at birth, political stability, and divorce rates (Economist Intelligence Unit, 2005). Furthermore, if people adapted to conditions, only change in conditions and not the long-term level of conditions would influence feelings of well-being. However, Diener and Biswas-Diener (2002) reviewed studies showing that national levels of wealth strongly predict the subjective well-being of nations, whereas change in wealth is inconsistent in its effects across studies.

This cross-sectional evidence that circumstances matter is supported by more definitive longitudinal studies examining individuals over time. For instance, Fujita and Diener (2005) used longitudinal data to determine whether long-term average levels of happiness ever change. They examined changes in baseline levels of well-being over a 17-year period in a large and representative sample from Germany. Although there was considerable stability in happiness reports, 24% of respondents changed significantly from their early baseline, comprising the first five years of the study, to the last five years. Nine percent changed by approximately two standard deviations or more. Thus, long-term levels of happiness do change for some individuals. The more intriguing question, then, is why happiness set points change for some individuals more than for others.

Using the same sample of Germans, we have examined the ways that specific life events influence happiness. In support of the initial adaptation model, people do seem to adapt to some life events. For instance, Lucas et al. (2003) showed that, on average, Germans did not get lasting boosts in happiness after marriage. Instead, they reported short-term increases in happiness that were followed by relatively quick adaptation. However, the extent of adaptation varies for different life events. Lucas et al. (2003) showed that widows and widowers, people who were laid off

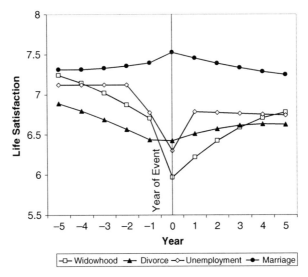

Fig. 2 Adaptation to good and bad events

from work (Lucas, Clark, Georgellis, & Diener, 2004), and individuals who divorced (Lucas, 2005b) all reported long-lasting changes in life satisfaction after these life events. The widows showed the greatest amount of adaptation (at least in terms of the absolute increase from their lowest level of happiness), but even this took about eight years and was not quite complete. Figure 2 shows life satisfaction levels before and after these four important life events.

Together these results suggest that happiness can and does change. What then should be made of the classic empirical findings of Brickman et al. (1978)? First, it should be noted that when Brickman et al.'s results are examined closely, the evidence for adaptation is not nearly as strong as many psychologists have tended to assume. In the case of individuals with spinal cord injuries, Brickman et al. did find that the participants who were disabled reported significantly less happiness than did controls. In fact, when we calculated standardized mean differences in general happiness from Brickman et al.'s data, we found that the difference between the spinal cord-injured and control groups was about 0.75 standard deviations—an effect that most psychologists would consider large. Similar effects have been found numerous times: Authors of a number of recent reviews have concluded that individuals with spinal cord injuries are less happy than are people in the general population, with effect sizes in the moderate to large range (Dijkers, 1997, 2005; Hammell, 2004). However, the studies cited in these reviews are often published in rehabilitation journals and are rarely cited in psychological literature on adaptation.

Finally, Lucas (2005a) used two large, nationally representative panel studies to examine adaptation to the onset of disability. Participants in this study (who were followed for an average of seven years before and seven years after onset) reported moderate to large drops in satisfaction and very little evidence of adaptation over

time. For instance, those individuals who were certified as being 100% disab
reported life satisfaction scores that were 1.20 standard deviations lower than th _...
nondisabled baseline levels. Thus, although people with paraplegia and other individuals with disabilities usually are not subjectively miserable, happiness levels
do seem to be strongly affected by this important life circumstance. When compared with the actual variability between individuals in happiness rather than with
the extreme endpoints of the scale, many of the group differences in happiness are
substantial.

It should no longer come as a surprise that people living in negative circumstances report well-being scores that are above neutral. This well-documented fact
is interesting and theoretically important, but it should not be used as evidence that
people inevitably adapt. Furthermore, it is not enough for researchers interested in
adaptation to show that people who have experienced a negative life circumstance
report well-being scores that are higher than what other people would think they
should report (e.g., Brickman et al., 1978; Riis et al., 2005). Such research findings tell more about the average person's affective forecasting errors than about
adaptation itself (Gilbert & Wilson, 2000). To determine whether adaptation has
occurred, it is necessary to compare individuals who have experienced an event or
life circumstance with those who have not, ideally following the same individuals
over time.

Revision 5: Individual Differences in Adaptation

An implicit assumption of the hedonic treadmill theory is that adaptation to circumstances occurs in similar ways for all individuals. If adaptation results from
automatic and inevitable homeostatic processes, then all individuals should return
to neutrality or at least to their own unique baseline. But we have found individual
differences in the rate and extent of adaptation that occurs even to the same event.
In our longitudinal studies, the size and even the direction of the change in life
satisfaction varied considerably across individuals. For example, Lucas et al. (2003)
found adaptation to marriage at the aggregate level, but there was a great deal of
variability in these effects. Individuals who reacted most positively to their marriage
tended to be above their baseline many years after the event, but these individuals
were counterbalanced by those who experienced a lasting decline in satisfaction
after their marriage. In fact, the standard deviation for the amount of change that
occurred after the event was almost as large as the standard deviation for baseline
levels.

Understanding individual differences in adaptation will help illuminate when
and why adaptation does or does not occur. For example, in our study on reaction
and adaptation to marriage (Lucas et al., 2003), we relied on laboratory studies
of emotional reactivity (e.g., Larsen & Ketelaar, 1991) to predict that the happiest
individuals should react most strongly to positive life events. However, the results
showed—somewhat surprisingly—that less satisfied individuals were more likely to

benefit from marriage in the long run. These individuals with initially low baselines reported more positive reactions to marriage, and these positive reactions persisted long into the marriage. One explanation for this effect is that the most satisfied individuals are more likely than less satisfied individuals to have strong social support even before the marriage. People who chronically experience many positive events may have less to gain from one more positive event. Likewise, people who chronically experience many bad events may not be strongly affected by the addition of one more negative life event. Therefore, deviations from a person's typical life events might produce the greatest changes in happiness set points (Headey & Wearing, 1992; Oishi, Diener, Choi, Kim-Prieto, & Choi, 2005).

Two important research traditions shed light on when people adapt or do not adapt to negative events. The first of these traditions focuses on the utility of specific coping strategies. The second focuses on personality characteristics that influence the specific coping strategies that people use. From these literatures, it is known that certain coping strategies are more effective than others and that individuals vary in their preferred strategies. For example, individuals who tend to use reappraisal strategies experience more positive emotions and fewer negative emotions than do individuals who use strategies such as suppression (Gross & John, 2003). Using reappraisal is also associated with having better interpersonal relationships, which are likely to translate into increased social support. Similarly, among older people, the endorsement of coping styles such as using humor, seeking information, and "keeping going" predicts adjustment to old age (Staudinger & Fleeson, 1996).

Personality researchers have shown that a number of stable individual differences predispose people to use certain coping strategies (Carver, Scheier, & Weintraub, 1989). For example, neurotic individuals often choose ineffective strategies for coping, which can lead to greater reactivity to a stressful event (Bolger & Zuckerman, 1995) and possibly a slower return to baseline levels of happiness. Similarly, Ferguson (2001) found that neuroticism and introversion were associated with relatively ineffective coping behaviors such as denial. However, optimistic individuals tend to engage in active coping or strategies that can actually change the situation that is causing negative affect (Aspinwall & Taylor, 1997; Chang, 1998; Scheier, Weintraub, & Carver, 1986). Such strategies often pay off by leading to a resolution of the stressful situation. Optimistic people also tend to seek out social support, engage in positive reappraisal of adverse events, and feel as if they have the resources to overcome stressful situations (Scheier, 1986)—all factors that help buffer against the long-term effects of negative life circumstances. For example, optimism has been shown to predict problem-focused coping and quicker recovery from surgery (Scheier et al., 2003). Thus, there appear to be individual differences in effective coping and adaptation to stressful events.

Research on individual differences in adaptation raises questions about the processes that underlie adaptation effects. If adaptation is an inevitable and automatic process, it should occur in similar ways for most people, much as homeostatic processes work to return all people to their body temperature set point. The fact that substantial individual differences in these effects exist argues against this type of inevitable habituation model. It also suggests that research into these individual differences may help psychologists understand exactly how adaptation occurs. However, at this point, it is unclear whether there is a relatively automatic core habituation process that can be modified by coping and other variables or whether adaptation and coping are synonymous. Future research must incorporate measures of coping (along with other potential moderators and process variables) into sophisticated longitudinal studies that allow for strict tests of adaptation effects.

Recent research has provided a much stronger test of the hedonic treadmill than earlier studies did because of methodological refinements. First and most important, by relying on very large samples, researchers in recent studies have been able to track individuals from before an event happens to the time of the event to many years after the event. By contrast, earlier researchers drew conclusions from cross-sectional data in which preevent levels of life satisfaction of groups such as lottery winners or people with paraplegia were unknown. Second, large longitudinal designs allow for more precise measurement of changes in happiness over time and more powerful statistical methods that go beyond examinations of group means to reveal individual differences in adaptation. Finally, recent studies have used large and often representative samples of participants, unlike early studies that frequently used small accidental samples.

Implications of the Revised Model

If revisions must be made to the original hedonic treadmill model, is adaptation still an important concept for psychological research? We answer with a resounding "yes." Although recent studies have challenged the idea that adaptation is inevitable, people do adapt to many life events, and they often do so within a relatively short period of time. Thus, adaptation processes can explain why many factors often have only small influences on happiness. People tend to adapt to these conditions over time.

However, recent findings do place limits on the types of psychological processes that can account for the adaptation that does occur. For instance, initial models that relied on automatic physiological systems to account for hedonic adaptation will likely not be able to fully account for all existing data. Instead, more flexible processes are likely involved, and these processes may vary across events and individuals or even within the same individual over time. The research on coping with adversity will be a useful starting point for investigations of adaptation. However, processes related to adaptation to positive events must also be explored.

Newer theories of adaptation (e.g., Kahneman & Thaler, 2006; Wilson & Gilbert, 2005) rely on individuals' attention to particular life circumstances in explaining the changes. Kahneman and Thaler, for instance, posited that various features of a specific life circumstance might influence whether it draws a person's attention. It is this attention that determines whether an individual can adapt. Thus, Kahneman and Thaler predicted that conditions that continue to draw attention can influence well-being but that the novelty of certain circumstances wears off and therefore they draw less attention over time. Wilson and Gilbert further suggested that people naturally seek to explain and make sense of life events and circumstances. Features of one's life that cannot be explained continue to draw attention and thereby affect one's emotions and overall well-being. Experience-sampling reports over time of the stimuli to which people attend are needed to test attention theories. Whether these attention theories can predict greater and less habituation has not yet been rigorously tested.

Our revisions to the hedonic treadmill model suggest that interventions to increase happiness can be effective, and research supports this conclusion. These changes might be targeted at the individual, organizational, or even societal level. For instance, in an early set of studies, Fordyce (1977, 1983) demonstrated in seminal studies that a multipronged program successfully raised individuals' happiness for an extended period of time. These gains in well-being persisted over a period of a year or more. Perhaps because of the widely accepted view that happiness could not be changed, however, few rigorous studies have been conducted to follow up on this work. Very recently, this has begun to change. For instance, Sheldon and Lyubomirsky (2004) demonstrated that changes in activities raised people's happiness. They found that when individuals performed several random acts of kindness on one day each week, their happiness improved. Seligman, Steen, Park, and Peterson (2005) reported a series of happiness interventions that were implemented via the Internet. They found that several of these interventions led to changes in happiness that persisted for at least six months. Finally, Emmons and McCullough (2003) found that interventions to increase thoughts of gratitude increased levels of positive affect. Although these experimental intervention studies are in the initial stages, they indicate that levels of happiness can be raised. Again, this contradicts the idea of an unchangeable baseline for happiness.

If interventions can cause lasting changes among individuals, it may also be possible for organizations to adopt macrolevel policies that raise well-being for larger groups. For instance, organizational psychologists strive to make the workplace engaging and interesting. These benefits might be worthwhile in themselves, or the increased happiness that they provide may lead to increases in organizational citizenship and productivity. Similarly, community psychologists strive to enhance the quality of life within neighborhoods and cities. Our findings that baseline happiness can change, along with new studies showing that interventions can raise levels of happiness, provide an optimistic foundation for the various fields of applied psychology.

Finally, if organizational policies can have an impact on the happiness of large groups, it may be possible to change the happiness of a society as a whole. Philosophers such as J. S. Mill and Jeremy Bentham maintained that the best society is one where the greatest numbers of citizens experience the most happiness. Echoing this sentiment, Diener and Seligman (2004) called for a system of national accounts of well-being in which people's happiness, meaning, and engagement are assessed over time and in various situations. The goal of such a program would be to help policymakers understand when and why people are miserable and when and why they are happy. This information would then allow policymakers to develop programs to reduce misery and enhance happiness. Furthermore, it is hoped that national accounts of well-being might lead to policies that would heighten the engagement, joy, trust, and affection of ordinary citizens who do not have extraordinary problems. Fortunately, our findings indicate that the goal of creating a happier society is not doomed by the hedonic treadmill.

Although the research reviewed in this article provides an optimistic picture of the possibility for change, the processes of adaptation must still be carefully considered when designing and assessing well-being interventions. People might initially react positively to interventions just as they do to naturally changing conditions, but over time they may adapt to the intervention and return to their former levels of well-being. Thus, effective interventions must change people's baseline well-being, and measurements must be repeated over a long period of time to rule out the possibility that the effectiveness of the intervention is only temporary. A strong understanding of adaptation theories will enable researchers to develop programs with a great likelihood of long-term success.

Future Research and Conclusions

Although researchers have made progress in understanding adaptation, several key issues remain. First, an overarching question concerns the factors that lead to lasting change. Why do adaptation effects appear to vary across different events and circumstances? Although some theories (e.g., Kahneman & Thaler, 2006) offer predictions about the differential adaptation across varying events, these theories do not seem to explain the full set of results. For instance, it is unclear why people seem to exhibit a lasting effect of unemployment on well-being even after they become reemployed. A corollary question concerns how much control people have over adaptation: Can people slow adaptation to good events and speed recovery from bad events? Another important challenge is differentiating passive acceptance of negative circumstances versus active coping and a positive resolution of events. Finally, our studies raise the issue as to whether some components of well-being adapt more readily than others. For instance, do cognitive evaluations such as satisfaction adapt more slowly than moods and emotions? These are exciting unanswered questions about adaptation, questions that will need to be answered before fully effective interventions can be designed.

The treadmill model of happiness posited by Brickman and Campbell (1971) represents a milestone in psychologists' understanding of happiness, and our longitudinal findings on marriage support the treadmill idea. Our findings also indicate that different types of well-being may change at different rates or even in different directions. Furthermore, both experimental and longitudinal studies now show that the strong form of the adaptation theory is untenable. Adaptation may proceed slowly over a period of years, and in some cases the process is never complete. Finally, there are individual differences in the rates of adaptation.

Those who provide interventions aimed at improving subjective well-being need to understand the patterns involved in adaptation so that successful interventions can be designed. Although some of the studies we described involve changes in life circumstances that are extreme, other studies suggest that smaller interventions can make a difference. Adaptation is a powerful force, but it is not so complete and automatic that it will defeat all efforts to change well-being. The exciting research challenge is to discover the factors that control the adaptation process. Fortunately, research on coping, personality traits, and the effectiveness of interventions all offer clues about factors that influence adaptation. With the understanding that adaptation may be incomplete and varies across persons, the efforts to understand adaptation should be amplified.

References

Aspinwall, L. G., & Taylor, S. E. (1997). A stitch in time: Self-regulation and proactive coping. *Psychological Bulletin, 121*, 417–436.

Biswas-Diener, R., Vittersø, J., & Diener, E. (2005). Most people are pretty happy, but there is cultural variation: The Inughuit, the Amish, and the Maasai. *Journal of Happiness Studies, 6*, 205–226.

Bolger, N., & Zuckerman, A. (1995). A framework for studying personality in the stress process. *Journal of Personality and Social Psychology, 69*, 890–902.

Bonanno, G. A., Wortman, C. B., Lehman, D. R., Tweed, R. G., Haring, M., Sonnega, J., et al. (2002). Resilience to loss and chronic grief: A prospective study from preloss to 18-months postloss. *Journal of Personality and Social Psychology, 83*, 1150–1164.

Bonanno, G. A., Wortman, C. B., & Nesse, R. M. (2004). Prospective patterns of resilience and maladjustment during widowhood. *Psychology and Aging, 19*, 260–271.

Brickman, P., & Campbell, D. T. (1971). Hedonic relativism and planning the good society. In M. H. Appley (Ed.), *Adaptation level theory: A symposium* (pp. 287–302). New York: Academic Press.

Brickman, P., Coates, D., & Janoff-Bulman, R. (1978). Lottery winners and accident victims: Is happiness relative? *Journal of Personality and Social Psychology, 36*, 917–927.

Campbell, A., Converse, P. E., & Rodgers, W. L. (1976). *The quality of American life.* New York: Russell Sage Foundation.

Carver, C. S., & Scheier, M. F. (1990). Origins and functions of positive and negative affect: A control-process view. *Psychological Review, 97*, 19–35.

Carver, C. S., Scheier, M. F., & Weintraub, J. K. (1989). Assessing coping strategies: A theoretically based approach. *Journal of Personality and Social Psychology, 56*, 267–283.

Chang, E. C. (1998). Dispositional optimism and primary and secondary appraisal of a stressor: Controlling for confounding influences and relations to coping and psychological and physical adjustment. *Journal of Personality and Social Psychology, 74*, 1109–1120.

Diener, E., & Biswas-Diener, R. (2002). Will money increase subjective well-being? A literature review and guide to needed research. *Social Indicators Research, 57*, 119–169.

Diener, E., & Diener, C. (1996). Most people are happy. *Psychological Science, 7*, 181–185.

Diener, E., Diener, M., & Diener, C. (1995). Factors predicting the subjective well-being of nations. *Journal of Personality and Social Psychology, 69*, 851–864.

Diener, E., & Lucas, R. E. (1999). Personality and subjective well-being. In D. Kahneman, E. Diener, & N. Schwarz (Eds.), *Well-being: The foundations of a hedonic psychology* (pp. 213–229). New York: Russell Sage Foundation.

Diener, E., Sandvik, E., Seidlitz, L., & Diener, M. (1993). The relationship between income and subjective well-being: Relative or absolute? *Social Indicators Research, 28*, 195–223.

Diener, E., & Seligman, M. E. P. (2004). Beyond money: Toward an economy of well-being. *Psychological Science in the Public Interest, 5*, 1–31.

Diener, E., Wolsic, B., & Fujita, F. (1995). Physical attractiveness and subjective well-being. *Journal of Personality and Social Psychology, 69*, 120–129.

Dijkers, M. (1997). Quality of life after spinal cord injury: A metaanalysis of the effects of disablement components. *Spinal Cord, 35*, 829–840.

Dijkers, M. P. J. M. (2005). Quality of life of individuals with spinal cord injury: A review of conceptualization, measurement, and research findings. *Journal of Rehabilitation Research and Development, 42*, 87–110.

Easterlin, R. (2005, June). *Life cycle happiness and its sources: Why psychology and economics need each other.* Paper presented at the International Conference on Capabilities and Happiness, Milan, Italy.

Economist Intelligence Unit. (2005). *The Economist Intelligence Unit's Quality-of-Life Index.* Retrieved July 17, 2005, from http://www.economist.com/media/pdf/QUALITY_OF_LIFE.pdf

Eid, M., & Diener, E. (2004). Global judgments of subjective well-being: Situational variability and long-term stability. *Social Indicators Research, 65*, 245–277.

Emmons, R. A., & McCullough, M. E. (2003). Counting blessings versus burdens: An experimental investigation of gratitude and subjective well-being in daily life. *Journal of Personality and Social Psychology, 84*, 377–389.

European Values Study Group, & World Values Survey Association. (2005). European and World Values Surveys Integrated Data File, 1999–2002, Release I (2nd ICPSR version) [Computer file]. Ann Arbor, MI: Inter-University Consortium for Political and Social Research.

Feinman, S. (1978). The blind as "ordinary people." *Journal of Visual Impairment and Blindness, 72*, 231–238.

Ferguson, E. (2001). Personality and coping traits: A joint factor analysis. *British Journal of Health Psychology, 6*, 311–325.

Fordyce, M. W. (1977). Development of a program to increase personal happiness. *Journal of Counseling Psychology, 24*, 511–520.

Fordyce, M. W. (1983). A program to increase happiness: Further studies. *Journal of Counseling Psychology, 30*, 483–498.

Fredrick, S., & Loewenstein, G. (1999). Hedonic adaptation. In D. Kahneman, E. Diener, & N. Schwarz (Eds.), *Well-being: The foundations of a hedonic psychology* (pp. 302–329). New York: Russell Sage Foundation.

Fredrickson, B. L. (1998). What good are positive emotions? *Review of General Psychology, 2*, 300–319.

Fujita, F., & Diener, E. (2005). Life satisfaction set point: Stability and change. *Journal of Personality and Social Psychology, 88*, 158–164.

Gilbert, D. T., & Wilson, T. D. (2000). Miswanting: Some problems in the forecasting of future affective states. In J. P. Forgas (Ed.), *Feeling and thinking: The role of affect in social cognition* (pp. 178–197). New York: Cambridge University Press.

Gross, J. J., & John, O. P. (2003). Individual differences in two emotion regulation processes: Implications for affect, relationships, and well-being. *Journal of Personality and Social Psychology, 85*, 348–362.

Hammell, K. W. (2004). Exploring quality of life following high spinal cord injury: A review and critique. *Spinal Cord, 42*, 491–502.

Headey, B., & Wearing, A. (1989). Personality, life events, and subjective well-being: Toward a dynamic equilibrium model. *Journal of Personality and Social Psychology, 57*, 731–739.

Headey, B., & Wearing, A. (1992). *Understanding happiness: A theory of subjective well-being.* Melbourne, Victoria, Australia: Longman Cheshire.

Helson, H. (1948). Adaptation-level as a basis for a quantitative theory of frames of reference. *Psychological Review, 55*, 297–313.

Helson, H. (1964). Current trends and issues in adaptation-level theory. *American Psychologist, 19*, 26–38.

Inglehart, R., & Klingemann, H.-D. (2000). Genes, culture, democracy, and happiness. In E. Diener & E. M. Suh (Eds.), *Culture and subjective well-being* (pp. 165–184). Cambridge, MA: MIT Press.

Kahneman, D., & Thaler, R. H. (2006). Anomalies: Utility maximization and experienced utility. *Journal of Economic Perspectives, 20*, 221.

Larsen, R. J., & Ketelaar, T. (1991). Personality and susceptibility to positive and negative emotional states. *Journal of Personality and Social Psychology, 61*, 132–140.

Lucas, R. E. (2005a). *Happiness can change: A longitudinal study of adaptation to disability.* Manuscript submitted for publication, Michigan State University, East Lansing.

Lucas, R. E. (2005b). Time does not heal all wounds: A longitudinal study of reaction and adaptation to divorce. *Psychological Science, 16*, 945–950.

Lucas, R. E., Clark, A. E., Georgellis, Y., & Diener, E. (2003). Reexamining adaptation and the set point model of happiness: Reactions to changes in marital status. *Journal of Personality and Social Psychology, 84*, 527–539.

Lucas, R. E., Clark, A. E., Georgellis, Y., & Diener, E. (2004). Unemployment alters the set point for life satisfaction. *Psychological Science, 15*, 8–13.

Lucas, R. E., Diener, E., & Suh, E. (1996). Discriminant validity of well-being measures. *Journal of Personality and Social Psychology, 7*, 616–628.

Lyubomirsky, S., King, L. A., & Diener, E. (2005). The benefits of frequent positive affect: Does happiness lead to success? *Psychological Bulletin, 131*, 803–855.

Myers, D. (1992). *The pursuit of happiness.* New York: Morrow.

Oishi, S., Diener, E., Choi, D. W., Kim-Prieto, C., & Choi, I. (2005). *The dynamics of daily events and well-being across cultures: The declining marginal utility of daily events.* Manuscript submitted for publication, University of Virginia, Charlottesville.

Okun, M. A., & George, L. K. (1984). Physician- and self-ratings of health, neuroticism, and subjective well-being among men and women. *Personality and Individual Differences, 5*, 533–539.

Riis, J., Loewenstein, G., Baron, J., Jepson, C., Fagerlin, A., & Ubel, P. A. (2005). Ignorance of hedonic adaptation to hemodialysis: A study using ecological momentary assessment. *Journal of Experimental Psychology: General, 134*, 3–9.

Scheier, M. F., Matthews, K. A., Owens, J. F., Magovern, G. J. S., Lefebvre, R. C., Abbott, R. A., et al. (2003). Dispositional optimism and recovery from coronary artery bypass surgery: The beneficial effects on physical and psychological well-being. In P. Salovey & A. J. Rothman (Eds.), *Social psychology of health* (pp. 342–361). New York: Psychology Press.

Scheier, M. F., Weintraub, J. K., & Carver, C. S. (1986). Coping with stress: Divergent strategies of optimists and pessimists. *Journal of Personality and Social Psychology, 51*, 1257–1264.

Scollon, C. N. (2004). *Predictors of intraindividual change in personality and well-being.* Unpublished doctoral dissertation, University of Illinois, Urbana-Champaign.

Scollon, C. N., & Diener, E. (2006). Love, work, and changes in extraversion and neuroticism over time. *Journal of Personality and Social Psychology, 91*, 1152–1165.

Seligman, M. E. P., Steen, T. A., Park, N., & Peterson, C. (2005). Positive psychology progress: Empirical validation of interventions. *American Psychologist, 60*, 410–421.

Sheldon, K., & Lyubomirsky, S. (2004). Achieving sustainable new happiness: Prospects, practices, and prescriptions. In P. A. Linley & S. Joseph (Eds.), *Positive psychology in practice* (pp. 127–145). Hoboken, NJ: Wiley.

Silver, R. L. (1982). *Coping with an undesirable life event: A study of early reactions to physical disability.* Unpublished doctoral dissertation, Northwestern University, Evanston, IL.

Staudinger, U. M., & Fleeson, W. (1996). Self and personality in old and very old age: A sample case of resilience? *Development and Psychopathology, 8*, 867–885.

Suh, E., Diener, E., & Fujita, F. (1996). Events and subjective well-being: Only recent events matter. *Journal of Personality and Social Psychology, 70*, 1091–1102.

Tellegen, A., Lykken, D. T., Bouchard, T. J., Wilcox, K. J., Segal, N. L., & Rich, S. (1988). Personality similarity in twins reared apart and together. *Journal of Personality and Social Psychology, 54*, 1031–1039.

Wilson, T. D., & Gilbert, D. T. (2005). *Making sense: A model of affective adaptation.* Manuscript submitted for publication, University of Virginia, Charlottesville.

Will Money Increase Subjective Well-Being?:
A Literature Review and Guide to Needed Research

Ed Diener and Robert Biswas-Diener

The happy man will need external prosperity.
Aristotle
It is difficult for a man laden with riches to climb the steep path that leads to bliss.
Islamic saying
People who claim that money can't buy happiness just don't know where to shop.
Anonymous

Abstract Four replicable findings have emerged regarding the relation between income and subjective well-being (SWB): 1. There are large correlations between the wealth of nations and the mean reports of SWB in them, 2. There are mostly small correlations between income and SWB within nations, although these correlations appear to be larger in poor nations, and the risk of unhappiness is much higher for poor people, 3. Economic growth in the last decades in most economically developed societies has been accompanied by little rise in SWB, and increases in individual income lead to variable outcomes, and 4. People who prize material goals more than other values tend to be substantially less happy, unless they are rich. Thus, more money may enhance SWB when it means avoiding poverty and living in a developed nation, but income appears to increase SWB little over the long-term when more of it is gained by well-off individuals whose material desires rise with their incomes. Several major theories are compatible with most existing findings: A. The idea that income enhances SWB only insofar as it helps people meet their basic needs, and B. The idea that the relation between income and SWB depends on the amount of material desires that people's income allows them to fulfill. We argue that the first explanation is a special case of the second one. A third explanation is relatively unresearched, the idea that societal norms for production and consumption are essential to understanding the SWB-income interface. In addition, it appears high SWB might increase people's chances for high income. We review the open issues relating income to SWB, and describe the research methods needed to provide improved data that will better illuminate the psychological processes relating money to SWB.

E. Diener (✉)
Department of Psychology, University of Illinois, Urbana-Champaign, Champaign, IL 61820, USA
e-mail: ediener@s.psych.uiuc.edu

Money is a fundamental aspect of human life throughout the world. People spend a large fraction of their time earning and spending money, and use market goods during all of their waking and sleeping moments. In wealthy and poor societies around the globe, there is now an enormous concern about economic development, and in most nations it is the foremost policy issue. Nation-states recently have crumbled when they have failed to "deliver the goods." The world economy in 1998 reached 24 trillion US dollars, or 4,000 US dollars per person, and continues to grow dramatically.

From 1974 to 1994 productivity in the United States increased so that it required 3 days of work for a wage earner to purchase a color T.V. compared to 3 weeks just 20 years earlier, and substantially less time to buy most other items such as food, leisure, and travel (Templeton, 1999). Economic development is not just occurring in a few wealthy nations, however; it is spreading to the majority of the nations of the world. From 1975 to 1993 the number of cars in the world almost doubled, and automobiles in developing countries increased threefold. Although industrialized societies still use a disproportional share of electricity, the amount consumed in the developing countries tripled between 1980 and 1995. Even in the poorest region of the world, sub-Sahara Africa, the availability of many commodities approximately doubled in the 20 year period from the 1970s to the 1990s: meat and cereal production, electricity use, and automobile purchases, for example (UN Development Programme, 1998). In the developing nations of the Pacific Rim and Southeast Asia, consumption increased 3 to 4 times during this period. Recent growth rates in economically developed and developing nations alike have exceeded the material growth rates that characterized earlier time periods (Easterlin, 1996).

In view of the current economic growth rates of several percentage points throughout the majority of nations in the world, it is natural to ask whether most people on earth will be happier in the decades to come? One flourishing area of study in the social and behavioral sciences is concerned with the effects of income on subjective well-being (SWB), to which this review is devoted. Many people ask whether money will make them happier, and this paper reviews the intricate answer to their question.

Wealth is related to many positive outcomes in life (Furnham & Argyle, 1998). For example, people with higher incomes tend to be given lighter prison sentences for the same crimes (Black, 1976), have better health and mental health (e.g., Langner & Michael, 1963; Mayer, 1997), have greater longevity (Wilkinson, 1996), lower rates of infant mortality (Smith, Brooks-Gunn, & Jackson, 1997), are less frequently the victims of violent crime (Mayer, 1997), and experience fewer stressful life events (Wilson, Ellwood, & Brooks-Gunn, 1995). Financial problems are a strong predictor of DSM depression (Wheaton, 1994). The children of the well-to-do are less likely to drop out of school or become pregnant as teens (Mayer, 1997). In addition, richer people score higher in characteristics such as interpersonal trust (Rosenberg & Pearlin, 1978). It should be noted that the correlates of higher incomes are not confined entirely to the benefits of not being poor; the richest group, for example, has better health than the second highest income category (Pamuk, Makuc, Heck, Reuben, & Lochner, 1998).

Given the multiplicity of positive variables that covary with income, we should not be surprised if wealthier people are substantially happier than others, but there are also reasons to question this prospect. Modern society appears to have mixed feelings about rich people, containing both respect and dislike. For example, although Dittmar (1992) found that rich people were perceived as more inteligent and successful, she also found that wealthy individuals were viewed as more unfriendly and cold. Another reason that income might not strongly predict higher SWB is that most people must earn their money, and wealthier people thus might be required to spend more of their time in work, and have less time available for leisure and social relationships. Also, wealthy people might adapt to their conditions, and have rising expectations and desires that counteract the effects of the desirable circumstances of their lives. Finally, a materialistic mind-set that leads to higher incomes might create lower feelings of well-being (e.g., Kasser & Ryan, 1993). Thus, it is not a foregone conclusion that the more benign life circumstances of people with higher incomes will necessarily translate into greater SWB.

Whether higher income will lead to greater happiness is not merely of academic interest or idle curiosity. Many individuals are personally concerned with this question because of the important implications it has for how they should structure their lives. In addition, governments and other institutions are also very interested in economic policies. Political parties and governments can rise and fall depending on the economic prosperity of the society. The impact of income on SWB is one important way we can judge the benefits of economic progress. Andrew Oswald (1997) argues that "Economic things matter only in so far as they make people happier" (p. 1815).

In the current paper we present a comprehensive picture of the existing research on income and SWB, and then review the theories that seek to explain the findings. The extant data are, however, inadequate to definitely test the theories, primarily because the key mediating psychological variables in the models have rarely been measured. For example, our hypothesis that income relates to SWB to the extent that it allows people to fulfill their current desires cannot be tested in a thorough way with existing survey data. In addition, a number of intriguing psychological questions that we review remain unexplored. Although broad surveys have yielded intriguing findings on income and SWB, we describe the methodologies and measures that are required to make further theoretical progress in this area. In the following section we review the various types of evidence related to money and the experience of well-being.

Analyses at the Individual Level

Cross-Sectional Correlations for Individuals

Frey and Stutzer (2000) report results within Switzerland that are typical for cross-cultural data of this type—significant but relatively small correlations between SWB and income within nations. In Table 1 we present cross-sectional correlations within

Table 1 Correlations within nations and cities between income and subjective well-being

Citation	Place	Correlations	Concept
Diener and Oishi (2000)	19 nations	0.13 (mean r, range −0.02 to 0.38)	Life satisfaction
Schyns (1998a)	W. Germany	0.06–0.15	Life satisfaction
	Russian Federation	0.17–0.27	Life satisfaction
Lachman and Weaver (1998)	United States	0.18 and 0.18	Life satisfaction
Blanchflower, Oswald, and Warr (1993)	US (Log income)	0.15	Men, happiness
		0.14	Women, happiness
Hagerty (2000)	United States	0.18	Happiness
E. Diener, Sandvik, Seidlitz, and M. Diener (1993)	United States	0.13 (Circa, 1973)	Affect balance
		0.12 (Circa, 1983)	Affect balance
Mullis (1992)	United States males	0.17	Happy with life & domains
Keith (1985)	US older divorced and separated	0.23	Women and Men; both "Satisfaction with level of living"
		0.21	
Connor et al. (1985)	Retired professors from Iowa, USA	0.24	Life satisfaction
Brinkerhoff, Fredell, and Frideres (1997)	Village in India	0.22	Happiness
		0.35	Aggregate satisfaction
Biswas-Diener and Diener (2000)	Poor areas of Calcutta	0.45	Life satisfaction

Note. Although some studies present more than one correlation, virtually all of the correlations shown are statistically significant because the low correlations are based on very large samples.

nations between income and SWB for 11 published studies. The World Value Survey II studied by Diener and Oishi (2000) was based on large probability samples of many nations. As can be seen, the correlations are consistent in showing mostly modest correlations between income and various forms of SWB (e.g., happiness, life satisfaction, and positive affect). The table shows that the relation between income and SWB is much stronger among a very poor sample in Calcutta. Other evidence confirms the positive correlation between money and happiness. For example, Diener, Horwitz, and Emmons (1985) found that super-rich individuals (sampled from the Forbes' list of wealthiest Americans), matched to a comparison group living in the same geographical area, were about 1 point higher on a 0–6 life satisfaction scale. Although this difference is not immense, neither is it trivial.

Table 2 gives another view of the differences in SWB between richer and poorer individuals, showing for 19 nations the percent of people in the highest and lowest income categories who scored above or below neutral on several SWB items (World Value Survey Group, 1994). Counting responses that are either above or below

Table 2 Percent above neutral in life satisfaction by nation in the wealthiest and poorest income categories

Nation	SWB variable							
	Life satisfaction		Positive affect balance		Negative affect balance		Financial satisfaction	
Income category	Low	High	Low	Hign	Low	High	Low	High
Austria	76	76	57	80	29	9	74	67
Belgium	78	91	64	82	20	9	66	91
Britain	74	93	49	87	40	6	38	83
Canada	83	95	65	90	16	4	49	95
Chile	73	87	49	81	37	12	27	93
Denmark	80	95	65	91	26	5	54	84
Germany (East)	67	70	58	75	28	16	43	82
Germany (West)	62	91	47	86	39	4	48	92
France	56	85	49	81	28	9	26	82
Ireland	84	96	53	89	25	5	56	88
Japan	49	84	35	46	29	20	41	82
Mexico	79	90	71	80	18	5	57	89
Netherlands	87	93	66	87	19	6	53	100
Nigeria	48	73	44	79	33	15	22	76
Norway	73	94	90	91	5	2	48	83
Portugal	55	88	46	85	38	10	35	90
Russia	42	54	46	58	42	25	13	59
Spain	64	90	37	72	35	13	40	83
Switzerland	88	95	71	81	14	3	74	95
Mean	69	86	56	80	27	9	45	85
Risk ratio for poor people	0.80		0.70		3.0		0.53	

Note. Nations in the World Value Survey II (1994) for which there were a minimum of 20 respondents in both the wealthiest and poorest income groups. Most surveys conducted in 1990–1991.

neutral has the advantage of not relying on differences in the reported intensity of SWB, which might be less reliable across respondents and nations because these reports require that people use scale numbers in an equivalent way. The percentage figures assume only that people can report whether they are primarily happy versus unhappy, or more satisfied than dissatisfied, and that this judgment is more likely to be made similarly across respondents. The poor income category in most nations had a very low upper bound, and thus represented true poverty. In contrast, the highest income category was not so extreme, and thus included upper middle incomes and above, not just truly wealthy people. As can be seen across nations, 17% more of the wealthiest group reported that they were satisfied with their lives. Stated differently, the likelihood that a poor person will be satisfied with her or his life is 0.80 as great as that of a richer person.

Several interesting conclusions can be drawn from Table 2 regarding life satisfaction. First, it appears that impoverished individuals score relatively better in social democratic nations with liberal welfare benefits, although Norway is an exception to this pattern. It is noteworthy, for example, that poor people were more satisfied in the former East Germany than in West Germany, whereas wealthier people were more satisfied in the former West Germany. Second, even wealthier respondents are dissatisfied in the unstable conditions of Russia (see Inglehart & Klingemann, 2000, for an explanation). Finally, poor people are substantially less satisfied than wealthier individuals in Portugal, Spain, Japan, West Germany, and France.

Although the correlations in Table 1 between income and life satisfaction may appear small, the data in Table 2 reveal that the relation has significance at a societal level. Projecting the data from Table 2 across the entire population of the world, for example, would equate to millions of more satisfaction individuals if the poor could move to the life satisfaction level of the richest income categories.

When we consider the other dependent variables, the effects of income appear larger. In Table 2 we show affect balance (pleasant affect minus unpleasant affect based on Bradburn's 1969 scale) for both positive and negative values, and financial satisfaction. Positive affect balance in Table 2 is when pleasant emotions exceed unpleasant emotions, and negative affect balance is when unpleasant emotions exceed the pleasant ones. As can be seen, the differences between richer and poorer respondents for these variables is larger than for life satisfaction. For instance, the poor are only 0.53 as likely to be satisfied with their incomes as the rich. They are 0.70 as likely to be satisfied with their incomes as the rich. They are 0.70 as likely to show a positive affect balance (more pleasant than negative affect reported). Finally, the risk ratio for the negative affect balance scores show that based on this index the poor are much more likely to report low SWB. We arrive at the same conclusion if we examine Bradburn's (1969) data drawn from large US cities. The poorest group reported being "not so happy" 36% of the time, but the richest group responded in this way only 5% of the time. Thus, the poor had about a sevenfold greater risk of suffering from unhappiness compared to the wealthiest category in Bradburn's data, and almost a threefold greater likelihood of a negative affect balance score in the World Value Survey II data shown in Table 2. Therefore, the risk ratios for unhappiness among the poor versus wealthier individuals are substantial.

Similar to the Table 2 data, Bradburn's findings revealed that the likelihood of the poorest group being "pretty happy" or "very happy" was 0.67 of the richest group, obviously a much less extreme ratio than the unhappiness data. This divergence in conclusions when examining positive versus negative SWB occurs because a preponderance of people report being happy (E. Diener & C. Diener, 1996), and thus the low base rates in unhappiness make possible larger risk ratios. Thus, it can be said that higher income corresponds to modest differences in happiness, but it substantially reduces the risk of the rarer experience of unhappiness.

Various types of SWB. Andrews and Withey (1976), Diener (1984), and others have argued that life satisfaction, pleasant affect, and lack of unpleasant affect are separable constructs that must be independently examined. In a re-analysis of Bradburn's (1969) data, Lane (1991) reported that NA decreased as one rose through the very lowest income levels, but not thereafter, whereas PA moved up throughout the entire range of income. In our international college sample (Suh,

Diener, Oishi, & Triandis, 1998) income correlated 0.19 with positive affect but only 0.03 with negative affect. However, there were not strong differences across dependent variables in the large World Value Survey Group II (World Value Survey, 1994). Across a large number of individuals and societies, after controlling mean-level nation differences, income correlated 0.13 with life satisfaction, 0.13 with positive affect and −0.10 with negative affect. In many nations positive affect showed a stronger correlation with income than did negative affect, but in some societies this pattern was reversed. Thus, it is likely that income influences positive affect and negative affect differently in distinct contexts, but we are as yet unable to clearly identify the moderating variables involved.

At first glance it might appear that the lack of a reliably higher relation between income and negative affect is at odds with our earlier conclusions about the greater risk ratio of poor people for low SWB. The risk ratios are about groups of individuals compared to one another, however, not about particular dependent variables. Poor people score lower on a variety of SWB measures, not just on measures of unhappiness. The risk ratio for negative affect balance shown in Table 2, for example, is high. If we reverse our analysis of life satisfaction, however, and examine the ratio for life dissatisfaction, we find a ratio of 2.4 (0.31 divided by 0.13; there was no neutral category), indicating that poor people are almost $2^1/_2$ times more likely to be dissatisfied with their lives than well-off people. Thus, the high risk ratios for low SWB experienced by the poor are not necessarily due disproportionately to greater negative affect, but probably reflect the relatively high percentage of poor people in the low SWB range across different types of measures.

Control and moderator variables. In order to determine the causal pathways of income on SWB, we must first examine how the relation survives controlling other variables that might underlie the relation, such as education. For instance, it might be that educated people earn more money, but that it is education rather that income that leads to heightened happiness. Similarly, married men earn more money than unmarried men (Nakosteen & Zimmer, 1997), and therefore one should control for marriage to understand income's effect because married people on average are happier (Diener, Suh, Lucas, & Smith, 1999). The correlation of income and SWB controlling for education has been examined in many studies, and usually it changes little from the zero-order correlation (e.g., Blanchflower & Oswald, 1999). Tomes (1986) found that income had small but significant correlations with reported happiness and satisfaction even after controlling for education (which had very small effects), marriage (which had moderate to large effects), unemployment (which had a large negative impact, especially for men), and other control variables. Similarly, Marks and Fleming (1999) found that income influenced an aggregated measure of happiness with aspects of life even after controlling for marital status, occupation, employment, age, and sex. Biswas-Diener and Diener (2000) found that income and life satisfaction correlated after satisfaction with various domains, such as family and friends, was controlled. These findings suggest a direct relation of income with SWB that is not due to many other variables.

Some variables appear to moderate the effect of income on SWB, for example sex. Adelmann (1987) found that income was significantly related to happiness for men but not for women. Similarly, a wife's personal earnings did not affect her likelihood of depression, whereas a husband's personal earnings directly decreased the probability of his depression (Ross & Huber, 1985). Keith and Schafer (1982) found that low income was a predictor of depression among single women, but not among married women. Pearlin and Johnson (1977) reported that economic strain predicted depression, but that marriage buffered this effect to some degree. George (1992) reported that the relation of income and SWB was weaker for the elderly. These findings suggest that the effects of money on SWB differ depending on one's life circumstances, roles, and values.

These moderator variables imply that the importance of factors such as desires and feelings of self-worth in the relation between money and SWB. The effect of income on happiness appears not to be an absolute one, but instead is one that depends on an individual's roles and relationships, as well as other factors.

An important moderator of the effects of income on SWB is the wealth of the society. Veenhoven (1991) found that the correlations between income and SWB were stronger in poorer nations, and this effect was largely duplicated among college students by Diener and Oishi (2000). E. Diener and M. Diener (1995b) found that among women financial satisfaction was more strongly related to life satisfaction in poorer versus richer nations, and this trend was of borderline significance for men. Schyns (1998a;1998b) also reproduced the finding that the relation between income and life satisfaction is largest in the poorer nations. Thus, there is evidence that income has a larger correlation with SWB in poor societies, although there remain several possible explanations of this finding—the greater variability in the fulfillment of biological needs in poor nations, the larger amount of social welfare protections in wealthy nations, and the greater income inequality that characterizes many poor nations are all viable explanations of the differences in correlations. The findings of Biswas-Diener and Diener (2000) in the slums of Calcutta that income was strongly related to life satisfaction indicates that where income differences are related to differences in meeting universal basic needs for food and shelter, the effects of income can be relatively strong.

Just as the correlations show a larger effect of income in poor nations, there is also evidence for the declining effects of money at upper income levels within societies. Diener et al. (1993) found a curvilinear effect between income and SWB within the USA, with ever higher income categories being related to smaller increments of SWB. This effect is disguised in many studies because income scales are used in which responses have increasingly larger ranges as one goes up the income ladder; the income categories increase in a nonlinear fashion. When actual income figures are used, the data are often subjected to a log transformation. Thus, when the income scale correlates in a linear fashion with SWB, it often hides a curvilinear effect.

Veenhoven (1995) and Diener and Oishi (2000) both report that income correlates less strongly with SWB for college student samples than for adult samples, which is to be expected considering that the life style of students and their elite status usually protects them to a degree against the most severe effects of poverty. Further, poverty during college is often seen as a temporary state. The college findings are important, however, in again reminding us that the influence of income is contextual, and depends on the life circumstances of the respondents we are studying.

Financial satisfaction as a mediator between income and global SWB. Are the effects of income mediated by financial satisfaction, or are there direct effects that perhaps come from the daily pleasures of greater income, not mediated by a judgment about one's income? First, it should be noted that the correlation of income with financial satisfaction is usually stronger than the correlation of income with global life satisfaction (e.g., Douthitt, MacDonald, & Mullis, 1992; Headey & Wearing, 1992). In Diener and Oishi's (2000) analysis of the World Value Survey II data (World Value Survey Group, 1994), for instance, financial satisfaction and income correlated across countries an average of 0.25, compared to the mean correlation of 0.13 for life satisfaction. This finding makes sense because life satisfaction can be influenced by many important factors that are relatively unrelated to income, whereas financial satisfaction should have income as a major input. This pattern suggests the possibility that financial satisfaction is closer in the causal chain to life satisfaction than is income. To assess this possibility, Schyns (2000) performed a mediational analysis for both West Germany and Russia, examining the direct and indirect paths of income's influence on life satisfaction. In Germany the path was indirect through financial satisfaction, whereas in Russia the direct effect was significant. These findings suggest that the effect of income on life satisfaction can come either from its influence on financial satisfaction, or more directly from the life circumstances of rich versus poorer people. George (1992) reviewed studies showing that financial satisfaction to some degree mediated the relation between income and more global SWB, but that there were direct effects as well.

Several conclusions can be drawn from the cross-sectional correlations within nations. The findings are incompatible with the idea that SWB flows automatically from higher income, because there are a number of moderators of this relation. These moderations indicate that psychological factors such as needs, desires, and role might play a critical role in the relation of money to SWB. It appears that income makes a larger difference to SWB within poorer societies than in rich ones. This finding might point to the importance of the fulfillment of basic needs in the income-SWB relation, because physical needs are more of an issue in poorer groups in most poor countries. Alternately, the findings might mean that in wealthier societies poor people more frequently have their material desires met because of welfare payments or because material desires are more flexible once more people move beyond the level of abject poverty. We now turn to other types of evidence on the income and SWB relation, which can shed greater light on the nature of the effects.

Changes in Individual Income, and the Causal Order of Variables

Income change. Do changes in income lead to changes in SWB? Answering this question will help us determine whether it is shifts in income rather than the absolute level of money that increases SWB, and will aid us in understanding the causal order of variables. In Table 3 we present both longitudinal and experimental studies in which income change was studied at the individual level. In the longitudinal studies the same respondents were followed over time, and both their incomes and their SWB were assessed more than once. Surprisingly, the longitudinal studies provide

Table 3 Income change and subjective well-being, individual level

Type of study and citation	Findings
Longitudinal studies	
Diener et al. (1993)	General well-being in US significantly different across income change groups, the income increase group was *lowest* in SWB
Schyns (2000)	Income change correlated nonsignficantly with life satisfaction in both Russia and W. Germany
Bradburn (1969)	Changes in income over a one-year period were not related to changes in affect balance
Marks and Fleming (1999)	Australian young adults, income change predicted by SWB, and SWB (happy with aspects of life) change predicted by income
Experimental or quasi-experimental studies	
Thoits and Hannan (1979)	Larger payments to welfare recipients led to *greater* stress
Brickman, Coates, and Janoff-Bulman (1978)	Nonsignificantly higher happiness among lottery winners compared to comparison group. Pleasure in mundane pleasant activities significantly *lower*
Smith and Razzell (1975)	Football pool winners reported higher levels of SWB than comparison group; 39% vs. 19% reported being very happy
Gardner and Oswald (2001)	Lottery winners and heirs receiving windfalls reported higher SWB

mixed evidence for the influence of income change on SWB. Diener et al. (1993) found that the group whose income declined were the happiest, and the group whose income increased reported the lowest well-being, a surprising finding that is consistent with the negative income tax study described below. The Schyns (2000) and Bradburn (1969) studies found nonsignificant effects for income change. In a study not shown in the table, Saris (2001) found stronger effects of income, after controlling for previous income, in Russia compared to in Germany, suggesting that the effect of income change might be stronger in poorer nations.

The experimental or quasi-experimental research includes lottery studies, a governmentally funded negative income tax experiment in which randomly selected welfare recipients were paid higher levels of benefits, and a study of people in a longitudinal study who received financial windfalls through a lottery or inheritance. In the case of the negative income tax studies, participants were randomly assigned to conditions, but only measures of stress were included and no positive well-being constructs were assessed. As can be seen, the negative income tax studies (Thoits & Hannan, 1979) found *higher levels of stress* among those receiving *higher welfare payments*.

In the lottery studies, Brickman and colleagues found that winners were nonsignificantly happier, and were significantly *less pleased* with everyday events; but the number of respondents was very small. In the study of football pool winners in England, Smith and Razzell (1975) found that the lucky individuals did report higher levels of well-being, and Gardner and Oswald (2001) found an increase in SWB among those whose financial life had brightened due to a lottery winning or to inheritance. These authors found that a windfall of about 75,000 US dollars led to a 0.1–0.3 standard deviation rise in SWB during the following year. In addition, there are data suggesting that increases in income do lead to higher satisfaction with one's job and one's income (Clark, 1999; Schyns, 2000; Schyns, 2001).

Problems faced by the lottery winners in the United Kingdom (Smith & Razzell, 1975) demonstrated that higher income is not invariably an unalloyed good, and can have costs and well as benefits. For example, many of the lottery winners quit their jobs and moved to new neighborhoods, thus losing some of their former friends. The social mobility of the lottery winners had the costs of possibly losing old friends and being despised by new neighbors. In addition, family and friends who wanted part of the earnings were often recipients of what they perceived as an inadequate amount of money, thus leading to interpersonal friction. A related finding is that people whose income rose have been found to be more likely to get divorced (Clydesdale, 1997), thus possibly offsetting the higher SWB that could possibly follow from having more money. These studies suggest the possibility that the effects of income on interpersonal relationships may be an important consideration, but there is little systematic longitudinal research on this topic. Despite the possible downsides of higher income, the large longitudinal study by Gardner and Oswald (2001) indicates that the net effects of income on SWB are often positive. Because winning the lottery and receiving an inheritance are somewhat random, the longitudinal data of Oswald indicates that the SWB-income relation is not entirely due to the fact that happy people make more money.

The theory of adaptation (Brickman et al., 1978) and Michalos's Multiple Discrepancy Theory (1985) predict that changes in income should influence SWB, and will do so more than a person's absolute level of income. However, the data present a mixed picture. Hamermesh (2001) found that changes in income produced short-term changes in job satisfaction especially among those with concrete skills where the income changes were less expected. In some cases increases in income produce *lower* SWB. The changes a person makes in his or her life in reaction to greater income (e.g., changing neighborhoods) might produce decreases in SWB. In addition, increases in income might often be accompanied by an even bigger increase in one's appetite for consumables, thus leading to a greater discrepancy between desires and possessions. Conversely, declines in income might not always be perceived in negative terms. In the Diener et al. (1993) study, many respondents were older and therefore the income-decline group might have been heavily populated by people who retired. When retiring, people usually expect their incomes to decline, and often have investment savings to offset the decline, as well as ownership of greater numbers of durable goods (e.g., a car and house). In addition, some declines in income occur because people voluntarily cut back on their work hours. Thus, some people with declining incomes might have chosen an alternative lifestyle with lower income, and this could produce very different levels of SWB compared to a lower income from being fired. Windfall increases in income can increase feelings of well-being, but also create some new stresses. Thus, the data on income change

do not indicate that there is an automatic rise in SWB following increases in one's
income, nor are declines in income always antecedents to lower SWB.

SWB influencing income. Not only might the correlation between income and
SWB indicate the influence of money on happiness, but as the discussion above
indicates, the causal arrow could point in the other direction: happy people might
on average earn more income. In a panel survey of young adults in Australia, Marks
and Fleming (1999) found that high SWB (happy feelings about nine aspects of life)
at an earlier time period preceded increasing income. For respondents who were two
standard deviations higher in SWB there was an 8–12% greater income increase
at the next time period compared to the lower group. In addition, current SWB
had a strong influence on later unemployment—with less happy respondents being
more likely to be unemployed later. Diener, Scollon, Oishi, Dzokoto, & Suh (2000)
analyzed cheerfulness reports from a large cohort of students entering college in
1976 (see Bowen & Bok, 1998), and data on the income of these individuals in
about 1993. Figure 1 shows that the respondents' parents' income moderated the
effects of cheerfulness on later income.

For individuals form economically advantaged backgrounds, a cheerful disposition was likely to be followed by substantially higher income in adulthood. For most
respondents, a cheerful disposition in late adolescence was followed by a somewhat
higher income in adulthood compared to those with a less cheerful disposition. For
respondents who had grown up in poor households, there was no effect of cheerfulness on later income. These studies indicate that SWB can influence later income.
Thus, the correlations between individual income and SWB must be interpreted in
light of the fact that some of the relation is likely due to the tendency of happier

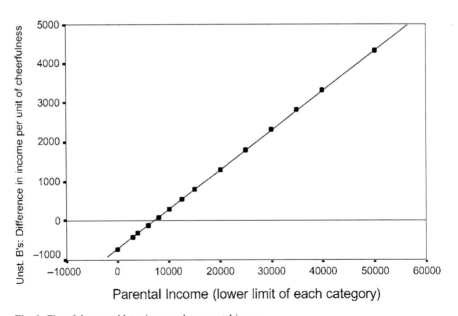

Fig. 1 Cheerfulness and later income, by parents' income

people to earn higher incomes than unhappy people. Thus, we have evidence that the relation between SWB and income is bidirectional.

Analyses at the National Level

Mean Income Per Person

In addition to the individual-level analyses presented above, we can also analyze whether people in wealthier societies are on average happier. Such analyses can reveal whether societal conditions rather than individual circumstances influence SWB. Again, we might assume that wealthier nations are higher in SWB because they are higher on a large number of desirable characteristics (E. Diener & C. Diener, 1995a) such as equality, literacy, longevity, health, human rights, lower crime, and democracy. Nevertheless, one can think of reasons that people in wealthy nations would not be happier, despite their resources—competitiveness, materialism, less time for leisure and socializing, and so forth. In what is the most extensive international study to date, Inglehart and Klingemann (2000) present recent SWB figures for a large number of nations, and a subset of these are presented in Table 4,

Table 4 Percent above neutral and wealth for selected nations

Nation	Percent above neutral on Life Satisfaction	Year of survey	Income
Netherlands	92	1990	13,281
Canada	90	1990	16,362
Switzerland	89	1996	15,887
Ireland	88	1990	9,637
Sweden	87	1990	13,986
USA	85	1995	17,945
New Zealand	84	1998	11,363
Mexico	83	1996	6,253
Portugal	76	1990	7,478
Japan	72	1990	15,105
France	72	1990	13,918
China	72	1995	1,493
Brazil	72	1996	3,882
Nigeria	71	1995	978
India	67	1996	1,282
Bangladesh	63	1997	1,510
Romania	57	1990	2,043
South Africa	56	1996	3,068
Hungary	52	1998	4,645
Bulgaria	33	1998	5,208
Russia	28	1995	7,741

Note. Source for SWB is Inglehart and Klingemann (2000), and for income is Sumners and Heston (1991).

along with per capita income figures for the year each survey was conducted. The relation between the wealth of nations and the SWB there is evident, although there are discrepancies from a perfect relation arising from additional factors such as political stability and cultural norms. Inglehart and Klingemann report that the correlation between per capita income and mean SWB across their entire sample of nations was 0.70.

Table 5 shows the correlations across studies between mean income in nations (usually assessed by gross domestic product per captia, or purchasing power parity) and the mean SWB of those societies. As can be seen, the correlations are consistently large, and much higher than the covariation we reported for individuals within nations. The mean correlation across studies is about 0.60. The first explanation that comes to mind for these large correlations is that the error term for these societal correlations might be much smaller than in the individual-level analyses because differences in temperament and other individual characteristics are likely to be averaged out of the means, resulting in the clearer covariation of income and SWB. Diener and Oishi (2000) examined this possibility by analyzing the unstandardized regression coefficients in a hierarchical linear model across nations. They found that income has a larger effect moving from nation than going from individual to individual, and this difference is not due merely to more variability at the individual level. Similarly, Schyns (1998b) found that national income substantially predicts individual SWB beyond the effects of individual income, again suggesting that additional variables such as human rights and equality might increase positive experience in wealthier nations.

One explanation for the greater correlations of income at the national level is that high income countries have a number of additional positive characteristics besides material goods—human rights, greater equality, and higher literacy, for example (Diener et al., 1995a; E. Diener, & C. Diener, 1995a). Wealthy nations also tend to be more individualistic. Although Diener, Diener and Diener attempted to separate the influence of these variables through partial correlation procedure is doubtful in

Table 5 Correlations across nations of income and mean subjective well-being

Reference	Number of nations	Correlations
Veenhoven (1991)	14	0.51
(Cantril's 1965 sample)		
(Based on Gallup sample)	9	0.59
E. Diener, M. Diener, and C. Diener (1995)	55	0.59
Inkeles and Diamond (1980) (Cantril's 1965 sample, controlled for education)	10	0.55–0.61
Ouweneel and Veenhoven (1991)	28	0.62
E. Diener and C. Diener (1995a)	34	0.64
Schyns (1998a)	40	0.64
Diener and Oishi (2000)	42	0.69
Inglehart and Klingemann (2000)	64	0.70

Note. All of the correlations are significant at $p < 0.05$ (one-tailed) or less.

light of the small number of nations and the high intercorrelations among predictors. However, it seems plausible that the abundance of shared public goods in wealthy nations (e.g., public schools, highways, water and sewage systems, hospitals, and parks) might heighten the SWB of both poorer and richer persons in them.

In considering the effects of income across nations, a natural question arises about the comparability of measures across countries. For example, one could suppose that respondents in individualistic nations might be more likely to report happiness to an interviewer than collectivists, who might want to appear humble and not stand out from the group. Diener, Scollon, Oishi, Dzokoto, and Suh (2000) found that a general positivity disposition varies across nations and is correlated with reports of SWB, and predicts SWB beyond national income. This finding suggests that although national income increases mean SWB, the positivity of the people in a society does so as well. Thus, the effects of national income on SWB will not be definitive until additional measures of well-being based on experience sampling, memory, and physiological reactions (e.g., cortisol levels) are also available. Yet another type of evidence regarding money and happiness is based on SWB and income *change* at the national level.

National Changes in Income

The increase in income was dramatic in the United States from World War II to 1995. For example, in 1988 the lowest fifth of the American population had per capita expenditures, adjusted for cost of living, higher than the median income in 1955! The amount of work time required to buy almost all goods has fallen substantially (Templeton, 1999) in recent decades. Today's poor were yesterday's middle-class in terms of income and consumption. Yet little or no change in SWB occurred during this period (Blanchflower and Oswald, 1999; Diener & Oishi, 2000).

Although the increase in income in the United States was dramatic in the decades following World War II, the rise in income in Japan was spectacular—one of the greatest economic growth periods in human history. Figure 2 shows the increase in income for Japan during the period from 1958 to 1987, along with the slope for SWB. It is important to note that the income figures are corrected for inflation. Japan in 1958 had an average per capita income of about 3,000 US dollars (in current dollars), an amount that is well below the present poverty level in the US. Thus, Japan started the period in a state of poverty and ended it one of the wealthiest nations in the world; yet, there is little discernible change in SWB.

Like the United States and Japan, many nations experienced rapid economic growth during the last several decades, and longitudinal SWB data are available for a number of the wealthier countries. As can be seen in Table 6, which presents SWB slope lines for countries experiencing economic growth, there is very little overall change.

Although not readily perceptible in Fig. 2, life satisfaction did increase 3% in Japan during the period shown. Based on small increases such as this, Hagerty and Veenhoven (1999) argue that SWB is increasing in economically developed nations

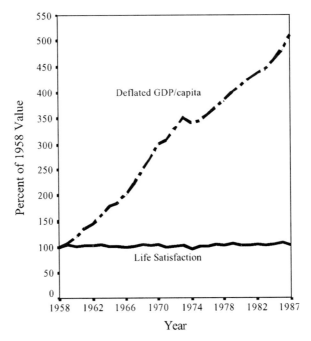

Fig. 2 Economic growth and SWB in Japan

as wealth makes them more livable. They found that increases in national income lead to increases in happiness especially in the short-term, when poor nations are included in the analyses. If the small upward slope is due to economic development, and not due to chance or some third variable influence, it implies that enormous increases in wealth in developed nations are required to produce tiny increments in happiness. Furthermore, the reasons for the small increases are unknown, and do not occur in all developed nations with growing economies. Diener and Oishi (2000) reported, however, that for poorer nations with high growth there was a clear increase in SWB, although the number of surveys was too small to reliably estimate the slopes for SWB. Thus, it is possible that poor nations undergoing economic growth are experiencing a greater increase in SWB.

Table 6 Time trends in SWB for nations

Source	Place	Slope
Blanchflower et al. (1993)	United States	−0.00004 Women 0.004 Men
Blanchflower and Oswald (1999)	United States Britain	−0.0027 0.0003
Diener and Oishi (2000)	15 nations	0.007 (Mean, range −0.04 to 0.09; Time trends about 1965–1990)

In addition to analyzing longitudinal changes in SWB in nations, we can also examine the cross-sectional studies in which past economic growth and current SWB are correlated. These correlations, reported by Diener and Oishi (2000), are quite inconsistent—the World Value Survey, $r = +0.49$; their international college sample, $r = -0.16$; the Michalos college sample, $r = -0.21$; Ouweneel and Veenhoven, $r = -0.15$; the Veenhoven (1993) data, $r = -0.24$. Similarly, Diener et al. (1995a) reported that across four surveys income growth correlated a nonsignificant -0.08 with SWB, and varied from -0.44 to $+0.40$ in individual surveys. These findings confirm the conclusions drawn from Tables 3 and 6—long-term trends in income do not have a necessary connection to changes in SWB. It seems likely that people's desires can change as fast or faster than their incomes, and thereby negate the salutary influence of increased money. The national longitudinal data, as well as the income growth data, strongly converge with the conclusions drawn from income change at the individual level—there is no necessary long-term relation between increases in income and higher SWB. Although increases in income might product short-term increases in SWB, it appears that over time people adapt as their material desires increase.

The data presented above on income changes in nations were based almost entirely on nations undergoing economic growth. Interestingly, decreases in income at the national level, due to recessions for instance, might with greater certainty cause declines in SWB. Inglehart and Rabier (1986) found that a declining income in Belgium after 1979 was followed by declining SWB. There are also data to indicate that people suffer more marital and mental health problems during recessions, although this effect is greater for people who already have lower SWB (Liker & Elder, 1983; Aldwin & Revenson, 1986). Thus, the national-level economic change data tentatively support Prospect Theory (Kahneman & Tversky, 1984) in which it is predicted that losses loom larger than gains. At least in the short-term, economic downturns might decrease SWB; possibly people do not reduce their material desires as quickly as they increase them.

Materialism

There is now convincing evidence at least within the United States that materialistic goals and values are inimical to high SWB (Ahuvia & Wong, 2001; Ahuvia & Wong, 2002; Kasser & Ryan, 1993; Richins & Dawson, 1992; Sirgy, 1997). This relation is shown in Fig. 3 for our international college student study, which covered over 7,000 respondents in 41 countries (Diener & Oishi, 2000). As can be seen, placing a high importance on money has an inverse relation with life satisfaction. In contrast, those who place a high value on love are more satisfied with their lives. At the nation level, we found that the mean value placed on money in countries correlated -0.53 with the average life satisfaction in those societies, with income controlled. A number of reasons can be hypothesized for why materialism correlates inversely with SWB. According to Kasser and Ryan (1993) it is because striving for material goods does

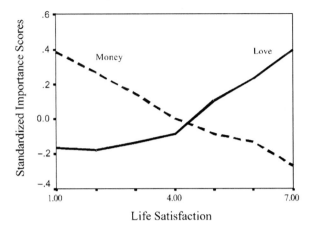

Importance values are standardized within
nations, and thus societal differences are controlled.

Fig. 3 The importance of love and money, and SWB

not fulfill intrinsic human desires. Another plausible reason is that people who are unhappy or low on other desirable resources such as close friends might seek solace in material goods; a phenomenon likened to "shopping therapy." One possible explanation can probably be rejected—that people are materialistic because they are poor, and therefore unhappy. When income is controlled, the inverse relation between materialism and SWB persists. For example, in our international college study the negative relation barely changed when family income was controlled.

Another plausible hypothesis explaining the toxic effects of materialism is that placing too much importance on material goods is detrimental owing to the fact that it is a goal that can never be fulfilled because there are always additional goods and services that one does not have, and probably that one cannot afford even if one were affluent. Partial support for the idea that the lack of fulfillment of material desires is one of the causes of discontent among materialistic people comes from Crawford, Diener, Oishi, and Wirtz (2000). In Fig. 4 we present the relation they report between income and life satisfaction for participants with less and more materialistic goals. Each of the adult respondents listed their five most important goals. Next they rated how relevant money was to achieving each of these goals, and their materialism score was the sum of these five ratings. As can be seen, materialistic people were much less satisfied with their lives if they were poor. Materialists were closer in happiness to nonmaterialists, however, if they were well-off. Langner and Michael (1963) found similar results; those who said that money is the most important thing in life were at greater risk for mental health problems, except in the wealthiest group. Similarly, Nickerson, Schwartz, Kahneman, and Diener (2001) found that those granting high importance to income were less happy except at very high levels of wealth. Interestingly, Nickerson et al. found that materialists were less satisfied with their social relationships. Thus, materialism may be most

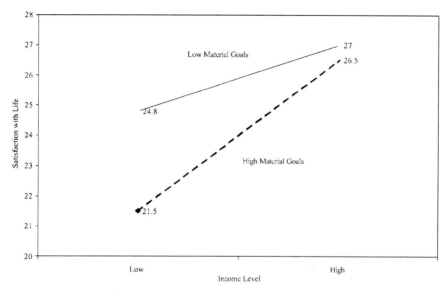

Fig. 4 Income, materialism, and life satisfaction

detrimental for the poor, but appears to have some negative effects even for the financially well-off.

One explanation for why materialistic people are less happy reverses the direction of causality discussed above; in this explanation feelings of inadequacy (and other motives that are incompatible with high SWB) lead to materialism. Crawford, in an unpublished study, found that after people had listed their inadequacies, they rated money as more important—as though being rich might compensate in part for feelings of low self-esteem. Similarly, Srivastava Locke, and Bartol (2001) found that the motives of seeking power and status, as well as overcoming self-doubt, mediated the inverse relation between materialism and SWB.

Theoretical Models of the Data

Several psychological conclusions can be garnered from the existing data on income and SWB. It is evident that there is not a simple input-output relation between money and happiness; the data are too complex for that. The relation of income to SWB is moderated by psychological variables such as level of desires and social comparisons. At the same time, the objective life conditions afforded by higher income do on average enhance SWB. The lower average levels of SWB among poor individuals and in poor nations indicates that poverty can and does lower SWB. It also appears that once people have high incomes (by current world standards), additional increases in wealth have a very small influence on SWB, suggesting that added income beyond modest affluence no longer helps answer important desires and needs. Finally, it appears that intensely desiring more money correlates inversely with SWB.

Several theoretical models have been advanced to explain the data on income and SWB: the Human Nature or Needs hypothesis, the Relative Standards model, and the Culture approach.

Human Nature

One explanation of the data is that there are certain universal human characteristics, such as basic biological needs, and that income will facilitate SWB to the extent that it allows people to meet these needs. For example, people have homeostatic needs for food, water, and thermoregulation, and therefore they will be happy to the extent that their incomes allow them to fulfill these needs with satisfactory nourishment, clothing, and housing. The human needs can be expanded beyond homeostatic ones to include self-respect, excitement seeking, status, self-actualization, and so forth. Accordingly, income might enhance SWB if it helps people, in addition to food and shelter, to also obtain security, status, and the development of their abilities. A modern version of this approach is the "Self-Determination Theory" of Deci and Ryan (1980), with an emphasis on well-being devolving from the expression of intrinsic and autonomous strivings. In his writings on happiness, Veenhoven (e.g., 1995) has called the human needs approach "livability theory" because some societies are considered to be more livable than others, fulfilling inherent human requirements. The Human Nature approach suggests that there will be an invariant relation between income and happiness to the degree that income can be used to purchase things that are truly pleasurable because they fulfill innate requirements.

The model appears to fit some of the existing data well. For example, the effects of income, at both the individual and societal levels, seem strongest at the lower levels of income. This finding is consistent with livability theory because needs are likely to be one of the first desires met with income. Similarly, the finding that students' income correlates at lower levels with their SWB is consonant with livability theory because university students are an elite group in which variations in income are probably not strongly related to the fulfillment of basic needs. The finding that there has been little gain in SWB in the economically developed nations over the last several decades is explained in livability theory by hypothesizing that basic human needs were met in these societies even in the early years after WW II when the first surveys were conducted.

On the negative side, the Human Nature theories have a number of limitations. They do not readily explain why the highest income group surpasses the second highest group in terms of SWB. For instance, Diener and Oishi (2000) found that even the top two income groups in the World Value Survey (1994) differed significantly in life satisfaction. Similarly, Easterlin (1999) found that eight percent more of the richest group said they were "very happy" compared to the second-richest group. If the highest group is still obtaining additional needs that cannot be met by the penultimate group, however, the needs account of why wealthy nations are not increasing in SWB does not seem plausible. Similarly, if one examines the Japanese data from the 1950s to the present, it appears that the Human Nature explanation may not be complete. With an income of $3,000 US a year in 1958, it appears that many Japanese would have been at a level insufficient to meet all of their needs, and yet there has been virtually no increase in SWB since that time, despite huge economic growth.

The Japanese case points to a major problem with the livability approach—the difficulty in defining when human needs have been met, and the lack of measures to assess this. One might argue that human needs were met in Japan in 1958, even with a low income equivalent to 3,000 US current dollars, because of the structure of the society at that time. We do not, however, know whether this is true or not. The lack of a clear definition and measurement of human needs leaves this approach open to post-hoc explanations in which each case can be fit to the model after the fact. Thus, a much more rigorous set of definitions of need fulfillment, and measures of it, are needed if this approach is to be tested in a definitive way.

Relative Standards

Relative standards or judgment models are based on the idea that people use various standards to evaluate their well-being (Campbell, Converse, & Rodgers, 1976; Michalos, 1985; Parducci, 1995)—standards such as how they did in the past, how others are doing, and their goals. Standards can vary from time to time and person to person, depending on what happens to be salient for that individual. Thus, a person might be happy or unhappy with a particular level of standing in an area, depending on the level of others in this domain, or depending on how he or she stood in the past in this domain.

In evaluation theory Diener and Lucas (2000) hypothesized that the fulfillment of desires, especially those desires that are adopted as active goals for which the person is working, will be chronically salient standards for most people, and therefore are the most ubiquitous standard influencing SWB. There are both experimental and survey data indicating that the fulfillment or nonfulfillment of material desires is related to people's level of satisfaction. In two experimental studies and several survey studies, Crawford et al. (2000) demonstrated that people's ability to meet their material goals influenced both their life satisfaction and financial satisfaction. Further, they found that the influence of past income on SWB was mediated by its influence on material desires. The effects of social comparison were mediated partly by their influence on desires, although social comparison also had a direct effect on satisfaction. Finally, Crawford et al. found that people's satisfaction with hypothetical incomes could be experimentally manipulated, suggesting that meeting basic needs does not completely explain income satisfaction.

In terms of the data on income and SWB reviewed earlier, the lack of increase in SWB over time in economically developed societies can be explained by the rise in desires there, which seems to offset the benefits of more goods and services. Brant et al. (1999) found that the majority of US college students now believe they will be able to retire before age 50, and 77% believe that they will be millionaires. The UN Development Report (1998) shows that the income needed to fulfill consumption aspirations doubled in the USA between 1986 and 1994!

Van Praag (1993) has extensively studied what he calls the "welfare function," in which people describe the level of income that they would call "excellent," "adequate," "very bad," and so forth. Across many studies he finds that wealthier respondents have higher welfare functions; they require greater levels of money to call an income "sufficient." Van Praag and his colleagues calculate that up to 80% of the benefit of increasing income disappears because of the rising welfare function as income increases (Kapteyn, Praag, & van Herwaarden, 1976).

Easterlin (1999) found that the number of material aspirations increases as people age. People acquired more goods as they aged, but middle and older age groups grew further from their aspirations over time because their desires increased more rapidly than did their possessions! Furthermore, Douthitt et al. (1992) found in a daily diary study that those who spent more money relative to their incomes showed lower global satisfaction.

Schor (1998) reviews survey evidence on what Americans believe is included in the "good life." Between 1975 and 1991, the percent checking "vacation home" increased 84%. During the period from 1987 to 1994 the income needed to "fulfill all your dreams" increased from $50,000 US dollars to $102,000, much more than the rate of inflation. Of those earning more than $100,000 a year in 1995, 27% responded that they cannot afford to buy everything they "really need," and 19% reported that they spend nearly all of their money on "basic necessities."

There is little doubt that those in industrial nations want more than they possess. Sixty-one percent of respondents said they *always* have something in mind that they are looking forward to buying, and 27% said they very often dream about things they do not own (Schor, 1998). The average respondent had 6.3 items on his or her wish list; for example 47% wanted a bigger or better house. The amount of money reported in surveys needed to live in "reasonable comfort" has remained several thousand dollars above the median income level, even as the latter figure doubled over two decades. Thus, the chronic salience of desires combined with increasing material aspirations, explains why increases in income at both the individual and national levels have not enhanced SWB. It may be that well-off people around the world serve as models of consumption for others, even people in poorer nations. Thus, although wealth does bring rising desires, it might be that the want-possession gap is greatest for poor individuals in less developed societies. Although there are findings that indirectly support the Fulfillment of Desires explanation of the income-SWB relation, as with the Human Needs theory, there are few studies that directly test the theory. For example, almost never is there an assessment of what people desire and what they possess, in conjunction with measures of income and SWB.

The relative standards model based on desires suggests that wealthier nations and individuals are happier because they possess more of the goods that everyone throughout the world wants. However, this explanation has not been tested in a definitive way; we do not have proof, for instance, that people in wealthier nations possess a greater percentage of the goods that they desire. Furthermore, the reason that increases in income do not produce enhanced SWB—because desires also increase—has not been directly tested in longitudinal studies in which possessions, desires, and SWB are simultaneously measured. In other words, although the goal approach to well-being has promise, many aspects of it have not been directly tested.

Culture

The major idea behind the cultural approach is that people are socialized in a culture to have certain values, goals, and behaviors. Carrying out the behaviors that are valued within the culture is likely to lead to feelings of well-being because the person has adopted the cultural goals and experiences emotions socialized to the cultural norms. Thus, people in industrial nations are socialized to work at a paid job and to feel worthwhile for doing so. People see the acquisition of goods and money as a desirable activity that reflects how well they are carrying out the cultural imperative, and respond with pleasant emotions when they are successful at this imperative.

In this approach, people engaged in work and consumption are seen as likely to experience SWB because they are behaving in ways that the society values. Even people with very different incomes or status can see themselves as participating in valued and respected activities. A person who earns more, however, might be seen as more successful at carrying out the cultural dictates, and therefore on average might be likely to have somewhat higher SWB than someone who is poorer. Similarly, people in wealthy nations might feel more successful on average at being efficient producers and consumers of goods, and therefore report higher SWB. In this approach, it is not just having copious amounts of money that counts, it is being involved in a responsible way in the daily production and consumption activities of the culture. A person can gain pleasure from the activities of the culture. A person can gain pleasure from the activities of work, and also might obtain pleasure from the purchasing, consuming, and gift-giving that are part of market economies.

The cultural approach allows for additional differences between societies. For instance, some cultures stress competition, others focus on efficiency, and yet others emphasize the ability to save. In each of these cases, success is defined somewhat differently, and therefore there are likely to be differences in how money is related to SWB. Furthermore, in some cultures there is an emphasis on avoiding failure and in others there is an emphasis on seeking rewards (Diener et al., 1999), and these differences could lead to variation in how income is connected to SWB. In a culture oriented to avoiding failures, being poor might be especially difficult, whereas in a culture oriented to approach behavior, greater recognition may be given to wealthy individuals. Alesina, DiTella, & MacCulloch (2001) found that inequality of incomes had an effect on reports of happiness in Europe but not in the USA. They discovered that both poverty and political ideology moderated the effects of inequality, suggesting that social mobility and ideological beliefs could influence the way in which social comparisons of income influence SWB.

The culture approach explains why even most relatively poor individuals report high SWB—because most of them are involved in productive activities that are respected in their cultures. However, most studies show that unemployed people are substantially less happy than others (e.g., Clark, Diener, and Georgellis, 2000; Clark & Oswald, 1994; Frey & Stutzer, 2000), and this effect is apparent even when income is controlled. It appears that unemployed people on average would be dissatisfied even if they had a relatively high income—presumably because they are not doing a task that is respected in the culture. Similarly, very poor people have a difficult time participating in the consumption culture and therefore are more likely to experience low SWB. In contrast, elderly retired people are told that it is acceptable to not be working at this point in their lives, and therefore retirement does not on average harm SWB.

There are very few studies testing the Culture Model. For example, we do not have measures of how cultural norms influence the effects of work and money on SWB. There is evidence, however, that higher incomes may result from one's socialization. McClelland and Franz (1992) found that an emphasis on achievement during early socialization led to higher need for achievement, as well as higher later income. This finding points to the fact that making money can signify achievement in western society, and is not invariably driven by the desire for consumption.

People may feel good about work, with income being secondary. Juster (1985) and Dow and Juster (1985) found that working activities were preferred to eating out, shopping, watching movies and T.V., playing sports, household chores, and reading books. Csikszentmihalyi (1997) presents evidence that people prefer working to not working, and can obtain pleasure out of even mundane jobs. Thus, the enjoyment of material culture might actually be as much about the pleasures of production as it is about consumption. Certainly, work cannot just be counted as a cost to be endured for the sake of consumption. Virtually no studies have considered the pleasure derived from work when evaluating the income-SWB relation.

Comparing and Combining the Three Approaches

In terms of describing the preconditions for SWB, the three approaches differ dramatically. In the Human Nature approach having one's biological needs met, engagement in interesting activities, and the presence of social support are seen as necessary and sufficient for high SWB. Thus, the conditions seen as prerequisites for high SWB are universal, relatively few in number, highly specifiable, and fulfillable with modest resources. In contrast, the culture approach predicts that the prerequisites for SWB are variable, depending on learning histories that lead to very different values and goals. In addition, there is a stress on how individuals with different roles in a society may find different activities to be fulfilling. Finally, the relative standards approach allows for even greater variability, with the relevant standards varying across time and situations. In the culture and relative standards approaches, how resources and goals are judged is complex, and therefore the relation of money to happiness seems more difficult to predict than in the Human Nature approach.

The three models can be integrated to explain the relation between income and SWB. People in industrial society are socialized to work, and to enjoy participating in the consumption of the culture. Individuals who are successful at this cultural imperative are somewhat happier, but all people can to some degree take pleasure in the activity. Desires arise both from innate needs (the Human Nature approach) and from cultural goals; those who can make greater progress toward their desires will tend to be happier because goals are frequently a salient judgment standard. However, having higher income is not an infallible indicator of the number of desires that can be met because some individuals with high incomes can develop lofty material aspirations. In addition, the effects of income must be considered within the framework of other human needs—such as for close social relationships and interesting activities—and within the cultural context. For example, the pleasures that can be purchased with a high income can be offset if materialism leads to instability in people's lives, to loneliness and poor social relationships, or to long hours of work at a boring job. Conversely, low income might not detract from SWB in a stable society such as the Amish where material desires are restricted. As of yet, there are so many unknowns in the available data that this integrated conceptual account is speculative. The report of existing findings in the first half of this paper reveals that in past studies too few variables were measured to fully test the integrated conceptual model.

Reverse Order of Causation

One other explanation of the income-SWB relation mentioned earlier is that happy people and societies are more likely to earn higher incomes. Lyubomirsky et al. (2001) review the extensive evidence that happiness leads to success in various domains, including the financial area. For example, the longitudinal data reported by Diener et al. (2000) indicates that people who are high in life satisfaction later earn more income. These data are difficult to interpret in terms of income causing satisfaction because the life satisfaction measures were collected many years before, prior to the respondents entering the working world. However, the data on wind-fall income (Gardner & Oswald, 2001) also indicates that greater wealth can produce higher SWB, at least in the short-run. In addition, the deterioration of SWB in the former communist nations is also difficult to interpret as an effect of a happy disposition on income (Inglehart & Klingemann, 2000). In sum, the causal arrow between income and SWB appears to go in both directions, but the interactions between personality dispositions and income are poorly understood.

A Guide to Needed Research

Although there are intriguing findings about the relation of money to happiness, the extant research leaves many important questions unanswered. The needed research involves repeating existing studies with better measures of SWB and income, adding measures of possible mediating variables such as desires and beliefs, and discovering more about how income affects people's actual everyday lives. Existing research findings are often compatible with all of the theoretical accounts described above, and for this reason more probing research is needed. In the following section we discuss several of the methodological innovations needed to further our theoretical understanding of the area, as well as describe additional questions that need to be explored.

Methods

Measuring income better. Might it be that the low individual correlations reported earlier are due to weak measures of income? Current measures of income suffer from serious limitations as valid indicators of individuals' material well-being, whereas indicators of income at the societal level are likely to be somewhat more accurate. Thus, the aggregated measures at the national level, although not perfect, might result in strong correlations, whereas the more faulty measures at the individual level might be so fraught with error of measurement that the individual level correlations are necessarily low.

There is misreporting of income, both deliberate and unintentional, as well as varying definitions of income across studies. Errors of memory also occur. For example, Herriott (1977) found that people report more income when it is broken into finer categories than they do when only a global report is requested, suggesting that certain income is not recalled when global income measures are employed. Furthermore, income measures are likely to be only modestly correlated with material well-being. Besides income, the material goods and services available to people also depend on their taxes, their savings, the availability of subsidized goods, the goods they already own (including housing), prices in their locale, their spending efficiency, the number of individuals in the household, gifts from relatives, and so forth. Mayer (1997) reported that annual consumption is more evenly distributed than annual income, in part because some people are only temporarily poor and because many have unreported income. It is noteworthy that Mullis (1992) found that current earnings correlated only 0.32 with a composite financial indicator (including long-term income and net worth), and that net worth and long-term income each made an independent contribution to the prediction of happiness beyond earned income.

The societal trend toward more women working at paid jobs reveals the problem of using earned income as the only measure of material welfare. Women on average in recent decades are working much more at paid jobs, and this work enters the national accounting system and increases the national GDP per person, as well as reports of household income. If families then eat out more, hire a house cleaner, send their children to daycare, and so forth, the payments for these services enter into the national accounts. Had the woman stayed home and worked full time as a homemaker, as was much more frequent in former days, however, none of her home services would have been counted toward national income, although her home production was likely to have been substantial. The woman's home production might have even surpassed the services now purchased in the marketplace. Thus, the increased family income (which will be taxed) due to a second wage earner in the family is likely to substantially overstate the rise in material standards of the family (Mayer, 1997). Similarly, retired people may have lower reported income than formerly, and yet retain much the same standard of living (George, 1992) because they own their home and car, have fewer debts, have no children to educate, have greater savings on which to rely, and pay fewer taxes on their retirement pensions. Thus, older adults can often experience the same material quality of life with less reportable income.

Because of the numerous limitations in the material well-being measures employed in SWB surveys, a necessary course for future study is determining how various types of measures improve the prediction of SWB. We need measures of the ownership, use, and consumption of goods and services, not just income. We need measures of the ownership, use, and consumption of goods and services that people produce for themselves or obtain through trade. Certainly, we need income measures that are calibrated for factors such as family size, regional cost of living, governmental services, and expenditures for the basic necessities such as health and food. In effect, we need measures of material quality of life, not just income per se.

Another important issue is how people spend their incomes. Some people buy luxury goods, whereas others give substantial amounts to charity; certainly it is plausible that income used in different ways might differentially influence SWB, and we need measures reflecting different patterns of saving and consumption. Finally, we must understand whether the means by which money is obtained (e.g., through luck, inheritance, investments, or wages) influences the effects it has on SWB. Thus, simple measures of a respondent's wages or household income, even when calibrated for household size, must be augmented with more detailed questions about his or her standard of living if we are to fully understand the relation of material welfare and SWB.

Measuring subjective well-being better. Just as the income measures have limitations, the SWB measures can also be improved. The large survey studies in which much SWB research is usually embedded have given us large and broadly representative samples, but are based on somewhat superficial measures. When a respondent indicates whether she is "very happy," "pretty happy," or "not so happy," much about her subjective experience of well-being is missed. Initial research work indicates that the global measures do have a degree of validity, correlating at moderate levels with other indicants of SWB such as informant reports, experience sampling measures, and interviewer ratings (Sandvik, Diener, & Seidlitz, 1993). With the current measures, however, we have little idea *when* rich and poor people feel happy and unhappy, satisfied and dissatisfied, and *why*. Furthermore, the global measures have clear shortcomings. Schwarz, Strack and their colleagues (e.g., 1999) showed in a series of important studies that chance situational factors can influence global reports of life satisfaction. Not only do the Strack and Schwarz studies reveal that there can be substantial random error in the global survey measures used in this field, but they also indicate that variables such as a person's circumstances in the past can have either positive *or* negative effects on reports of SWB, depending on how the question is framed. Because many of the situational factors affecting global reports of well-being may vary somewhat haphazardly across surveys (e.g., the weather and current events at the time of the survey), random error might be reducing relation between income and SWB. Thus, additional measurement methods are required in addition to cross-sectional surveys.

A promising approach is to use experience sampling to measure SWB across income groups. In the experience sampling method, researchers obtain mood and satisfaction reports from respondents at random times in everyday life, often for a period of one or two weeks. In this way, we hope to obtain a more accurate representation of people's feelings, which is not influenced by memory biases and scaling artifacts. In addition, we can obtain reports of how people spend their time, and how various activities contribute to SWB.

There is evidence that the experience sampling method will not produce the exact same conclusions as the global survey method that has dominated the field. Existing research has demonstrated discrepancies in the findings of the two methods. For example, Oishi and Diener (2000) showed in a series of studies that Asian-Americans have similar emotional experiences "on-line" (recorded at the moment) to European-American respondents, but that European Americans recall being happier and more satisfied in retrospective global measures. Mitchell, Thompson, Peterson, and Cronk (1997) found that people recalled their vacations as being better than was reported during the vacation, presumably because people have a belief that vacations are fun and this belief distorted their recall. Wirtz, Scollon, Kruger, and Diener (2001) found that the moods of spring break were misremembered by college student participants, but that the misrecalled moods were a better prediction of choosing to repeat the vacation than were actual online moods. There is also evidence indicating that global measures of well-being compared to more specific measures can be influenced by temperament (e.g., happy people weight good circumstances more, and weight bad factors less in global reports, Diener, Lucas, Oishi, & Suh, 2002) and by people's norms about whether they believe it is good to be satisfied (Diener et al., 2000). Diener et al. found that global reports show systematic discrepancies from more specific satisfaction reports and these discrepancies appear to stem from a global positivity disposition. Thus, poor and wealthy people's memories of their happiness may or may not accord well with their actual on-line hedonic experiences. It could be that global reports of satisfaction are influenced by people's expectations of how happy they think they should be, and do not faithfully reproduce on-line feelings of pleasure versus displeasure (Kahneman, 1999).

The one study in which on-line recordings of mood were related to socioeconomic status did *not* find a large positive influence of income on SWB. Csikszentmihalyi and Schneider (2000) report SWB data based on experience sampling of 849 adolescents several times a day for a week in each of three consecutive years (over 33 responses on average per respondent). They found a small but significantly *decreasing* trend in happiness across respondents in higher SES communities: poor, 5.4; lower middle-class, 5.4; middle-class, 5.3; upper middle-class,

4.8; and upper-class, 5.2 (on a 1–7 scale). Although this declining trend is not large, it indicates that even with sophisticated experience sampling data we might not find large positive effects of money on happiness. Indeed, these data suggest that there may be high expectations for achievement, or relationship difficulties, that can make wealthier youth less happy than other adolescents.

Despite the fact that the initial experience sampling study in which socioeconomic status was related to SWB did not show a positive effect of money, this does not indicate that different conclusions might be reached when experience sampling measures are used with working adults. Not only might the experience sampling measures lead to different conclusions compared to the global survey scales, but they should reveal more intricate patterns of how income influences behavior and affect. In addition, we should supplement the experience sampling method with biological indicators of well-being (e.g., measures of cortisol and eye-blink response). One of the hopes, albeit untested, is that the biological and experience-sampling measures might reveal whether the differences between rich and poor are larger at the level of momentary experience than they are in global reports, because people adjust their scale responses to the global reports to fit their situation (Kahneman, 1999). By finding out when wealthy and impoverished people are feeling pleasant versus unpleasant emotions, we should gain a firmer understanding of the effects of income. In addition to experience sampling, the global surveys should be supplemented with biological measures (e.g., cortisol), memory recall for good and bad life events, qualitative measures, and reports by informants.

Longitudinal research. One of the advantages of experience sampling is that the researcher gains measures over time, and therefore can examine the time-sequencing of variables. When more global measures are employed, it would be very helpful if they were also used much more often in panel designs that longitudinally span a period of time. The cross-sectional survey studies that rule the field leave open questions of causal direction and mediating processes. The few published longitudinal studies provide stronger conclusions than the cross-sectional studies, and thus the addition of sampling over time is a research imperative for the future.

Measures of mediating processes. A difficulty with making theoretical conclusions in this field is that the data are so sparse in terms of measures of psychological processes and behavior. Thus, we have correlations of income and SWB, but are left guessing as to the mediating psychological processes. For instance, we can make conjectures about rising aspirations, but measures of desires must be included in the studies, and their effects ascertained, in order to test these ideas. Similarly, we can make conjectures about the social relationships, fulfillment of needs, time pressures, stressors, social comparisons, and daily behaviors of the rich and poor, to explain the existing patterns of data, but we very much need measures of these putative intervening variables. If these possible mediating variables are measured over time, we will be in a much stronger position to create meaningful theoretical models.

In the above section we outline the research methods needed to make progress in developing adequate psychological theories in this area. In the following section we outline several important questions that need to be answered.

Why are People in Richer Nations Happier?

A question that is central to policy considerations is why individuals in wealthy nations report higher SWB than people in poorer nations. This question bears directly on the issue of the extent to which governments should continue to aggressively pursue policies to stimulate economic growth. Equality, education, literacy, longevity, human rights, and subjective well-being are higher in wealthier nations (E. Diener, & C. Diener, 1995a), but which direction does the causal arrow point between income and these variables? Does wealth cause these other valuable characteristics or is it a result of democracy and SWB? Policy makers can, to varying degrees, temper economic aims with other values (e.g., environmental or equality goals), and therefore the question of why wealthy nations are happier is a central one relevant to creating economic policies.

One possibility for explaining the higher SWB of wealthier nations is that they set the standard for material fulfillment. Thus, wealthy nations exhibit a lifestyle that is desired in poorer nations, but that is only achieved in wealthier ones. If so, it might be that people in wealthier countries are happier because they are closer to the standard to which people throughout the world aspire. It is also possible, however, that affluence has little or nothing to do with the high SWB in wealthy nations. It might be that the wealthier nations had more stability, greater democracy, freedoms, human rights, equality, and a culture emphasizing approach behavior, and these variables led to both greater happiness and higher incomes. Political stability and security in particular may have caused more productive economies and higher SWB, without any direct influence of money on happiness. If it were the case that political stability and so forth produced both happiness and higher incomes in the wealthy nations, economic development would not be so clearly necessary in terms of producing higher levels of SWB. Research on economically developing nations, especially those with political stability and so forth, but less economic growth, will shed light on this issue.

Why Do People Want More Money?

An increase in income among well-off people in wealthier nations appears not to substantially enhance happiness, at least as assessed with existing measures. Within most economically developed nations richer people are only slightly happier than most others. Why do people desire a higher income if it will not make them much happier? One possible reason is that people do not realize that money will not raise their SWB. Because money is such a central topic of concern in modern society, scripts and beliefs attaching it to happiness may be firmly entrenched in our belief network, regardless of our actual experiences. This reason is to some extent, however, cast in doubt by the fact that most people claim that money is not that important in their hierarchy of values (e.g., Diener & Oishi, 2000), thus suggesting that they know money is not crucial to their happiness. Nonetheless, it could be that people believe more money will make them happier, but do not readily admit this in surveys. A related hypothesis is that people feel good working for the goal of higher income, regardless of whether attaining a high income is ever reached.

Another reason that people may seek money is that it produces short-term spurts in positive affect even if it does not enhance people's long-term levels of well-being. In other words, people may be reinforced for earning and spending money by positive emotional feelings, regardless of whether these feelings continue for long periods. Yet another factor may be that people may feel a need to acquire money, goods, and services because of societal pressure. That is, individuals may feel that they must buy cars and so forth to gain status and good standing in the community, and to not be perceived as failures.

Conclusions

In the title of this review we raise the question of whether money will make us happy. What can we conclude? It appears that a higher income might help if we are very poor. Living in a wealthy society appears to be beneficial. On the other hand, strongly desiring large amounts of money appears likely to hinder our chances for high SWB. Gaining more income if we are middle-class or upper-class and are living in a wealthy nation is unlikely to substantially bolster our SWB on a long-term basis. Thus: our advice is to avoid poverty, live in a rich country, and focus on goals other than material wealth. What of individuals then, who reside in poor nations or who live in rich nations but remain poor despite their efforts? To these individuals we owe public policies, as well as private initiatives, to enhance their incomes in a time when the material wealth of the world is growing at a rapid pace.

A fundamental finding of the present review is that for middle-and upper-income people in economically developed nations, acquiring more income is not likely to strongly enhance SWB. Indeed, some studies find that rising wages predict less well-being. For example it has been found that rising income led to higher divorce rates (Clydesdale, 1997), greater stress (Thoits & Hannan, 1979), lower global well-being (Diener et al., 1993), and less enjoyment of small activities (Brickman et al., 1978). It thus appears that some reorientation is needed in material goals, from acquiring money to enjoying the process of work and contributing to society. People should understand that placing great emphasis on the acquisition of wealth can be counterproductive to happiness, and that gaining increased income has dangers as well as pleasures. As the world enters a new era of material abundance, a new paradigm is needed in which greater emphasis is placed on fulfilling vocations that benefit society, and on preventing the involuntary poverty that is associated with a higher risk of unhappiness.

References

Adelmann, P. K. (1987). Occupational complexity, control, and personal income: Their relation to psychological well-being in men and women. *Journal of Applied Psychology, 72,* 529–537.

Ahuvia, A. C., & Wong, N. Y. (2002). Personality and values based materialism: Their relationship and origins. *Journal of Consumer Psychology, 12,* 389–402.

Ahuvia, A. C., & Wong, N. (2001). *Cognitive and affective antecedents of materialism: Implications for the development of materialism as a political orientation.* Unpublished Manuscript.

Aldwin, C. M., & Revenson, T. A. (1986). Vulnerability to economic stress. *American Journal of Community Psychology, 14,* 161–175.

Alesina, A., DiTella, R. & MacCulloch, R. (2001). *Inequality and happiness: Are Europeans and Americans different?* Manuscript submitted for publication, Harvard University.

Andrews, F. M., & Withey, S. B. (1976). *Social indicators of well-being: America's perception of life quality.* New York: Plenum Press.

Aristotle. (1969). *The Nichomachean Ethics.* (R. Williams, Trans.). Green, London: Longmans.

Biswas-Diener, R., & Diener, E. (2001). Making the best of a bad situation: Satisfaction in the slums of Calcutta. *Social Indicators Research, 55,* 329–352.

Black, D. (1976). The behavior of law New York: Academic Press.

Blanchflower, D. G., and Oswald, A. J. (1999). *Well-being over Time in Britain and the USA.* (NBER Working Papers 7487). National Bureau of Economic Research, INC.

Blanchflower, D. G., Oswald, A. J., & Warr, P. B. (1993). *Well-being over time in Britain and the USA.* Paper presented at the CEP Conference on the Economics and Psychology of Happiness and Fairness.

Bowen, W. G., & Bok, D. C. (1998). *The shape of the river: Long-term consequences of considering race in college and university admissions.* Princeton, NJ: Princeton University Press.

Bradburn, N. M. (1969). *The structure of psychological well-being.* Chicago: Aldine.

Brant, M., Stone, B., Joseph, N., Gegax, T. T., Underwood, A., Arora, A., & Davis, A. (1999, July 5). They're rich and you're not. *Newsweek, 134,* 36–43.

Brinkerhoff, M. B., Fredell, K. A., & Frideres, J. S. (1997). Basic minimum needs, quality of life and selected correlates: Exploration in villages in northern India. *Social Indicators Research, 42,* 245–281.

Brickman, P., Coates, D., & Janoff-Bulman, R. (1978). Lottery winners and accident victims: Is happiness relative? *Journal of Personality and Social Psychology, 36,* 917–927.

Campbell, A. (1981). *The sense of well-being in America.* New York: McGraw-Hill.

Campbell, A., Converse, P. E., & Rodgers, W. L. (1976). *The quality of American life.* New York: Russell Sage.

Clark, A. (1999). Are wages habit forming? Evidence from micro data. *Journal of Economic Behavior and Organization, 39,* 179–200.

Clark, A., Diener, E., & Georgellis, Y. (2000, July). *Lags and leads in life satisfaction: A test of the baseline hypothesis.* Paper presented at the German Socio-Economic Panel Conference 2000, Berlin.

Clark, A. E., & Oswald, A. J. (1994). Unhappiness and unemployment. *Economic Journal, 104,* 648–659.

Clark, A. E., & Oswald, A. J. (1996). Satisfaction and comparison income. *Journal of Public Economics, 61,* 359–381.

Clydesdale, T. T. (1997). Family behaviors among early U.S. baby boomers: Exploring the effects of religion and income change, 1965–1982. *Social Forces, 76,* 605–635.

Connor, K., Dorfman, L., & Tompkins, J. (1985). Life satisfaction of retired professors: the contribution of work, health, income, and length of retirement. *Educational Gerontology, 11,* 337–347.

Crawford, E., Diener, E., Oishi, S., & Wirtz, S. (2000). *Desires as a standard explaining income satisfaction.* Manuscript submitted for publication, University of Illinois.

Csikszentmihalyi, M. (1997). *Finding flow.* New York: Basic Books.

Csikszentmihalyi, M., & Schneider, B. (2000). *Becoming adults: How Teenagers prepare for work.* New York: Basic Books.

Deci, E. L., & Ryan, R. M. (1980). Self-determination theory: When mind mediates behavior. *Journal of Mind and Behavior, 1,* 33–43.

Diener, E. (1984). Subjective well-being. *Psychological Bulletin, 95*, 542–575.

Diener, E., & Biswas-Diener, R. (2000). New directions in subjective well-being research: The cutting edge. *Indian Journal of Clinical Psychology, 27*, 21–33.

Diener, E., & Diener, C. (1995a). The wealth of nations revisited: Income and quality of life. *Social Indicators Research, 36*, 275–286.

Diener, E., & Diener, C. (1996). Most people are happy. *Psychological Science, 7*, 181–185.

Diener, E., & Diener, M. (1995b). Cross cultural correlates of life satisfaction and self-esteem. *Journal of Personality and Social Psychology, 68*, 653–663.

Diener, E., Diener, M., & Diener, C. (1995). Factors predicting the subjective well-being of nations. *Journal of Personality and Social Psychology, 69*, 851–864.

Diener, E., Horwitz, J., & Emmons, R. A. (1985). Happiness of the very wealthy. *Social Indicators Research, 16*, 263–274.

Diener, E., & Lucas, R. E. (2000). Explaining differences in societal levels of happiness: Relative standards, need fulfillment, culture, and evaluation theory. *Journal of Happiness Studies, 1*, 41–78.

Diener, E., Nickerson, C., Lucas, R. E., & Sandvik, E. (2000). *Do happy people earn more money? The causal relation of income and subjective well-being*. Manuscript submitted for publication, University of Illinois.

Diener, E., & Oishi, S. (2000). Money and happiness: Income and subjective well-being across nations. In E. Diener & E. M. Suh (Eds.), *Subjective well-being across cultures*. Cambridge, MA: MIT Press.

Diener, E., Lucas, R. E., Oishi, S., & Suh, E. M. (2002). Looking up and looking down: Weighting good and bad information in life satisfaction judgments. *Personality and Social Psychology Bulletin, 28*, 437–445.

Diener, E., Sandvik, E., Seidlitz, L., & Diener, M. (1993). The relationship between income and subjective well-being: Relative or absolute? *Social Indicators Research, 28*, 195–223.

Diener, E., Scollon, C., Oishi, S., Dzokoto, V., & Suh, E. M. (2000). Positivity and the construction of life satisfaction judgments: Global happiness is not the sum of its parts. *Journal of Happiness Studies, 1*, 159–176.

Diener, E., Suh, E. M., Lucas, R. E., & Smith, H. L. (1999). Subjective well-being: Three decades of progress. *Psychological Bulletin, 125*, 276–302.

Dittmar, H. (1992). Perceived material wealth and first impressions. *British Journal of Social Psychology, 31*, 379–391.

Douthitt, R. A., MacDonald, M., & Mullis, R. (1992). The relationship between measures of subjective and economic well-being: A new look. *Social Indicators Research, 26*, 407–422.

Dow, G. K., & Juster, F. T. (1985). Goods, time, and well-being: The joint dependence problem. In F. T. Juster & F. P. Stafford (Eds.), *Time, goods, and well-being*. Ann Arbor, MI: Institute for Social Research.

Easterlin, R. A. (1996). *Growth triumphant: The twenty-first century in historical perspective*. Ann Arbor: University of Michigan Press.

Easterlin, R. A. (1999). *Life cycle welfare: Evidence and conjecture*. Unpublished paper, University of Southern California.

Frey, B. S., & Stutzer, A. (2000). Happiness, economy and institutions. *The Economic Journal, 110*, 918–938.

Furnham, A., & Argyle, M., (1998). *The psychology of money*. London: Routledge.

Gardner, J., & Oswald, A. (2001). *Does money buy happiness? A longitudinal study using data on windfalls*. Manuscript submitted for publication.

George, L. K. (1992). Economic status and subjective well-being: A review of the literature and an agenda for future research. In N. E. Cutler, D. W. Gregg, & M. P. Lawton (Eds.), *Aging, money, and life satisfaction: Aspects of financial gerontology*. New York: Springer.

Hagerty, M. R. (2000). Social comparisons of income in one's community: Evidence from national surveys of income and happiness. *Journal of Personality and Social Psychology, 78*, 764–771.

152   E. Diener and R. Biswas-Diener

Hagerty, M. R., and Veenhoven, R. (1999). *Wealth and happiness revisited: Growing wealth of nations does go with greater happiness.* Unpublished manuscript, University of California, Davis.

Hamermesh, D. S. (2001). The changing distribution of job satisfaction. *The Journal of Human Resources, 36,* 1–30.

Headey, B., & Wearing, A. (1992). *Understanding happiness: A theory of subjective well-being.* Melbourne, VIC: Longman Cheshire.

Herriott, R. A. (1977). Collecting income data on sample surveys: Evidence from split-panel studies. *Journal of Marketing Research, 14,* 322–329.

Inglehart, R., and Klingemann, H. D. (2000). Genes, culture, and happiness. In E. Diener & E. M. Suh (Eds.), *Subjective well-being across cultures.* Cambridge, MA: MIT Press.

Inglehart, R., & Rabier, J. R. (1986). Aspirations adapt to situations – But why are the Belgians so much happier than the French? A cross-cultural analysis of the subjective quality of life. In F. M. Andrews (Ed.), *Research on quality of life.* Ann Arbor, MI: Survey Research Center.

Inkeles, A., & Diamond, L. (1980). Personal development and national development: A cross-national perspective. In A. Szalai & F. M. Andrews (Eds.), *The quality of life: Comparative studies.* Beverly Hills, CA: Sage.

Juster, F. T. (1985). Preferences for work and leisure. In F. T. Juster & F. P. *Stafford (Eds.), Time, goods, and well-being.* Ann Arbor, MI: Institute for Social Research.

Kahneman, D. (1999). Objective happiness. In D. Kahneman, E. Diener & N. Schwarz (Eds.), *Well-being: The foundations of hedonic psychology.* (pp. 3–25). New York: Russell Sage Foundation.

Kahneman, D., & Tversky, A. (1984). Choices, values, and frames. *American Psychologist, 39,* 341–350.

Kapteyn, A., Praag, B. M. S., & van Herwaarden, F. G. (1976). Individual welfare functions and social reference spaces. *Economic Letters, 1,* 173–178.

Kasser, T., & Ryan, R. M. (1993). A dark side of the American Dream: Correlates of financial success as a central life aspiration. *Journal of Personality and Social Psychology, 65,* 410–422.

Keith, P. M. (1985). Financial well-being of older divorced/separated men and women: Findings from a panel study. *Journal of Divorce, 9,* 61–72.

Keith, P. M., & Schafer, R. B. (1982). A comparison of depression among employed single-parent and married women. *Journal of Psychology, 110,* 239–247.

Lachman, M. E., & Weaver, S. L. (1998). The sense of control as a moderator of social class differences in health and well-being. *Journal of Personality and Social Psychology, 74,* 763–773.

Lane, R. E. (1991). *The market experience.* Cambridge, UK: Cambridge University Press.

Langner, T. S., & Michael, S. T. (1963). *Life stress and mental health.* New York: Free Press.

Liker, J. K., & Elder, G. H. (1983). Economic hardship and marital relations in the 1930's. *American Sociological Review, 48,* 343–359.

Lyubomirsky, S., Tucker, K.L., & Kasri, F. (2001). Responses to hedonically conflicting social comparisons: Comparing happy and unhappy people. *European Journal of Social Psychology, 31,* 511–535.

Marks, G. N., & Fleming, N. (1999). Influences and consequences of well-being among Australian young people: 1980–1995. *Social Indicators Research, 46,* 301–323.

Mayer, S. E. (1997). Indicators of children's economic well-being and parental employment. In R. M. Hauser, B. V. Brown, & W. R. Prosser (Eds.), *Indicators of children's well-being.* New York: Russell Sage Foundation.

Mayer, S. E. (1997). *What money can't buy: Family income and children's life chances.* Cambridge, MA: Harvard University Press.

McClelland, D. C., & Franz, C. E. (1992). Motivational and other sources of work accomplishments in mid-life: A longitudinal study. *Journal of Personality, 60,* 679–707.

Michalos, A. C. (1985). Multiple discrepancies theory (MDT). *Social Indicators Research, 16,* 347–413.

Mitchell, T. R., Thompson, L., Peterson E., & Cronk, R. (1997). Temporal adjustments in the evaluations of events: The "rosy view". *Journal of Experimental Social Psychology, 33,* 421–448.

Mullis, R. J. (1992). Measures of economic well-being as predictors of psychological well-being. *Social Indicators Research, 26*, 119–135.

Nakosteen, R. A., & Zimmer, M. A. (1997). Men, money, and marriage: Are high earners more prone than low earners to marry? *Social Service Quarterly, 78*, 66–82.

Nickerson, C., Schwartz, N., Kahneman, D., & Diener, E. (2001). *The American dream: The dark side is in the wish, not the realization.* Manuscript submitted for publication.

Oishi, S., & Diener, E. (2000). *Remembering versus experiencing well-being: The case of Asian-Americans and European-Americans.* Manuscript in preparation, University of Illinois.

Oswald, A. J. (1997). Happiness and economic performance. *The Economic Journal, 107*, 1815–1831.

Ouweneel, P., & Veenhoven, R. (1991). Cross-national differences in happiness: Cultural bias or societal quality. In N. Bleichrodt & P. J. Drenth (Eds.), *Contemporary issues in cross-cultural psychology.* Amsterdam: Swets & Zeitlinger.

Pamuk, E., Makuc, D., Heck, K., Reuben, C., & Lochner, K. (1998). *Socioeconomic status and health chartbook: Health, United States, 1998.* Hyattsville, MD: National Center for Health Statistics.

Parducci, A. (1995). *Happiness, pleasure, and judgment: The contextual theory and its applications.* Mahwah, NJ: Erlbaum.

Pearlin, L. I., & Johnson, J. S. (1977). Marital status, life strains and depressions. *American Sociological Review, 42*, 704–715.

Richins, M. L., & Dawson, S. (1992). A consumer values orientation for materialism and its measurement: Scale development and validation. *Journal of Consumer Research, 19*, 303–316.

Rosenberg, M., & Pearlin, L. E. (1978). Social class and self-esteem among children and adults. *American Journal of Sociology, 84*, 54–58.

Ross, C. E., & Huber, J. (1985). Hardship and depression. *Journal of Health and Social Behavior, 26*, 312–327.

Sandvik, E., Diener, E., & Seidlitz, L. (1993). Subjective well-being: The convergence and stability of self-report and non-self report measures. *Journal of Personality, 64*, 319–341.

Saris, W. E. (2001). The relationship between income and satisfaction: The effect of measurement error and suppressor variables. *Social Indicators Research, 53*, 117–136.

Schor, J. B. (1998). *The overspent American.* New York: Basic Books.

Schwartz, B. (1994). *The costs of living: How market freedom erodes the best things in life.* New York: W.W. Norton.

Schwarz, N., & Strack, F. (1999). Reports of subjective well-being: Judgmental processes and their methodological implications. In D. Kahneman, E. Diener & N. Schwarz (Eds.), *Well-being: The foundations of hedonic psychology* (pp. 61–84). New York: Russell Sage Foundation.

Schyns, P. (1998a, December 3–6). *Nation wealth, individual income and life-satisfaction in 42 countries: A multilevel approach.* Paper presented at the Second Annual ISQOLS conference, Williamsburg, VA.

Schyns, P. (1998b, July 26–August 1). *The relationship between wealth of countries, individual income and life-satisfaction: A multilevel approach.* Paper presented at ISAXIV World Congress of Sociology, Montreal, Canada.

Schyns, P. (2000). The relationship between income, changes in income and life satisfaction in West Germany and the Russian Fedration: Relative, absolute, or a combination of both? In E. Diener & D. R. Rahtz (Eds.), *Advances in quality of life theory and research* (Vol 1, pp. 83–109). Dordrecht, Netherlands: Kluwer.

Schyns, P. (2001). Income and satisfaction in Russia. *Journal of Happiness Studies, 2*, 173–204.

Sirgy, M. J. (1997). Materialism and quality of life. *Social Indicators Research, 43*, 227–260.

Smith, J. R., Brooks-Gunn, J., & Jackson, A. (1997). Parental employment and children. In R. M. Hauser, B. V. Brown, & W. R. Prosser (Eds.), *Indicators of children's well-being.* New York: Russell Sage Foundation.

Srivastave, A., Locke, E. A., & Bartol, K. M. (2001). Money and subjective well-being: It's not the money, it's the motives. *Journal of Personality and Social Psychology, 80*, 959–971.

Smith, S., & Razzell, P. (1975). *The pools' winners*. London: Calibon Books.

Suh, E. M., Diener, E., Oishi, S., & Triandis, H. (1998). The shifting basis of life satisfaction judgments across cultures: Emotions versus norms. *Journal of Personality and Social Psychology, 74*, 482–493.

Summers, R., & Heston, A. (1991). Penn World Table (Mark 5): An expanded set of international comparisons, 1950–1988. *Quarterly Journal of Economics, 106*, 327–368.

Tepleton, J. M. (1999). A worldwide rise in living standards. *The Futurist 33*, 17–22.

Thoits, P., & Hannan, M. (1979). Income and psychological distress: The impact of an income-maintenance experiment. *Journal of Health and Social Behavior 20*, 120–138.

Tomes, N. (1986). Income distribution, happiness, and satisfaction: A direct test of the interdependent preferences model. *Journal of Economic Psychology 7*, 425–446.

Van Praag, B. M. S. (1993). The relativity of the welfare concept. In M. Nussbaum & A. Sen (Eds.), *The quality of life*. Oxford: Clarendon.

Veenhoven, R. (1991). Is happiness relative? *Social Indicators Research, 24*, 1–34.

Veenhoven, R. (1993). *Happiness in nations: Subjective appreciation of life in 55 nations* 1996–1990. Rotterdam: RISBO.

Veenhoven, R. (1995). The cross-national pattern of happiness: Test of predictions implied in three theories of happiness. *Social Indicators Research, 34*, 33–68.

United Nations Development Programme. (1998). *Human development report – 1998*. New York: Oxford University Press.

Wheaton, B. (1994). Sampling the stress universe. In W. R. Avison & I. H. Gotlib (Eds.), *Stress and mental health* (pp. 77–114). New York: Plenum Press.

Wilkinson, R. G. (1996). *Unhealthy societies: The afflictions of inequality*. London: Routledge.

Wilson, J. B., Ellwood, D. T., & Brooks-Gunn, J. (1995). Welfare-to-work through the eyes of children. In P. L. Chase-Lansdale & J. Brooks-Gunn (Eds.), *Escape from poverty*. New York: Cambridge University Press.

Wirtz, D., Scollon, C., Kruger, J. & Diener, E. (2001). *Selecting a spring break: Online versus recalled mood of the last one*. Manuscript submitted for publication, University of Illinois.

World Value Survey Group. (1994). *World values survey, 1981–1984 and 1990–1993*. Ann Arbor, MI: Institute for Social Research, ICPSR.

The Well-Being of Nations: Linking Together Trust, Cooperation, and Democracy

William Tov and Ed Diener

Abstract The theme of this chapter is that cooperative and trusting social relationships tend to enhance people's subjective well-being (happiness and life
satisfaction), and that in turn positive feelings of well-being tend to augment cooperation and trust. Extensive empirical work now supports the fact that sociability,
interpersonal warmth, community involvement, and interpersonal trust are heightened by positive emotions. New analyses based on the World Value Survey show
that nations that are high on subjective well-being (SWB) also tend to be high on
generalized trust, volunteerism, and democratic attitudes. Additional analyses indicate that the association of SWB to volunteerism and democratic attitudes is not
fully accounted for by GDP per capita, freedom, or filial piety. The implications of
SWB for promoting greater cooperation and trust within society and across nations
is considered.

In his book, *Nonzero*, Robert Wright (2000) argues that the basic direction of human
history is towards greater social and technological complexity and an increasing
realization that all people are linked in a fundamental web of interdependence. That
is, across every province and nation, the fact remains that we all live in the same
world, navigating the course of humanity in the same proverbial boat. This basic fact
of interdependence comes with an important implication: that the ultimate survival
of all societies rests on finding solutions to social, political, and economic issues
that are *non-zero-sum*.

In game theory, a zero-sum approach is one in which winning comes at the ex-
pense of others. In contrast, a non-zero-sum solution is one in which all parties gain
something so that everyone is better off than before. For example, in the *tragedy
of the commons*, a public resource is only sustainable to the extent that everyone
uses it responsibly. If several individuals exploit too much of the resource for their
own benefit, it is lost and *everyone* suffers. If individuals take only what they need,
the resource is replenishable and in the long run, everyone benefits. Non-zero-sum

W. Tov (✉)
Department of Psychology, University of Illinois, Urbana-Champaign,
Champaign, IL 61820, USA
e-mail: williamtov@smu.edu.sg

E. Diener (ed.), *The Science of Well-Being: The Collected Works of Ed Diener*, Social
Indicators Research Series 37, DOI 10.1007/978-90-481-2350-6_7,
© Springer Science+Business Media B.V. 2009

solutions call for cooperation and trust among all parties. To preserve the resource for future use, people must be cooperative in fulfilling their needs. At the same time, in order to curb the impulse to hoard, individuals must trust that others will not hoard for themselves. The benefits are not only material resources as implied by the tragedy of the commons; there are also consequences for the happiness and contentment of individuals and entire communities. Wright's central thesis is that long-term *global* well-being depends heavily on cooperation and trust at the supra-national level. There is a utilitarian ethic that undergirds the appeal of non-zero-sumness. That is, by regulating impulsive self-interest, the happiness of all people can be maximized. Although scholars debate how well people are able to follow this principle, the logic is intuitive: a society in which people can trust and cooperate with each other is likely to be happier and more productive than a society paralyzed by rampant distrust and fear. The implication is that trust and cooperation provide the conditions for subjective well-being. Slightly less intuitive is the possibility that happiness causes and facilitates interpersonal trust and cooperation. In this chapter, we argue that subjective well-being both influences and is influenced by cooperation and trust. This bi-directional relationship is supported by empirical research. After reviewing this literature, we explore the association between national levels of subjective well-being and cooperation in our analyses of the World Values Survey. First, we briefly discuss the concepts of cooperation, trust, and subjective well-being.

Cooperation and Trust

Cooperation involves working together toward a common goal. As we discuss later, cooperation is not necessarily opposed to competition. In competitive contexts such as sports, the interaction between competing teams requires that everyone observe the rules governing fair play. Thus, cooperation and competition can function together in a single activity. As Wright (2000) notes, zero-sumness on one level can even foster non-zero-sumness on another level. Competition between teams necessitates cooperation among members *within* a team. Cooperation is not inherently good or bad; people can work together to accomplish harmful, anti-social acts. However, any well-functioning society requires cooperation among its citizens.

What sort of factors facilitate cooperation in society? How do people decide to cooperate with others—especially those they do not know well? Wright (2000) points to two critical factors: communication and trust. Communication enables people to reach an understanding of common goals and an agreed upon means of attaining those goals. Trust provides people with assurance that their cooperation will not be exploited. Both communication and trust are more likely in enduring social relationships so that people are more likely to trust and cooperate with close friends and relatives than a stranger. Putnam (2000) draws a distinction between the *thick* trust that exists among close associates, and the *thin* trust that may be felt for most people in general. He argues that greater community involvement can increase social capital, thereby fostering trust in one's fellow citizens. However, there are two forms of social capital that Putnam (2000) refers to as *bonding* and *bridging*.

Bonding social capital refers to exclusive forms of relationships such as when people associate with each other to reinforce shared identities (e.g., support groups based on gender or ethnicity). In contrast, bridging social capital refers to more inclusive relationships based on certain causes (e.g., civil rights) or professional networks that emphasize broader identities. Bridging social capital can broaden one's social networks and expand one's sources of information, but the social ties are often weak. On the other hand, bonding social capital can provide emotional support and foster solidarity, but strong in-group loyalty can be accompanied by more hostility toward outgroups.

Thus, bonding and bridging both have advantages and disadvantages. Based on this distinction, one might expect bridging but not bonding social capital to increase generalized trust. However, Uslaner (2002) argues that voluntary associations may not always foster generalized trust because they often bring together people with similar interests and perspectives. Such groupings seem to provide little basis for generalizing trust to anonymous others who are more likely to be different from ourselves. Instead, Uslaner proposes that generalized trust reflects an optimistic worldview. Optimistic people are less concerned with being exploited and are more resilient in their efforts to trust and cooperate with others. Optimism also remains positively associated with well-being, even after controlling for education and income (Uslaner, 1998). Whether cooperation and trust are fostered by social connections or optimism, it is important to note that the latter two are both associated with subjective well-being.

Subjective Well-Being

The field of subjective well-being (SWB) refers to the scientific study of happiness and life satisfaction. SWB consists of emotional and cognitive components (Diener, Suh, Lucas, & Smith, 1999). Emotional well-being is reflected in frequent experiences of pleasant emotions and infrequent experiences of unpleasant emotions. The cognitive component of SWB refers to a global evaluation of one's life, often assessed as life satisfaction. The cognitive and emotional components are often correlated so that people with high life satisfaction tend to report more frequent pleasant emotions than those with low life satisfaction (Diener & Fujita, 1995).

SWB is an important value for many societies and is not limited to Western or industrialized nations (Diener, 2000). Over the past two decades, research has illuminated a number of important determinants of SWB. These include differences among individuals in their personalities or emotional predispositions. For example, extraversion is frequently associated with pleasant affect, and neuroticism with unpleasant affect (Costa & McCrae, 1980). Some people are simply more likely to experience pleasant or unpleasant emotions in part because they pay more attention to pleasant or unpleasant stimuli (Derryberry & Reed, 1994). SWB is also affected by the fulfillment of basic needs. When basic needs are not met, the well-being of individuals and societies tends to decrease (E. Diener, M. Diener, & C. Diener, 1995). However, once basic needs are regularly met, other factors become important such as self-development and social relationships. This might explain why income leads to stronger increases in SWB in poorer countries, but has a smaller impact on well-being as the wealth of a nation increases (E. Diener & M. Diener, 1995; Oishi, Diener, Lucas, & Suh, 1999). Money and material resources *do* increase SWB—even beyond the level required for basic subsistence (Diener et al., 1995). After a yearly income of roughly $10,000, however, increases in SWB begin to level off.

Aside from personality and material resources, one of the most important determinants of SWB is having social relationships. Diener and Seligman (2002) compared the happiest (top 10%) of a college student sample with the unhappiest individuals (bottom 10%). The happiest individuals reported stronger relationships with friends, family, and romantic partners than those who were unhappy. Even more telling, the unhappiest 10% reported spending more time alone and less time with friends and family. Experience sampling studies in which participants provide reports of their emotions at random moments during the day reveal that people tend to experience more pleasant emotions when they are with others than when they are alone (Oishi, Diener, Scollon, & Biswas-Diener, 2003). Close relationships provide us with opportunities to experience love, joy, and affection, and married individuals consistently report being happier than those who are not married (Myers, 2000). In contrast, the experience of widowhood has a lasting negative impact on happiness. In a 15-year longitudinal study, those who were widowed did not return to prior levels of happiness until eight years later, on average (Lucas, Clark, Georgellis, & Diener, 2002). There is also some evidence that social isolation and loneliness are detrimental to long-term health, and some of these effects have been measured physiologically. Compared to socially integrated individuals, lonely individuals possess higher levels of cortisol (a sign of stress) and poorer immune system functioning (Cacioppo et al., 2000).

In sum, personality, material resources, and social relationships all are critical determinants of SWB. The last finding is of special relevance for our discussion because it highlights the relation between social capital and SWB. According to Putnam (2000), another reason why social capital might increase volunteerism is that individuals with rich social networks are more likely to be *asked for help* by others in their network. If this is correct, an association between SWB and increased sociability would have important implications for cooperation and trust. Indeed, previous researchers found SWB to be a strong correlate of generalized trust, even after controlling for demographic factors (Brehm & Rahn, 1997; Rahn & Transue, 1998). Next, we review evidence of mutual influence between SWB on the one hand, and cooperation and trust on the other.

The Effects of Cooperation and Trust on SWB

Cooperation and trust can have both short-term and long-term effects on SWB. Cooperative interactions may have short-term effects by evoking positive affect and attitudes. When participants engaged in a structured cooperative activity with a member of a stigmatized social group (former mental patients), they developed more positive attitudes of the group in general than when they worked individually in the presence of the stigmatized person (Desforges et al., 1991). Tasks that are performed within cooperative contexts rather than competitive or individualistic contexts result in better performance as well as increased self-esteem (Stanne, Johnson, & Johnson, 1999). However, the way competition is structured is also important. For instance, Tauer and Harackiewicz (2004) found that youth enjoyed shooting free throws in the context of *intergroup* competition more than they did in an individually competitive context. Intergroup competition involves elements of *both* cooperation and competition: *cooperation with* team members to shoot a joint number of free throws *in competition with* the performance of an opposing team. Thus, cooperation and competition can be combined to enhance task enjoyment.

Cooperation and trust also have long-term implications for well-being. Compared to individualistic efforts, cooperative tasks more effectively increase social support (Stanne et al., 1999). Such cooperative efforts may promote positive relationships with others in working toward common goals and help individuals to build upon their social resources, which are among the strongest correlates of SWB (Diener & Fujita, 1995). By facilitating the development of social relationships, then, trust and cooperation can contribute to SWB. In contrast, *pervasive* distrust of others can interfere with the development of rewarding relationships. Consistent with this argument, college females who were taught to not trust strangers in their childhood also reported greater loneliness and fear of intimacy than students who were not taught to be distrustful (F. Terrell, I. S. Terrell, & Von Drashek, 2000). Loneliness, in turn, is associated with stress (Cacioppo et al., 2000). Although more research is needed, these findings support the possibility of a causal relation from trusting attitudes to reduced loneliness and greater SWB.

Trust also facilitates cooperation with others. High trusters were more responsive to cooperative messages than competitive messages from other participants in a social dilemma (Parks, Henager, & Scamahorn, 1996). Trust may encourage cooperation by reducing the fear of being taken advantage of. However, even when one experiences fear, strong trust may override it. For example, Yamagishi and Sato (1986) operationalized trust by comparing friends with strangers in a public goods dilemma. Among strangers, contributions to public goods were reduced when participants either feared exploitation or were motivated by greed. However, among friends, fear and greed were less predictive of contributions. The researchers proposed that even when fear and greed are experienced among friends, people are more likely to retain their mutual trust or decide not to free-ride on their friends.

Organizational research attests to the importance of a trusting, cooperative work environment for productivity and job satisfaction. By relying on a tacit understanding that employees and supervisors operate in a trustworthy manner, organizations can avoid the costs of monitoring the behaviors of all employees (Kramer, 1999). Such measures not only cost time and money, but they may lead employees to feel distrusted, and to infer that their co-workers must be untrustworthy as well. Feeling distrusted, in turn, can undermine intrinsic motivation, with negative implications for job satisfaction and performance. Enzle and Anderson (1993) found that when participants were surveillanced for controlling reasons (e.g., to make sure they followed instructions), they were less engaged with a free-play activity. Not only is it important for employees to feel that they are trusted, it is also important for them to trust their employers. Positive emotions are enhanced when people feel they are being evaluated by a trustworthy authority figure who is using accurate methods (De Cremer, 2004). When an authority is perceived as untrustworthy, people report lower positive emotions regardless of accuracy.

Finally, Lu and Argyle (1991) found that positive attitudes toward group leisure activities predicted greater happiness six months later, even after controlling for prior levels of extraversion and happiness. These findings suggest that attitudes that support positive social interactions like cooperation may also promote and sustain happiness over time.

The Effects of SWB on Cooperation and Trust

A consistent finding in psychological research is that positive moods promote helping behavior and cooperation (Eisenberg, 1991). Much of the evidence relies on experiments that manipulate mood, suggesting that positive moods lead to prosocial behavior. However, *dispositional* positive affect also exhibits similar effects (for a review see Lyubomirsky, King, & Diener, 2005). We review the effects of positive mood and positive affectivity at the individual and group level, and then consider the potential benefits of happiness at the societal level.

Individual Level Effects

In a classic study, Isen and Levin (1972) induced positive mood by leaving a dime in a phone booth. People who found the dime after using the phone were more likely than those who did not to help a nearby confederate who dropped papers on the ground. People in a positive mood were also more willing to help co-workers (Baron & Bronfen, 1994), more likely to volunteer for future experiments (Aderman, 1972; Isen & Levin, 1972), and more likely to prefer cooperation over competition (Aderman, 1972; Barsade, 2002; Forgas, 1998) than people in neutral or negative moods. Although, negative moods occasionally induce helping, the findings are more consistent for positive mood (Eisenberg, 1991; however, see Eisenberg & Eggum, 2008, for an analysis of how sympathy contributes to helping behavior). Dispositional happiness (or trait positive affectivity) is also associated with greater helping. Happy people report more helping behavior in the past (Krueger, Hicks, & McGue, 2001), as well as greater willingness and intention to help others (Williams & Shiaw, 1999).

Why might positive mood facilitate helping and cooperation? One possibility is that positive mood increases positive thoughts, which may lead to more favorable evaluations of others. Participants who were exposed to a positive newscast were not only more cooperative in a subsequent task, they also *expected* others in the group to cooperate compared to participants who watched a negative newscast (Hornstein,

LaKind, Frankel, & Manne, 1975). Positive mood also enhances interest in social and prosocial activities (Cunningham, 1988b), increases liking for other people, and leads to more intimate self-disclosures in social interactions (Cunningham, 1988a). These findings suggest that individuals who experience positive affect are more inclined to trust others, and this is supported by research (Dunn & Schweitzer, 2005).

However, not only might happy people be more trusting, but others might be more likely to trust *them*. Dispositionally happy people tend to be more likeable than depressed individuals (Lyubomirsky et al., 2005). Women who smiled in their yearbook photo were rated as more affiliative and less hostile by observers who interacted with them, as well as by coders who only saw their photos (Harker & Keltner, 2001). Compared to unhappy people, happy people were rated as morally good and more likely to go to Heaven (King & Napa, 1998). When negotiating, people in positive moods were more likely to not only make deals, but to *honor* those deals in an interpersonal setting (Forgas, 1998). Thus, happy people may behave in ways that communicate their trustworthiness, and this can encourage others to be more cooperative with them.

Organizational and Group Level Effects

The relations among happiness, trust, and cooperation may yield important benefits in the workplace. Diener, Nickerson, Lucas, and Sandvik (2002) found that cheerfulness in college predicted job satisfaction and income nineteen years later. The helpfulness of happy people also appears to generalize to the workplace. Reviews of organizational citizenship behaviors (OCB) find a modest correlation between positive affectivity and altruistic behaviors at work (Borman, Penner, Allen, & Motowidlo, 2001; Organ & Ryan, 1995), and both trait and mood measures of positive affect separately predict intentions to engage in OCB (Williams & Shiaw, 1999).

However, happy people do not blindly and invariably trust and cooperate with others. Rather, the effects of positive mood on cooperation may depend on contextual factors such as current goals (Sanna, Parks, & Chang, 2003) or perceived social norms (Hertel, Neuhof, Theuer, & Kerr, 2000). For example, in a public goods game, Hertel et al. (2000) manipulated participants' expectancies about the average contribution of other players so that perceived norms were either cooperative (high average contribution) or uncooperative (low average contribution). In the cooperative norm condition, positive mood led to greater cooperation than negative mood after the first block of trials. In contrast, no effect of mood was found in the *uncooperative* norm condition. Hertel et al. suggested that in a positive mood, people might rely on social heuristics (such as group norms) to guide their behavior.

Thus, happy individuals do not function in a bubble; the surrounding work environment can facilitate or reduce mood effects. Consistent with this idea, Forgas (1998) found that negotiation was most cooperative when two bargaining groups were *both* in a positive mood. In contrast, a happy group that negotiates with a sad group tends to cooperate less. This trend may be due to the strong preference of sad groups for competition over cooperation. However, sad groups were still more likely to cooperate with happy groups than with another sad group—another indication that happy people may invite trust and cooperation from others.

The above research suggests that a positive work environment may be just as important as individual happiness. Management teams with high average trait positive affect reported greater cooperativeness and less conflict on group projects (Barsade, Ward, Turner, & Sonnenfeld, 2000). Greater cooperation among happy work groups might explain the greater productivity and lower turnover rates in such groups (see Diener & Seligman, 2004).

Implications for Society

Inglehart and colleagues (2000; Inglehart & Klingemann, 2000) have argued that life satisfaction may be necessary (though not sufficient) for the sustainability of democracies. Although democratic countries generally exhibit a higher quality of life, it is also important to consider that no society can function well when most of its citizens are discontent. High life satisfaction may not only indicate that people's needs are fulfilled, it might also help legitimize the government in the eyes of its citizens. Indeed, life satisfaction has been associated with greater confidence in the government (Brehm & Rahn, 1997).

However, the benefits of a happy citizenry might extend beyond the mere fact of stability to the *flourishing* of entire communities. Thoits and Hewitt (2001) suggested that high well-being may be an important resource for individuals to draw upon, enabling them to contribute more time to volunteering. They found that well-being predicted the amount of volunteer work three years later, and that this relation was fully mediated by involvement with community organizations. The authors suggested that well-being may facilitate social integration, which in turn provides individuals with greater opportunities for volunteering. The reciprocal relation was also found. That is, volunteer work at Time 1 predicted well-being three years later. Thus, the relation between well-being and volunteerism may be bi-directional (cf. Piliavin, 2008).

Analyses from the World Value Survey

Using data from the second (1990–1991) and third (1995–1997) waves of the World Value Survey (WVS; Inglehart et al., 2003), we examined the relation among subjective well-being, trust, and cooperation at the nation level. Our analyses include 13 nations from the second wave, and 45 nations from the third wave of the WVS (see Appendix).

Main Variables

All items were averaged across participants within each nation. We computed *SWB* by averaging two items measuring happiness and life satisfaction; scores range from

1 (dissatisfied and not at all happy) to 7 (satisfied and very happy). *Trust* scores reflect the percentage of respondents within a nation who believe that most people can be trusted. Previous analyses of the WVS have included trust and life satisfaction in a composite measure of "self-expression values" (Inglehart & Welzel, 2003). Values such as life satisfaction, trust, and tolerance reflect a regard for individual integrity. In our analyses, we dissect these self-expression values in order to more fully explore the relation of SWB and trust to cooperation.

We examined cooperation at the nation level in two ways. First, we examined mean levels of *volunteerism* (both the level of involvement and the number of voluntary associations). Second, we examined democratic attitudes and beliefs because such attitudes may reflect a cooperative orientation towards governance, political participation, and civic life. These measures included two indices of tolerance. The first is the percentage of respondents in a nation who believe that *tolerance is an important quality* for their children to possess. The WVS also presented respondents with a list of commonly stigmatized groups (e.g., homosexuals, people of different race, etc.) and asked them to indicate which, if any, they would not like to have as a neighbor. Thus, our second measure was an index of *intolerance* created by summing up the number of groups that were mentioned as undesirable neighbors.

We also created two overall measures of positive and negative attitudes towards democratic systems. *Positive attitudes* were the average of two items: the extent to which democracy was viewed as a "good way of governing" one's country, and the belief that democracy is "better than any other form of government." *Negative attitudes* were the average of three items assessing the belief that democracies have poor economic systems, are characterized by indecision and squabbling, and are not good at maintaining order. Other items we examined concerned attitudes toward *competition*, *autocracy* (government by a strong leader with no elections), *preference for a cooperative leader*, and *perceived democracy* (the percent of respondents who believe the country is run for all people instead of just a "few big interests").

Respondents were also asked to prioritize a list of goals for their nation (e.g., fighting crime). These items have been used previously to measure postmaterialist values. According to Inglehart (2000), as wealth increases in a society, the emphasis shifts from economic growth to quality of life concerns. In our analyses, we concentrate on three of these goals: building a more humane society, giving people more say in their jobs and communities, and giving people more say on important government issues. Scores on these items reflect the percentage of respondents who selected the item as a major priority for their country for the next ten years.

Finally, we included three variables as economic, political, and cultural indicators. For each nation, we obtained data on real *GDP per capita* in constant 1996 dollars from the Penn World Tables (Heston, Summers, & Aten, 2002). We also obtained ratings of civil liberties and political rights for each nation from the *Freedom in the World* surveys (Freedom House, 2005). These ratings range from 1 (*highest level of freedom*) to 7 (*lowest level of freedom*). We reversed scored these ratings and averaged them so that high scores reflect societies with greater *freedom*. As a measure of social culture, we adapted a forced-choice item from the WVS assessing attitudes toward respect for parents. Respondents indicated whether they believed either that one should always love one's parents regardless of their faults, or that one is not obligated to love one's parents if they have not earned it through their attitudes and behaviors. We averaged these responses within nations, and normalized the distribution by applying an inverse transformation so that high scores reflected greater *filial piety*. In societies where filial piety is emphasized, close familial bonds may be highly valued and a stronger distinction might be made between ingroups and outgroups (Triandis, 1989). Thus, filial piety can be seen as a type of bonding social capital (Putnam, 2000) and might be associated with less generalized trust. When appropriate, data were transformed in order to normalize the distribution. For all analyses, we used an alpha level of 0.05 to evaluate statistical significance.

Results

SWB and trust were positively correlated ($r = 0.39$; see Table 1) as found in previous analyses of the WVS (Inglehart, 1999). SWB and trust were both associated with greater value placed on tolerance, less intolerance of neighbors, higher GDP per capita, greater freedom, and lower levels of filial piety. Both the level of volunteer involvement and the number of voluntary memberships were positively associated with SWB, but not with trust. However, the *nature* of volunteer involvement may also be important. Putnam (1993) maintained that interpersonal trust is likely to arise from involvement in *horizontal* organizations where members participate as equals. The exact nature of involvement is unclear from the WVS data. We examined specific voluntary memberships and found that the level of trust in a nation correlated with the level of involvement in unions ($r = 28$, $p = 0.05$). To the extent that unions often rely on collective action in the interest of all members, this may support Putnam's arguments (see also Radcliffe, 2008). In contrast, memberships in other types of organizations (e.g., church, arts, political parties, etc.) were mostly unrelated to trust.

Interestingly, neither SWB nor trust were associated with attitudes toward competition. Nor were positive attitudes toward competition associated with volunteering or valuing tolerance. Thus, as other researchers have argued (Stanne et al., 1999; Tauer & Harackiewicz, 2004), competition is not inherently opposed to cooperation. The form that competition takes is an important consideration. The WVS asks respondents whether competition is good because it motivates hard work and new ideas, but it does not specify the type of competition. This might explain why societies that value tolerance do not necessarily oppose competition. In contrast, in those societies where *intolerance* is high, competition tends to be viewed more positively ($r = 0.36$). Perhaps in these societies, zero-sum competition is emphasized because it justifies inequities and intolerant attitudes. On the other hand those countries in which intolerance is high also tend to be less wealthy, have less freedom, and greater filial piety. Thus intolerance and competition might follow from conditions in which resources are scarce, and relationships with one's family or ingroup become tighter as a matter of survival.

Table 1 Intercorrelations among SWB, volunteering, attitudes, and societal variables

Variable	1	2	3	4	5	6	7	8	9	10
1. SWB	–									
2. Trust	0.39**	–								
3. Vol. Inv.[a]	0.46***	0.16	–							
4. Vol. No.[a]	0.37**	0.20	0.96***	–						
5. Tolerance Imp.	0.53***	0.39**	0.24†	0.25†	–					
6. Intolerance	-0.61***	-0.37**	-0.10	-0.11	-0.63***	–				
7. Competition	-0.07	-0.03	0.16	0.18	-0.06	0.36**	–			
8. GDP/capita[a]	0.50***	0.49***	-0.04	-0.03	0.65***	-0.71***	-0.32*	–		
9. Freedom	0.43**	0.38**	0.01	0.00	0.58***	-0.57***	-0.30*	0.79***	–	
10. Filial Piety	-0.42**	-0.72***	-0.04	-0.10	-0.64***	0.52***	-0.01	-0.69***	-0.50***	–

[a] Data were transformed via natural log.

† $p < 0.10$.

* $p < 0.05$.

** $p < 0.01$.

*** $p < 0.001$.

Note. N = 58. SWB = average of life satisfaction and happiness; Vol. Inv. = level of volunteer involvement; Vol. No. = number of voluntary memberships; Tolerance Imp. = importance of one's child possessing tolerance.

Table 2 Correlations of SWB, Trust, and GDP/capita with democratic attitudes

Variable	SWB	Trust	GDP/cap.[a]	N
Democracy (Positive Attitude)	0.51**	0.26[†]	0.05	43
Democracy (Negative Attitude)	−0.23	−0.34*	−0.04	41
Autocracy	−0.52***	−0.35*	−0.37*	42
Cooperative Leader	−0.03	0.27[†]	0.13	42
Perceived Democracy	0.44**	0.28[†]	0.14	41
Value More Humane Society	0.42**	0.43**	0.63***	57
Value More Say in Job/Community	0.51***	0.43**	0.69***	58
Value More Say in Government[b]	0.40**	0.14	0.59***	58

[a] Data were transformed via natural log.
[b] Data were transformed via arcsine of the square root.
[†] $p < 0.10$.
* $p < 0.05$.
** $p < 0.01$.
*** $p < 0.001$.

Table 2 presents the correlations of SWB and trust with various democratic attitudes. Here, trust and SWB show an interesting divergent but supportive pattern of correlations. For instance, SWB is associated with more positive attitudes toward democracy, greater *perceived* democracy, and more importance placed on giving people more say on important government decisions. Trust but not SWB was significantly associated with less negative attitudes toward democracy. Preference for a cooperative leader was not correlated with SWB and had only a weak positive association with trust. Nevertheless, *both* SWB and trust were correlated with less approval of autocratic governance, and greater importance placed on building a more humane society and giving people more say in one's job and community. Taken together these findings suggest that national levels of SWB and trust are associated with a greater preference for participatory and cooperative approaches in government and civic life.

Interestingly, GDP per capita was not associated with either positive or negative attitudes toward democracy. However, several other attitudes do correlate with the wealth of a nation. As GDP per capita also correlates with SWB and trust, it is possible that some of the observed relations among SWB, trust, and cooperative behaviors and attitudes are due to the wealth of a nation, rather than its level of SWB or trust *per se*. Therefore, we conducted a series of regression analyses predicting volunteering and democratic attitudes from SWB and trust, after controlling for wealth, freedom, and filial piety. These analyses are presented in Table 3.

SWB and trust were no longer significant predictors of tolerance after controlling for other variables. For example, valuing tolerance appears to be strongly predicted by filial piety. In societies where filial piety is high and ingroup bonds are presumably stronger, people are less likely to mention tolerance as an important quality for their child to possess. This may mean that tolerance is not a salient value in these societies, rather than that tolerance is negatively regarded. In terms of intolerance, per capita GDP seems to account for much of the variance previously associated with trust and SWB. A number of explanations are possible. Diener et al. (1995)

Table 3 Regression analyses predicting volunteering and democratic attitudes

Dependent variable	Standardize regression coefficients (β)					R^2	N
	GDP/cap.[a]	Freedom	Filial piety	Trust	SWB		
Vol. Inv.[a]	−0.46[†]	0.09	0.14	0.22	0.62***	0.34	54
Vol. No.[a]	−0.45[†]	0.07	0.01	0.22	0.48**	0.24	54
Tolerance Imp.	0.07	0.24	−0.52**	−0.18	0.18	0.54	53
Intolerance	−0.53**	−0.01	−0.06	−0.05	−0.32**	0.59	54
Pos. Dem	−0.72**	0.15	−0.62**	−0.01	0.58***	0.51	41
Neg. Dem	0.42	0.13	0.63*	−0.09	−0.21	0.34	40
Autocracy	0.11	−0.05	0.38	−0.01	−0.41*	0.38	40
Perceived Dem	−0.29	0.20	0.03	0.25	0.44**	0.26	44
Humane Soc.	0.56*	−0.03	0.00	0.12	0.09	0.44	55
More Say (J/C)	0.20	0.46**	−0.11	−0.01	0.21*	0.69	55
More Say (Govt)[b]	0.37	0.26	−0.05	−0.25	0.18	0.40	55

[a] Data were transformed via natural log.
[b] Data were transformed via arcsine of the square root.
[†] $p < 0.10$.
* $p < 0.05$.
** $p < 0.01$.
*** $p < 0.001$.
Note. Vol. Inv. = level of volunteer involvement; Vol. No. = number of voluntary memberships; Tolerance Imp. = importance of one's child possessing tolerance; Dem. Pos. = positive attitudes toward democracy; Dem. Neg. = negative attitudes toward democracy; Autocracy = approval of strong leader with no elections; Perc. Dem. = perceived democracy; Humane Soc. = value more humane society; More Say (J/C) = value more say in jobs and community; More Say (Gov) = value more say on important government decisions.

found that wealthier nations tended to have greater equality in terms of income and access to education. Education in turn might reduce stereotypic beliefs about stigmatized groups. Alternatively, intolerance may be a reflection of security needs. In wealthy nations, basic needs are better met and people are more likely to feel safe and secure. As a result, they might also feel less threatened by neighbors who are different from them.

After controlling for filial piety, trust was no longer significantly associated with negative attitudes toward democracy. Societies that value filial piety appear to hold more negative attitudes toward democracy (β = 0.63, $p < 0.05$). However, mean level attitudes for most nations fall between 2 and 3 on a 4-point Likert scale. This suggests that countries that are high on filial piety agree only slightly that democracies are flawed and inefficient, while countries that are lower on filial piety only *disagree* slightly with these beliefs. Thus, few countries fully despise democracy. Rather, these associations may be due to greater sense of empowerment among individualistic nations (e.g., the Scandinavian countries), which tend to be lower on filial piety.

After controlling for wealth, freedom, filial piety, and trust, SWB was no longer predictive of the importance placed on either building a more humane society or giving people more say on important government matters. However, SWB continued to show a strong relation with several other variables. For instance, the relation between SWB and volunteering does not appear to be fully accounted for by GDP per capita. These findings are consistent with those of Thoits and Hewitt's (2001), who found evidence for a bi-directional relation between well-being and volunteering, even after controlling for family income. Thus, in countries, where SWB is high, people may be more likely to possess the psychological resources (e.g., optimism, resilience, sociability) to engage in volunteer work. At the same time, increasing volunteer involvement may also increase social capital and subsequently, well-being.

After controlling for wealth and freedom, countries that are high on SWB continue to have higher mean levels of perceived democracy, positive attitudes toward democracy, greater disapproval of autocratic rule, and less intolerant attitudes. Moreover, wealth and freedom do not fully account for the relation between SWB and the increasing value placed on giving people more say in one's job and community, although freedom remained a significant predictor.

Although more research is needed, the findings above generally support our contention that SWB and cooperation have important social implications. In societies where SWB is high, people tend to prefer a government and civic life in which all people can participate. Just as well, in societies where community participation (i.e., volunteerism) is high, people tend to be happier. Although we did not find consistent relations between trust and democratic attitudes after controlling for other variables, it should be noted that many of these variables are intercorrelated. For example, societal levels of generalized trust were strongly linked to the endorsement of filial piety ($r = -0.72$). If societal levels of trust reflect cultural beliefs about human nature or social relations that are strongly embodied in filial attitudes, then the substantive meaning of trust could be lost when controlling for filial piety. Cultural knowledge can have important influences on trust and cooperation (Wong & Hong, 2005; Yuki, Maddux, Brewer, & Takemura, 2006). Thus, in some cases, we may be over-controlling for these variables in the regression models. Given the strong link between GDP per capita and SWB then, it is interesting that SWB should maintain strong links with several democratic and cooperative attitudes after controlling for wealth. These findings support previous arguments that SWB plays an important role in sustaining and legitimizing participatory forms of government such as democracy (Inglehart & Klingemann, 2000).

Discussion

Recent analyses indicate troubling social trends in the US. According to several researchers, generalized trust has declined over the past few decades among American teenagers and adults (Rahn & Transue, 1998; Putnam, 2000; Uslaner, 2002). Various causes have been proposed from increases in materialistic values (Rahn & Transue, 1998) to decreasing social capital (Putnam, 2000) to greater economic inequality (Uslaner, 2002).

Our analyses indicate that societies that are high on SWB are also higher on trust, volunteerism, and several democratic attitudes—even after controlling for GDP per capita and freedom. Although attitudes are subjective, it is worth pointing out that volunteer involvement is a fairly objective behavioral indicator. It is therefore impressive that national SWB should manifest strong relations to the number of associations that people join in a society. A critical implication of our results is that SWB accompanies both attitudes *and* behaviors that are conducive to building a more trusting, cooperative society. Although our analyses do not speak to causality, both directions of influence are supported by research. Experimental data suggest that positive emotions and greater SWB play a causal role by fostering greater sociability, trust, and cooperation. In positive moods, people tend to view others and be viewed *by* others more positively, show increased preference for cooperation, and are more likely to be active and involved in their communities. At the same time, trust and cooperation are important tools for building social connections, which are key ingredients for sustained happiness.

We do not argue that increasing SWB is the panacea for all our social ills. Positive emotions do not invariably lead to more trust and cooperation; social norms (Hertel et al., 2000) are also important. However, we do contend that SWB is a *necessary* condition for a flourishing society. No society can count on sustaining trust and cooperation when its citizens are discontented. The strong relation between national levels of SWB and cooperation underscore this point.

As nations around the world press on with economic development and establishing political stability, greater cooperation must occur on the international stage. This will entail the recognition and acceptance of common goals that all countries must work toward. Promoting subjective well-being should be one of these goals. If all countries are fundamentally interdependent, then sustaining the well-being of any single nation should be in the interests of all other nations. To the extent that SWB facilitates trust and cooperation, the promotion of SWB through international acts of goodwill is the quintessential non-zero-sum solution.

To this end, it will be necessary to develop national indicators that move beyond economic indices (Diener, 2000; Diener & Seligman, 2004; Diener & Tov, 2005). Traditionally, economic measures have been used as a proxy for well-being—and with good reason. Economic development is strongly linked to SWB. Particularly when an economy is developing and the fulfillment of basic needs are at risk, GDP per capita has a clear impact on SWB. However, as societies become wealthier, the utility of objective economic indicators of well-being diminishes. As Radcliffe (2008) shows, other structural aspects of society such as welfare provisions and union organization are also associated with aggregate levels of SWB. We agree with him that social institutions can be structured in ways that optimize cooperation and well-being. In order for this to happen, local and national governments need to be involved, and changes in well-being must be monitored in ways that can inform policy decisions. National measures of trust, community feelings, life satisfaction, pleasant and unpleasant affect need to be developed and implemented over successive periods of time. Consequently, room must be made on national agendas for maximizing well-being in addition to the maximizing economic output.

Acknowledgments This work was supported by a National Science Foundation Graduate Fellowship awarded to William Tov.

Appendix

Analyses of the World Values Survey includes nations from the 1990–1993 wave (Austria, Belgium, Canada, Czech Republic, Denmark, France, Iceland, Ireland, Italy, Netherlands, Portugal, Romania, Slovakia) and the 1995–1997 wave (Argentina, Armenia, Australia, Azerbaijan, Bangladesh, Belarus, Bosnia and Herzegovina, Brazil, Britain, Bulgaria, Chile, China, Columbia, Croatia, Dominican Republic, Estonia, Finland, Georgia, Ghana, India, Japan, Latvia, Lithuania, Macedonia, Mexico, Moldova, Nigeria, Norway, Peru, Philippines, Poland, Russia, South Africa, Serbia and Montenegro, Slovenia, Spain, Sweden, Switzerland, Taiwan, Turkey, Ukraine, Uruguay, United States, Venezuela, Germany).

References

Aderman, D. (1972). Elation, depression, and helping behavior. *Journal of Personality and Social Psychology, 24*, 91–101.

Barsade, S. G. (2002). The ripple effects: Emotional contagion and its influence on group behavior. *Administrative Science Quarterly, 47*, 644–675.

Baron, R. A., & Bronfen, M. I. (1994). A whiff of reality: Empirical evidence concerning the effects of pleasant fragrances on work-related behavior. *Journal of Applied Social Psychology, 24*, 1179–1203.

Barsade, S. G., Ward, A. J., Turner, J. D. F., & Sonnenfeld, J. A. (2000). To your heart's content: A model of affective diversity in top management teams. *Administrative Science Quarterly, 45*, 802–836.

Borman, W. C., Penner, L. A., Allen, T. D., & Motowidlo, S. J. (2001). Personality predictors of citizenship performance. *International Journal of Selection and Assessment, 9*, 52–69.

Brehm, J., & Rahn, W. (1997). Individual-level evidence for the causes and consequences of social capital. *American Journal of Political Science, 41*, 999–1023.

Cacioppo, J. T., Ernst, J. M., Burleson, M. H., McClintock, M. K., Malarkey, W. B., Hawkley, L. C., Kowalewski, R. B., Paulsen, A., Hobson, J. A., Hugdahl, K., Spiegel, D., & Berntson, G. G. (2000). Lonely traits and concomitant physiological processes: The MacArthur social neuroscience studies. *International Journal of Psychophysiology, 35*, 143–154.

Costa, P. T., & McCrae, R. R. (1980). Influence of extraversion and neuroticism on subjective well-being: Happy and unhappy people. *Journal of Personality and Social Psychology, 54*, 296–308.

Cunningham, M. R. (1988a). Does happiness mean friendliness? Induced mood and heterosexual self-disclosure. *Personality and Social Psychology Bulletin, 14*, 283–297.

Cunningham, M. R. (1988b). What do you do when you're happy or blue? Mood, expectancies, and behavioral interest. *Motivation & Emotion, 12*, 309–331.

De Cremer, D. (2004). The influence of accuracy as a function of leader's bias: The role of trustworthiness in the psychology of procedural justice. *Personality and Social Psychology Bulletin, 30*, 293–304.

Derryberry, D., & Reed, M. A. (1994). Temperament and attention: Orienting toward and away from positive and negative signals. *Journal of Personality and Social Psychology, 66*, 1128–1139.

Desforges, D. M., Lord, C. G., Ramsey, S. L., Mason, J. A., Van Leeuwen, M. D., West, S. C., & Lepper, M. R. (1991). Effects of structured cooperative contact on changing negative attitudes toward stigmatized social groups. *Journal of Personality and Social Psychology, 60*, 531–544.

Diener, E. (2000). Subjective well-being: The science of happiness and a proposal for a national index. *American Psychologist, 55*, 34–43.

Diener, E., & Diener, M. (1995). Cross-cultural correlates of life satisfaction and self-esteem. *Journal of Personality and Social Psychology, 68*, 653–663.

Diener, E., Diener, M., & Diener, C. (1995). Factors predicting the subjective well-being of nations. *Journal Personality and Social Psychology, 69*, 851–864.

Diener, E., & Fujita, F. (1995). Resources, personal strivings, and subjective well-being: A nomothetic and idiographic approach. *Journal of Personality and Social Psychology, 68*, 926–935.

Diener, E., Nickerson, C., Lucas, R. E., & Sandvik, E. (2002). Dispositional affect and job outcomes. *Social Indicators Research, 59*, 229–259.

Diener, E., & Seligman, M. E. P. (2002). Very happy people. *Psychological Science, 13*, 81–84.

Diener, E., & Seligman, M. E. P. (2004). Beyond money: Toward an economy of well-being. *Psychological Science in the Public Interest, 5*, 1–31.

Diener, E., Suh, E. M., Lucas, R. E., & Smith, H. E. (1999). Subjective well-being: Three decades of progress. *Psychological Bulletin, 125*, 276–302.

Diener, E., & Tov, W. (2005). National accounts of well-being. In K. C. Land (Ed.), *Encyclopedia of social indicators and quality-of-life studies*. New York: Springer.

Dunn, J. R., & Schweitzer, M. E. (2005). Feeling and believing: The influence of emotion on trust. *Journal of Personality and Social Psychology, 88*, 736–748.

Eisenberg, N. (1991). Meta-analytic contributions to the literature on prosocial behavior. *Personality and Social Psychology Bulletin, 17*, 273–282.

Eisenberg, N., & Eggum, N. D. (2008). Empathy-eelated and prosocial responding: Conceptions and correlates during development. In B. A. Sullivan, M. Snyder & J. L. Sullivan (Eds.), *Cooperation: The political psychology of effective human interaction*. Malden, MA: Blackwell Publishing.

Enzle, M. E., & Anderson, S. C. (1993). Surveillant intentions and intrinsic motivation. *Journal of Personality and Social Psychology, 2*, 257–266.

Forgas, J. P. (1998). On feeling good and getting your way: Mood effects on negotiator cognition and bargaining strategies. *Journal of Social and Personality Psychology, 74*, 565–577.

Freedom House. (2005). *Freedom in the World country ratings*. Retrieved September 6, 2005 from, http://www.freedomhouse.org/ratings/allscores2005.xls

Harker, L., & Keltner, D. (2001). Expressions of positive emotions in women's college yearbook pictures and their relationship to personality and life outcomes across adulthood. *Journal of Personality and Social Psychology, 80*, 112–124.

Hertel, G., Neuhof, J., Theuer, T., & Kerr, N. L. (2000). Mood effects on cooperation in small groups: Does positive mood simply lead to more cooperation? *Cognition and Emotion, 14*, 441–472.

Heston, A., Summers, R., & Aten, B. (2002). *Penn World Table Version 6.1*, Center for International Comparisons, University of Pennsylvania.

Hornstein, H. A., LaKind, E., Frankel, G., & Manne, S. (1975). Effects of knowledge about remote social events on prosocial behavior, social conception, and mood. *Journal of Personality and Social Psychology, 32*, 1038–1046.

Inglehart, R. (1999). Trust, well-being, and democracy. In M. E. Warren (Ed.), *Democracy and trust* (pp. 88–120). Cambridge, UK: Cambridge University Press.

Inglehart, R. (2000). Globalization and postmodern values. *Washington Quarterly, 23*, 215–228.

Inglehart, et al. (2003). *World values surveys and European values surveys, 1981–1984, 1990–1993, and 1995–1997* [Computer file, ICPSR02790-v1]. Ann Arbor, MI: Institute for Social Research.

Inglehart, R., & Klingemann, H.-D. (2000). Genes, culture, democracy, and happiness. In E. Diener & E. M. Suh (Eds.), *Culture and subjective well-being* (pp. 185–218). Cambridge, Massachusetts: MIT Press.

Inglehart, R., & Welzel, C. (2003). Political culture and democracy: Analysing cross-level linkages. *Comparative Politics, 36*, 61–79.

Isen, A. M., & Levin, P. F. (1972). Effect of feeling good on helping: Cookies and kindness. *Journal of Personality and Social Psychology, 21*, 384–388.

King, L. A., & Napa, C. K. (1998). What makes a life good? *Journal of Personality and Social Psychology, 75*, 156–165.

King, L. A., & Napa, C. K. (1998). What makes a life good? *Journal of Personality and Social Psychology, 75*, 156–165.

Kramer, R. M. (1999). Trust and distrust in organizations: Emerging perspectives, enduring questions. *Annual Review of Psychology, 50*, 569–598.

Krueger, R. F., Hicks, B. M., & McGue, M. (2001). Altruism and antisocial behavior: Independent tendencies, unique personality correlates, distinct etiologies. *Psychological Science, 12*, 397–402.

Lu, L., & Argyle, M. (1991). Happiness and cooperation. *Personality and Individual Differences, 12*, 1019–1030.

Lucas, R. E., Clark, A. E., Georgellis, Y., & Diener, E. (2002). Reexamining adaptation and the set point model of happiness: Reactions to changes in marital status. *Journal of Personality and Social Psychology, 84*, 527–539.

Lyubomirsky, S., King, L., & Diener, E. (2005). The benefits of frequent positive affect: Does happiness lead to success? *Psychological Bulletin, 131*, 803–855.

Myers, D. G. (2000). The funds, friends, and faith of happy people. *American Psychologist, 55*, 56–67.

Oishi, S., Diener, E. F., Lucas, R. E., & Suh, E. M. (1999). Cross-cultural variations in predictors of life satisfaction: Perspectives from needs and values. *Personality and Social Psychology Bulletin, 25*, 980–990.

Oishi, S., Diener, E., Scollon, C. N., & Biswas-Diener, R. (2003). Cross-situational consistency of affective experiences across cultures. *Journal of Personality and Social Psychology, 86*, 460–472.

Organ, D. W., & Ryan, K. (1995). A meta-analytic review of attitudinal and dispositional predictors of organizational citizenship behavior. *Personnel Psychology, 48*, 775–802.

Parks, C. D., Henager, R. F., & Scamahorn, S. D. (1996). Trust and reactions to messages of intent in social dilemmas. *Journal of Conflict Resolution, 40*, 134–151.

Piliavin, J. A. (2008). Long-term benefits of habitual helping: Doing well by doing good. In B. A. Sullivan, M. Snyder & J. L. Sullivan (Eds.), *Cooperation: The political psychology of effective human interaction*. Malden, MA: Blackwell Publishing.

Putnam, R. D. (1993). *Making democracy work: Civic traditions in modern Italy*. Princeton, NJ: Princeton University Press.

Putnam, R. D. (2000). *Bowling alone: The collapse and revival of American community*. New York: Simon & Schuster.

Radcliff, B. (2008). The politics of human happiness. In B. A. Sullivan, M. Snyder & J. L. Sullivan (Eds.), *Cooperation: The political psychology of effective human interaction*. Malden, MA: Blackwell Publishing.

Rahn, W. M., & Transue, J. E. (1998). Social trust and value change: The decline of social capital in American youth, 1976–1995. *Political Psychology, 19*, 545–565.

Sanna, L. J., Parks, C. D., & Chang, E. C. (2003). Mixed-motive conflict in social dilemmas: Mood as input to competitive and cooperative goals. *Group Dynamics: Theory, Research, and Practice, 7*, 26–40.

Stanne, M. B., Johnson, D. W., & Johnson, R. T. (1999). Does competition enhance or inhibit motor performance: A meta-analysis. *Psychological Bulletin, 125*, 133–154.

Tauer, J. M., & Harackiewicz, J. M. (2004). The effects of cooperation and competition on intrinsic motivation and performance. *Journal of Personality and Social Psychology, 86*, 849–861.

Terrell, F., Terrell, I. S., & Von Drashek, S. R. (2000). Loneliness and fear of intimacy among adolescents who were taught not to trust strangers during childhood. *Adolescence, 35*, 611–617.

Thoits, P. A., & Hewitt, L. N. (2001). Volunteer work and well-being. *Journal of Health and Social Behavior, 42*, 115–131.

Triandis, H. C. (1989). The self and social behavior in differing cultural contexts. *Psychological Review, 96*, 506–520.

Uslaner, E. M. (1998). Social capital, television, and the 'mean world': Trust, optimism, and civic participation. *Political psychology, 19,* 441–467.

Uslaner, E. M. (2002). *The moral foundations of trust.* Cambridge, UK: Cambridge University.

Williams, S., & Shiaw, W. T. (1999). Mood and organizational citizenship behavior: The effects of positive affect on employee organizational citizenship behavior intentions. *Journal of Psychology, 133,* 656–668.

Wong, R. Y., & Hong, Y. (2005). Dynamic influences of culture on cooperation in the prisoner's dilemma. *Psychological Science, 16,* 429–434.

Wright, R. (2000). *Nonzero: The logic of human destiny.* New York: Pantheon Books.

Yamagishi, T., & Sato, K. (1986). Motivational bases of the public goods problem. *Journal of Personality and Social Psychology, 50,* 67–73.

Yuki, M., Maddux, W. W., Brewer, M. B., & Takemura, K. (2005). Cross-cultural differences in relationship- and group-based trust. *Personality and Social Psychology Bulletin, 31,* 48–62.

The Optimum Level of Well-Being: Can People Be Too Happy?

Shigehiro Oishi, Ed Diener, and Richard E. Lucas

Abstract Psychologists, self-help gurus, and parents all work to make their clients, friends, and children happier. Recent research indicates that happiness is functional and generally leads to success. However, most people are already above neutral in happiness, which raises the question of whether higher levels of happiness facilitate more effective functioning than do lower levels. Our analyses of large survey data and longitudinal data show that people who experience the highest levels of happiness are the most successful in terms of close relationships and volunteer work, but that those who experience slightly lower levels of happiness are the most successful in terms of income, education, and political participation. Once people are moderately happy, the most effective level of happiness appears to depend on the specific outcomes used to define success, as well as the resources that are available.

Despite the fact that most people are already satisfied with their lives (Diener & Diener, 1996), many people aspire to be even happier. There are hundreds of self-help books, motivational speakers, and life coaches whose primary goal is to improve subjective well-being. In light of these attempts to boost well-being, it is necessary to question whether being happier is always better. Is it sensible for a society to encourage already happy people to aspire to even higher levels of well-being?[1] The present article focuses on the differences between moderately happy and very happy people to address questions about the optimal level of happiness.

The issues of optimal happiness are not merely academic. In recent years, psychologists and economists have increasingly called for large-scale projects that track national levels of well-being over time. The ultimate goal of these proposed national indexes of well-being is to enable decision-makers to use information about a population's well-being to guide public policy (Diener & Seligman, 2004; Kahneman,

S. Oishi (✉)

Department of Psychology, University of Virginia, P.O. Box 400400, Charlottesville, VA 22904–4400, USA

e-mail: soishi@virginia.edu

[1] There is a similar debate on the dark side of excessively high self-esteem (see Baumeister, Campbell, Krueger, & Vohs, 2003; Crocker & Park, 2004; Pyszczynski & Cox, 2004).

E. Diener (ed.), *The Science of Well-Being: The Collected Works of Ed Diener*, Social Indicators Research Series 37, DOI 10.1007/978-90-481-2350-6_8, © Springer Science+Business Media B.V. 2009

Krueger, Schkade, Schwarz, & Stone, 2004). However, these proposals implicitly raise the question of how happy nations should be. Policies may be put in place that reliably increase positive emotions and life satisfaction, but if these increases result in negative consequences for the individuals who experience them, then the policies would not effectively fulfill their original purpose. Similarly, issues regarding optimal levels of happiness affect individual decision makers. People often make important life decisions (such as the decisions to get married, divorce their current partner, change jobs, or more across the country) based in part on the predicted level of life satisfaction that would result. Numerous studies have shown that these predictions can be wrong (Wilson & Gilbert, 2003). But an even more basic question concerns the practicality of the initial desire. Can people's expectations for happiness sometimes be set too high, and can these expectations lead to negative outcomes for the individual?

We will begin our review by addressing the concept of happiness. We will also summarize why people seek happiness and discuss its various benefits. Then, we will develop the argument that although happiness has positive consequences in general, being happier is not always better. Once a moderate level of happiness is achieved, further increases can sometimes be detrimental. In support of our argument, we report empirical findings from a large cross-sectional project, an intense data collection study, and four large longitudinal studies.

The Concept of Happiness

Philosophers have debated the definition of happiness for millennia without reaching a definitive consensus (see Sumner, 1996, for review). The concept of happiness differs, sometimes substantially, across theorists. For Aristotle, the realization of one's potential was a critical ingredient of happiness, or *eudaimonia* (Waterman, 1990), whereas for Bentham, happiness consisted of the presence of pleasure and absence of pain (Tatarkiewicz, 1976). Similarly, according to some contemporary theorists, happiness emerges when several specific life conditions are met, such as self-acceptance, environmental mastery, personal growth, and relatedness (Ryan & Deci, 2001; Ryff, 1989). Others, however, fall in line with the tradition of Bentham by defining happiness as the average online experience of pleasure and pain, (Kahneman, 1999). In this article, we use the term *happiness* interchangeably with subjective well-being or the subjective evaluation of one's life. We conceptualize happiness as being hierarchically organized to emphasize complexity of the concept (see Diener, Scollon, & Lucas, 2003, for more detail). The highest level of the abstraction is happiness, which is a summary judgment of one's life. That is, we do not use the term *happiness* to refer to the momentary feeling state of happiness. Rather, we use this term to refer to a relatively stable feeling of happiness one has towards his or her life. Although we review the studies on the momentary mood of happiness below, when doing so, we will note this fact to distinguish it from the relatively stable feeling of happiness. At the next level of hierarchy, there are four components of happiness: pleasant emotions, unpleasant emotions, life satisfaction, and domain satisfaction. Each of these can be further dissected into specific aspects of life experiences (e.g., love, worry, meaning, health). Although these four components are correlated with one another (e.g., individuals who often feel pleasant emotions tend to be satisfied with their lives as a whole), they are distinguishable from one another (e.g., Lucas, Diener, & Suh, 1996). Similarly, none of the individual components can be equated with overall happiness or subjective well-being. However, because we analyzed data that had been already collected, we use specific components of happiness as proxies to the concept of happiness in the empirical part of this article.

Happiness as the Objective of Life: Why Do People Pursue Happiness?

People seek happiness for a multiplicity of reasons. In his chapter on "The Objective of Life," Aristotle reasoned that happiness is the ultimate goal of life because "we choose it for itself, and never for any other reason" (Thomson, 1953, p. 73). In contrast, all other aspirations (e.g., money, health, reputation, friendship) are instrumental goals pursued in order to meet higher goals, including happiness. Thus, according to Aristotle, it is only rational that happiness is the ultimate objective in life. Once we have happiness, we have all that we want. Although it is possible to debate the extent to which Aristotle's concept of eudaimonia maps on to modern ideas of happiness, it is certainly the case that he included felicitous spirits as one component of the state (i.e., when an individual has fulfilled one's potentials, she is likely to feel happy as well). In addition, later philosophers explicitly equated pleasurable experience with well-being and quality of life. In particular, the utilitarian theorists, such as Jeremy Bentham and J.S. Mill, went so far as to suggest that the principle of promoting the greatest amount of pleasure for the greatest number of people should be the bedrock of morality.

   Yet there are also more practical reasons why people pursue happiness. For instance, happiness is believed to reflect the extent to which one's life is going well (Sumner, 1996). Being happy implies success, whereas not being happy implies failure (King & Napa, 1998). It is no surprise then that many Americans strive for happiness and even feel pressure to be happy (Suh & Koo, in press). There are also hedonic reasons to value happiness. Ordinary citizens, including many who have not read Aristotle, recognize that happiness is pleasant and that unhappiness is unpleasant (Diener, 2000). People consider happiness and pleasantness to be conceptually similar, and indeed, they usually experience these two emotions together (Schimmack, 2006). It simply feels good to be happy, and all organisms are motivated to approach things that bring pleasure and to avoid things that bring pain. Not surprisingly, lay people also recognize the importance of the emotion in their lives. In a recent large international survey led by Ed Diener and with over 10,000 respondents from 48 nations (Diener & Oishi, 2006), the average importance rating of happiness was the highest of the 12 possible attributes, with a mean of 8.03 on a 1–9 scale (compared with 7.54 for "success," 7.39 for "intelligence/knowledge," and 6.84 for "material wealth").

Because both moral philosophers and lay people point to happiness as the ultimate goal that drives more immediate desires, initial research in the area focused on identifying the factors that would allow people to achieve this important goal. Specifically, early research focused on identifying predictors of high subjective well-being (see Diener, Suh, Lucas, & Smith, 1999, for review). Yet more recently, psychologists have begun to acknowledge that happiness is not just an end state that results when things go well. Instead, happiness may also be functional. On the basis of this theory, researchers have begun to systematically examine the consequences of happiness beyond simply feeling good. Lyubomirsky, King, and Diener (2005) conducted a meta-analysis of 225 papers on diverse life outcomes in the domains of work, love, and health and found that, in all three domains, happy people did better on average than did unhappy people. For instance, happy people receive higher job performance assessments from their supervisors (Cropanzano & Wright, 1999) and have more prestigious jobs (Roberts, Caspi, & Moffitt, 2003). In addition, happy people earn higher incomes than do unhappy people, even many years after the initial assessment (Diener, Nickerson, Lucas, & Sandvik, 2002). Happy people are more likely to get married than are their unhappy counterparts (Lucas, Clark, Georgellis, & Diener, 2003), and they are also more satisfied with their marriages (Ruvolo, 1998). Psychologists even live longer if they express more positive emotions and humor in their autobiographies (Pressman, Cohen, & Kollnesher, 2006).

Optimal Levels of Happiness: Is Happier Always Better?

As summarized above, happiness is associated with many desirable life outcomes (Lyubomirsky et al., 2005). However, is happier always better? Emotions likely evolved to solve specific problems that humans faced in their lives (Damasio, 1994; Darwin, 1872; Frijda, 1988; Schwarz, 1990). For example, fear helps people avoid danger (Mowrer, 1939) and prepare for stressful situations (Janis, 1968), anxiety can motivate people to work harder and to perform better (Norem & Cantor, 1986; Svanum & Zody, 2001), and guilt and shame can motivate people to avoid moral transgressions (Baumeister, Stillwell, & Heatherton, 1994). Indeed, although negative affect is unpleasant and often avoided, individuals who experience an absence of negative affect often suffer negative consequences. For instance, it has been suggested that psychopaths (who show little startle reflex; Patrick, Bradley, & Lang, 1993) may have a deficit of certain negative emotions, which leads to moral deficiencies and poor social functioning.

Even when we move beyond specific emotions, it is possible to find examples where unpleasant states motivate beneficial action. Consider the work domain. Job dissatisfaction can be thought of as a signal that the work environment does not fit one's personality and skills. Thus, job dissatisfaction might motivate job change. In fact, a longitudinal study in Switzerland showed that work dissatisfaction predicted job turnover (Semmer, Tschan, Elfering, Kälin, & Grebner, in press) and that those who changed jobs experienced a subsequent increase in job satisfaction in their new job. This study suggests that individuals who are dissatisfied but make efforts to change their life circumstances can improve their satisfaction. Conversely, individuals who consistently experience positive affect and never experience dissatisfaction might be less likely to make a change to improve their life circumstances. Thus, a very high level of satisfaction might lead individuals to fail to attain their full potential.

Although positive moods induced in the laboratory are generally associated with more creativity and better cognitive performance (see Fredrickson, 2001; Isen, 1999, for review), in some circumstances, positive moods are associated with inferior cognitive performance. For instance, in a syllogism task, participants in a positive mood condition performed significantly worse than did participants in the control condition (Melton, 1995). Participants in a positive mood condition also performed more poorly at a moral reasoning task than did those in neutral or sad mood conditions (Zarinpoush, Cooper, & Moylan, 2000). Similarly, participants in a positive mood condition performed worse than did participants in control or negative mood conditions in an estimation of correlation task (Sinclair & Marks, 1995). Finally, participants in a positive mood condition were repeatedly shown to use stereotypes in a person-perception task more frequently than did those in a neutral mood condition (e.g., Bodenhausen, Kramer, & Süsser, 1994).

It is clear that positive moods can occasionally have an adverse influence on life outcomes. In addition, negative moods can help individuals deal with specific problems that require distinct cognitive approaches to arrive at an optimal solution (see Schwarz, 2002, for review). Thus, these studies suggest that people who experience appropriate amounts of negative affect can adopt their cognitive strategy to the task at hand. The question then becomes whether these short-term effects of induced mood translate into long-term differences among those who tend to experience very high levels of these feelings. For instance, in the mood studies, there is an experimentally induced change in participant's affect (e.g., from neutral to happy or from neutral to sad). Thus, the effect of induced mood can be driven mainly by the shift in one's mood. Because individual differences in stable levels of happiness do not involve the temporary shift in mood, the translation of these induced mood effects to individual differences in chronic levels of happiness is problematic. Indeed, few studies have addressed this complex issue explicitly. However, several have provided results that support the idea that very high levels of happiness could be detrimental if they produce positive moods in situations where those feelings provide inappropriate cues to thought and action. For instance, although positive affect has been found to be predictive of longevity among nuns (Danner, Snowdon, & Friesen, 2001), psychologists (Pressman et al., 2006), and numerous other populations (Pressman & Cohen, 2005), a longitudinal study of the intellectually gifted participants in the Terman project showed that childhood cheerfulness rated by teachers and parents was inversely associated with risk of mortality (Friedman et al., 1993). Specifically, individuals who were in the 75th percentile of cheerfulness when they were 10 or 11 years old were estimated to be 21% more likely to die at any given time than were those who were in the 25th percentile. Moreover, childhood cheer-fulness in this sample was associated with more drinking, cigarette smoking, and risky hobbies and activities in adulthood (Martin et al., 2002).

In the only study we know of that has directly addressed the detrimental effects of high levels of positive affect, Fredrickson and Losada (2005) found that students who were flourishing experienced more positive emotions than negative ones at a ratio of 3.2 to 1 in one study and 3.4 to 1 in a second sample. However, these researchers also cautioned that positive-to-negative ratios that were too high were also detrimental. According to their computer simulation based on Lorenz's (1993) chaos theory, ratios above 11.6 led to performance that is suboptimal. Specifically, behavioral repertoires became more and more rigid. This study points to potential undesirable outcomes associated with an excessive amount of positive affect com-bined with an extreme lack of negative affect (see also Schwartz, 1997; Schwartz & Garamoni, 1989, for a similar idea).

In addition, it is not difficult to find anecdotes that could be explained by this account of the detrimental effect of overly positive evaluations. For instance, an active 77-year-old California woman went out to bike during a deadly heat wave, even though her family begged her not to go. She was later found dead of heat stroke (Steinhauer, 2006). Similarly, Maurice Wilson, a man with no mountain climbing experience decided to climb Mount Everest by first crashing a plane on the side of the mountain and then making his way to the top. However, he was later found frozen with his tent wrapped around him, and experts seriously doubt that he made it to the peak. In short, although positive affect and optimism are generally associated with positive outcomes, extreme levels of happiness might have a detrimental effect. These findings and anecdotes point to the possibility that the benefits of positive af-fect may vary, depending on individuals' life circumstances and the life outcome in consideration (see Kaufman & Baer, 2002, for the link between bipolar depression and poetry). Moreover, the literature summarized above suggests that the relation between happiness and various life outcomes may be nonlinear; that is, happier is not always better.

When Should Happier Be Better?

To gain a better understanding of the optimal level of happiness, we first exam-ine the positive consequences of happiness for in various life domains. Accord-ing to most models of ideal functioning, successful individuals are characterized as those who have loving relationships and contribute to society via their work and civic engagements (e.g., Allport, 1961; Keyes & Haidt, 2002; Maslow, 1971; Peterson & Seligman, 2004; Rogers, 1961; Ryan & Deci, 2001; Ryff & Singer, 1998; Sheldon, 2004). Although no perfect measures of success in these domains exist, numerous proxy variables can be obtained. Close relationships, volunteer work, and political participation are believed to capture loving relationships and the civic engagement of well-functioning individuals. Personal income and educational achievement can be thought of as imperfect proxies for the degree to which society values a person's work.

We first predict that a moderate level of happiness is best for life outcomes that require self-improvement motivation and analytical skills. These include such outcomes as academic achievement, job performance, and income. In these domains, slight dissatisfaction with the current situation can serve as motivation to achieve more, earn more money, and obtain more education. For instance, individuals who are completely satisfied with their current job situations might be less likely to acquire additional schooling to improve their credentials or apply for a new, more challenging job that has higher pay. Furthermore, being moderately happy may allow for optimal flexibility when dealing with novel situations. For example, the moderately happy individual may more readily experience worry when a mental heuristic is not working. Thus, he or she may adapt more quickly to new tasks when old strategies do not succeed. We also predict that outcomes related to political participation and civic engagement will be highest when happiness is moderate. Because political participation is motivated in part by dissatisfaction with current political situations (Klandermans, 1989), those who are completely satisfied may feel little motivation to effect change. Similarly, volunteer work is motivated by the desire to improve the status quo. Thus, we predict that the optimal level of happiness in this domain will not be the highest level of happiness, but a moderate level of happiness.

In contrast, we predict that the optimal level of happiness for a stable intimate relationship is the highest level of happiness (rather than a more moderate level). Individuals who are not completely satisfied with their current lives are more likely to actively change their life circumstances, such as by searching for alternative partners, than are those who are extremely satisfied with their lives (e.g., Rusbult, 1980). Indeed, positive illusions about one's partner are instrumental in establishing and maintaining intimacy and relationship stability (Murray, Holmes, & Griffin, 2003). Thus, it might be that the highest levels of happiness lead to the best social relationships.

One other possibility that we explore is whether the optimal level of happiness depends not just on the domain, but on one's circumstances. A happy person in relatively bad circumstances could experience very different outcomes than would a happy person in desirable circumstances. Being very happy in a relatively bad environment might lead to complacency, just as happy workers in less-than-ideal working conditions did not seek to improve their situations (Semmer et al., in press). Because happiness signals that things are going well (Schwarz, 1990), happy individuals are less likely to initiate changes in life circumstances. When life conditions are indeed ideal, this situation is not a problem. However, if life circumstances are far from ideal and some of the circumstances can be changed, too much happiness might become an impediment to positive changes in life.

Few, if any, studies have been specifically designed to explore optimal level of happiness (however, see Maslow, 1971; Rogers, 1961; Sheldon, 2004, for insightful discussions). The current investigation extends previous work on the benefits of happiness (such as Lyubomirsky et al., 2005) by asking for the first time the question "How much happiness is optimal?" (however, see Oishi & Koo, in press, for a preliminary effort). We will next analyze several data sets that allow us to empirically test the optimal level of happiness for various life domains.

Optimal Level of Happiness for Current Success

World Values Survey Data

To examine optimal levels of happiness in broad samples, we first analyzed the World Values Survey, which was administered in 1981, 1990, 1995, and 2000. The sample included 118,519 respondents from 96 countries and regions around the world (see www.worldvaluessurvey.org for more information about the survey questions and samples). Respondents rated their overall life satisfaction on a 10-point scale (in response to the question, "All things considered, how satisfied are you with your life as a whole these days?"). They also indicated their income (in deciles from the lowest 10% in the nation to the highest 10% of the nation), highest education completed, their relationship status (i.e., whether they were currently in a stable long-term relationship), volunteer work they participated in (respondents indicated which, if any, of the 15 types of volunteer work they were involved in), and political actions they had taken (e.g., signing a petition, joining in boycotts). These questions were embedded in more than 200 questions about values and beliefs. Here, we consider income, highest education completed, relationship status, volunteer work, and political participation. Despite imperfections, these measures provide indicators of success and successful functioning (see Lyubomirsky et al., 2005, for similar criteria).

For analysis of these data, we used a regression analysis in which each outcome variable was predicted from the linear well-being score (i.e., the original responses provided by participants) and a dummy variable that tests nonlinearity at the highest end of happiness. Specifically, the dummy variable was coded such that the highest level of well-being is 1 and the rest are coded 0. In the World Values Survey, the linear well-being score was the 10-point life satisfaction score, ranging from 1 to 10. The key dummy code here treated scores of 1–9 as 0 and 10 as 1. If the dummy variable is significantly lower than 0, this indicates that extremely satisfied individuals scored significantly lower than expected based on the linear model.

Our predictions concerning income, education, and political participation were supported, as the highest levels of income, education, and political participation were reported not by the most satisfied individuals (10 on the 10-point scale), but by moderately satisfied individuals (8 or 9 on the 10-point scale, see Table 1). Our prediction regarding close relationships was also supported, as the highest proportion of respondents in a stable intimate relationship was observed among both the very satisfied (10 on the 10-point scale) and satisfied individuals (9 on the 10-point scale). Contrary to our prediction, the highest level of volunteer activities was observed among the very satisfied individuals. This suggests that the motivations that drive

Table 1 The optimal level of happiness

Life satisfaction rating	Men			Women		
	N	M	SD	N	M	SD
Income						
1	2,815	3.25	2.142	2,887	3.09	2.040
2	2,034	4.20	2.379	2,167	3.99	2.343
3	3,039	3.82	2.137	2,975	3.64	2.141
4	3,043	4.06	2.150	2,997	3.88	2.194
5	7,259	4.22	2.120	7,600	4.02	2.181
6	4,812	4.65	2.312	5,063	4.34	2.286
7	6,748	5.07	2.418	6,400	4.73	2.400
8	8,516	5.37	2.532	8,472	5.03	2.526
9	5,406	**5.58**	2.568	5,623	**5.23**	2.581
10	6,620	4.88	2.530	7,355	4.61	2.531
Total	50,292	4.71	2.457	51,540	4.44	2.442
Education						
1	3,092	3.90	2.110	3,192	3.82	2.180
2	2,233	4.06	2.303	2,398	3.68	2.269
3	3,279	4.19	2.258	3,266	3.91	2.286
4	3,321	4.32	2.190	3,306	4.16	2.255
5	8,066	4.38	2.262	8,610	4.05	2.270
6	5,432	4.53	2.203	5,788	4.20	2.253
7	7,733	4.75	2.222	7,475	4.49	2.268
8	9,824	**4.82**	2.198	10,011	**4.66**	2.252
9	6,242	4.79	2.285	6,709	4.56	2.321
10	7,565	4.22	2.272	8,756	4.05	2.252
Total	56,786	4.49	2.251	59,512	4.25	2.283
Political action						
1	2,935	0.5373	0.97701	2,995	0.3846	0.79472
2	2,128	0.5787	0.94007	2,251	0.4505	0.78661
3	3,068	0.6888	1.09811	3,006	0.4298	0.84078
4	3,115	0.6400	1.02667	3,108	0.4933	0.86507
5	7,596	0.5964	1.01525	8,087	0.4535	0.84837
6	5,131	0.6963	1.02778	5,440	0.5286	0.87792
7	7,372	0.8070	1.07284	7,096	0.6298	0.92708
8	9,501	**0.8682**	1.09412	9,597	0.7190	0.97449
9	6,094	0.8603	1.08530	6,483	**0.7401**	0.96393
10	7,313	0.6718	1.01723	8,407	0.5480	0.88636
Total	54,254	0.7257	1.05330	56,468	0.5721	0.90592
Volunteer work						
1	2,105	0.9610	2.09955	2,217	0.7432	1.77238
2	1,051	0.6681	1.46975	1,206	0.5965	1.41521
3	2,180	0.6835	1.55950	2,256	0.5212	1.31047
4	2,114	0.7174	1.47918	2,182	0.5144	1.16532
5	5,282	0.8270	1.76464	5,658	0.6468	1.47731
6	3,602	0.7200	1.49506	3,817	0.5546	1.22231
7	5,493	0.7576	1.54235	5,295	0.5955	1.24198
8	6,736	0.7668	1.38692	6,957	0.6590	1.28102

Table 1 (continued)

Life satisfaction rating	Men			Women		
	N	M	SD	N	M	SD
9	3,704	0.7920	1.33510	4,075	0.7514	1.38403
10	4,452	**1.0145**	1.83718	5,306	**0.8187**	1.58798
Total	36,719	0.8026	1.59975	38,968	0.6566	1.39065
	Relationship status					
1	868	0.68	0.468	1,055	0.52	0.500
2	506	0.67	0.471	642	0.50	0.500
3	973	0.66	0.474	1,121	0.55	0.498
4	992	0.68	0.467	1,132	0.58	0.493
5	2,192	0.70	0.459	2,543	0.63	0.483
6	1,769	0.67	0.471	2,036	0.62	0.487
7	3,014	0.70	0.460	3,022	0.64	0.481
8	4,278	0.73	0.442	4,345	0.69	0.463
9	2,407	**0.76**	0.429	2,747	**0.72**	0.447
10	2,259	**0.76**	0.428	2,770	**0.72**	0.449
Total	19,258	0.71	0.452	21,413	0.65	0.478

Note. Data from World Values Surveys. Income was assessed with the self-report item. "Please indicate your income on the 10-point scale, ranging from 1 = the lowest 10% in the nation to 10 = the highest 10% of the nation." The highest education attained was assessed with the following scale: 1 = *don't know/not applicable*, 2 = *no formal education*, 3 = *inadequately completed elementary school*; 4 = *completed (compulsory) elementary school*; 5 = *incomplete secondary school: technical, vocational type*; 6 = *complete secondary school; technical, vocational type*; 7 = *incomplete secondary school; university prep type*; 8 = *complete secondary school: university prep type*; 9 = *some university without degree*; 10 = *university with degree or higher*. Political action was assessed by taking the sum of the following type of political actions taken by respondents: signing a petition, joining in boycotts, attending lawful demonstrations, joining unofficial strikes, and occupying buildings or factories (range = 0–5). Volunteer work was assessed by summing the number of the unpaid work conducted by respondents for the following types of organizations: social welfare service for elderly, church organization, cultural activities, labor union, political parties, local political organization, human rights, environment, conservation, animal rights, professional associations, youth work, sports or recreation, women's group, peace movement, health-related, or other groups (range = 0–15). Relationship status was assessed by 0 (*not in a stable relationship*) or 1 (*in a stable relationship*). Values in bold face indicate highest level of life satisfaction

volunteer work may be more similar to those that drive relationship variables than to those the drive political action (see Discussion for more detail).

We next tested the linear and nonlinear models by the regression analysis described above. As predicted, respondents who were very satisfied with their lives (10 on the 10-point scale) earned significantly less money than expected based on a pure linear model, $B = -0.92$, $SE = 0.03$, $\beta = -0.13$, $t(101860) = -35.70$, $p < 0.001$. In addition, very satisfied individuals completed significantly less education than expected based on the linear model, $B = -0.78$, $SE = 0.02$, $\beta = -0.12$, $t(116330) = -34.30$, $p < 0.001$. Furthermore, very satisfied respondents engaged in political activity significantly less than expected based on the linear model,

$B = -0.24$, $SE = 0.01$, $\beta = -0.09$, $t(110759) = -24.09$, $p < 0.001$. In contrast, the nonlinear effect of happiness on stable intimate relationship was not significant, $B = -0.01$, $SE = 0.01$, $\beta = -0.004$, $t(40677) = -0.78$, $p = 0.44$. Likewise, the respondents who were very satisfied with their lives engaged in even more volunteer activities than expected based on the linear model, $B = 0.20$, $SE = 0.02$, $\beta = 0.04$, $t(75721) = 10.31$, $p < 0.001$. In sum, the highest possible level of life satisfaction was superior in terms of volunteer work and relationship status, whereas moderately high levels of life satisfaction were best in terms of income, education, and political participation.

Illinois Data

As a second approach to testing the optimal level of happiness, we turned to a semester-long intensive data collection project conducted with students from the University of Illinois. As in the World Values Survey, participants completed a number of measures related to achievement and conscientiousness. In addition, they completed a variety of measures in the social relationships domain. Finally, respondents reported their affect on a daily basis over a period of approximately 7 weeks. Using these reports, we divided participants into groups based on affect balance—the degree to which positive affect was experienced more frequently than negative affect. The very happy subjects reported feeling positive emotions most of the time and rarely feeling negative emotions, whereas the unhappy respondents reported feeling negative emotions more frequently than positive ones. Unhappy respondents were defined as individuals with a negative affect balance score (reporting feeling more negative emotions than positive ones), and this group was only 5% of the sample. The slightly happy group comprised individuals whose positive emotion score exceeded their negative emotion score by 0 or 1 point. Similarly, the preponderance of positive to negative feelings for the other groups was as follows: moderately happy = 1.01–2.00 points; happy = 2.01–3.00 points; and very happy = above 3.00 points (12% of the sample).

We replicated the findings from the World Values Survey in this college data set. As expected, the second happiest group (labeled "Happy" in Table 2) performed best on all four achievement/conscientiousness measures such as grades and number of missed classes. In contrast, the happiest group (labeled "Very happy" in Table 2) scored highest in all five social measures such as time spent dating and the number of close friends. Significance testing mostly confirmed the visual inspection of the data above, showing that the nonlinear pattern for the highest affect-balance group held for three of the four achievement/conscientiousness measures but did not hold for any of the social measures. Grade point average (GPA) showed a significant linear trend for affect balance, $B = 0.18$, $SE = 0.05$, $\beta = 0.32$, $t(191) = 3.40$, $p < 0.001$, as well as a significant non-linear trend for the happiest group, $B = -0.43$, $SE = 0.16$, $\beta = -0.25$, $t(191) = 2.64$, $p < 0.01$. Namely, general affect balance was positively associated with GPA except at the highest end of happiness. Very happy people did not receive as high a GPA as expected

Table 2 College student success

	Affect balance				
Outcome	Unhappy ($N=8$)	Slightly happy ($N=43$)	Moderately happy ($N=75$)	Happy ($N=42$)	Very happy ($N=25$)
Grade point average	3.2 (0.6)	3.9 (0.5)	3.9 (0.6)	**4.1** (0.5)	3.8 (0.7)
Missed class	0.8 (0.9)	0.4 (0.3)	0.5 (0.4)	**0.3** (0.3)	0.4 (0.3)
Event balance	0.6 (2.8)	0.4 (2.5)	1.5 (3.1)	**2.9** (3.6)	1.3 (2.5)
Conscientiousness	15.6 (2.9)	17.5 (4.1)	19.3 (4.8)	**20.7** (3.7)	18.6 (4.7)
Gregarious	18.8 (4.9)	17.2 (5.2)	19.8 (4.3)	18.7 (4.3)	**20.5** (3.7)
Close friends	4.4 (1.6)	4.7 (1.3)	5.1 (1.2)	5.5 (1.3)	**5.8** (1.0)
Self-confidence	3.9 (1.7)	4.2 (1.6)	4.9 (1.4)	5.0 (1.3)	**5.6** (0.8)
Energy	4.0 (2.0)	4.2 (1.1)	4.7 (1.0)	5.1 (1.1)	**5.3** (1.0)
Time dating	2.8 (1.5)	3.1 (1.8)	4.1 (2.1)	4.3 (1.9)	**5.3** (2.0)

Note. Data are means with standard deviations in parentheses. Affect balance was the frequency of five positive affects (joy, affection, contentment, happy, and satisfaction) minus the frequency of negative emotions (anger, anxiety, sadness, guilt, and boredom). Grade point average was a 5-point scale (where $5 = A$). Missed class was the average number of classes missed on class days, where students had an average of about three classes per day. Event balance was the number of 20 specific objective positive events experienced minus the number of 29 objective negative life events experienced, with scores ranging from -9 to $+10$. Examples of positive events were "getting into graduate school" and "got a car," whereas examples of negative events were "got a traffic ticket" and "had an operation." Conscientiousness and gregariousness were the NEO scale and facet scores for these concepts. Close friends, self-confidence, and energy were self-ratings of these resources on a 7-point scale. Time dating was the amount of time spent socializing with date or romantic partner, where 2.8 indicates about 4 min and 5.3 is about 40 min per day

from the linear model. Similarly, affect balance was positively associated with the event balance score (i.e., how many objectively positive relative to negative events participants experienced), $\beta = 0.38$, $t(191) = 4.34$, $p < 0.001$, except at the highest end of happiness, $\beta = -0.24$, $t(191) = 2.78$, $p < 0.01$. Very happy people did not experience as many positive events relative to negative events as expected from the linear model. Likewise, affect balance was positively associated with the Big Five factor of Conscientiousness, $B = 1.75$, $SE = 0.37$, $\beta = 0.41$, $t(191) = 4.73$, $p < 0.001$, except at the highest end of happiness, $B = -3.60$, $SE = 1.20$, $\beta = -0.26$, $t(191) = -3.01$, $p < 0.01$. Very happy people were not as conscientious as expected from the linear model. The extent to which participants missed class showed a significant linear trend, $B = -0.12$, $SE = 0.04$, $\beta = -0.30$, $t(191) = -3.35$, $p < 0.001$, but not a significant nonlinear effect. In terms of the social variables, there was an expected significant linear trend for close friends, $B = 0.36$, $SE = 0.11$, $\beta = 0.29$, $t(191) = 3.28$, $p < 0.001$, self-confidence, $B = 0.48$, $SE = 0.12$, $\beta = 0.36$, $t = 4.16$, $p < 0.001$, energy, $B = 0.50$, $SE = 0.09$, $\beta = 0.45$, $t(191) = 5.28$, $p < 0.001$, and time spent dating, $B = 0.52$, $SE = 0.17$, $\beta = 0.26$, $t(191) = 3.03$, $p < 0.01$. In short, the happier person tended to score high on social domain measures but did not always score high on achievement/conscientiousness measures.

Optimal Levels of Happiness for Future Success

Although the World Values Survey and the University of Illinois data provide initial support for our hypotheses, the data on life satisfaction and outcome measures were measured concurrently. Thus, it is unclear whether a particular level of happiness is predictive of later success. To address this limitation, we review four longitudinal studies in which well-being was initially assessed and life outcomes were obtained many years later.

College and Beyond Data and American Freshman Data

Diener et al. (2002) analyzed a large set of longitudinal data from participants who had entered one of 25 mostly elite colleges in 1976. In this study, participants reported their cheerfulness when they were incoming college freshman, on a 5-point scale (1 = *lowest* 10%, 2 = *below average*, 3 = *average*, 4 = *above average*, 5 = *highest* 10%). Nineteen years later, at about age 37, these participants reported their annual income. The effects of a cheerful disposition on income were substantial. As seen in Table 3, the participants in the highest 10% of cheerfulness in 1976 earned an average of \$62,681 in 1995, whereas the participants in the lowest 10% of cheerfulness in 1976 earned an average of \$54,318. Furthermore, the most cheerful students at college entry were approximately two thirds as likely to ever be unemployed as were the least cheerful participants. Thus, cheerfulness was associated with both increased earnings later in life and a lower likelihood of unemployment. In keeping with our predictions, however, we found that those who were moderately cheerful (rated above average on cheerfulness) earned the most (\$66,144; see Table 3). Thus, if we use income as a criterion, the best level of cheerfulness was not the highest level, but a more moderate level. We next tested the linear and nonlinear models with a regression analysis similar to that described earlier. As predicted, respondents who reported being in the highest 10% in cheerfulness in 1976 earned significantly less money in 1995 than was expected from the linear model, $B = -6,063.92$, $SE = 2,178.08$, $\beta = -0.04$, $t(7889) = -2.78$, $p < 0.01$. However, in terms of unemployment history, there was no nonlinear effect.

It is also interesting to note that Diener et al. (2002) found a significant interaction between cheerfulness and parental income, such that the association between cheerfulness upon entering college and later income was stronger among individuals

Table 3 Nineteen-year longitudinal study of cheerfulness and income

Cheerfulness in 1976	Income in 1995
1 (*lowest 10%*)	\$54,318
2 (*below average*)	\$61,664
3 (*average*)	\$63,509
4 (*above average*)	\$66,144
5 (*highest 10%*)	\$62,681

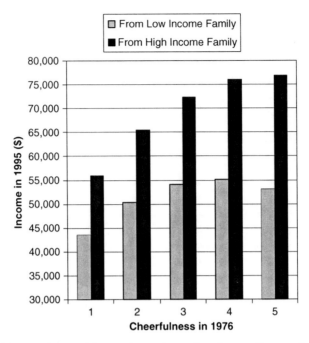

Fig. 1 Cheerfulness and parental income interaction on later income. Data are from individuals from low income families (one standard deviation below mean) and high income families (one standard deviation above mean)

from affluent families than those from poor families. Figure 1 shows the income by cheerfulness interaction for those with the poorest and most affluent parents. For instance, among individuals from well-off families (whose parental income was one standard deviation above the mean), the difference between the least cheerful individual and the most cheerful individual was more than $20,000: that is, those who rated themselves in the lowest 10% in cheerfulness earned \$55,951,[2] whereas those who rated themselves in the highest 10% earned \$76,948. In contrast, among individuals from poor families (whose parental income was one standard deviation below the mean), the difference in income between the very cheerful and the least cheerful people was less than $10,000; those who rated themselves in the lowest 10% in cheerfulness earned \$43,589, whereas those who rated themselves in the highest 10% earned \$53,097. In addition, when examined separately, the optimal level of cheerfulness for income among individuals from wealthy families was the highest 10%, whereas the optimal level was above average among individuals from poor families. In sum, the interaction between cheerfulness of the participants and their family background nicely illustrates that the effect of cheerful disposition on future income varies depending on individuals' life circumstances. High parental

---

[2] The incomes described in this paragraph are based on a regression equation (i.e., estimated income for those who were one standard deviation above or below the mean).

income suggests a benevolent environment. In a benevolent environment, boldness often results in positive outcomes. Cheerfulness is adaptive in a benevolent environment perhaps because optimism and sociability associated with cheerfulness help individuals to be bold. In contrast, low parental income suggests a harsh environment. Cheerfulness in a harsh environment might not be as adaptive, because it could lead individuals to be content with their less-than-ideal conditions and does not motivate them to improve their life circumstances. The interaction between cheerfulness and parental income on the future income seems to illustrate that the maximal success is obtained when one's level of cheerfulness is matched with their circumstances.

Australian Youth Data

The Australian Youth in Transition study, a longitudinal study of nationally representative cohorts of young people in Australia, also showed that life satisfaction predicts later earning (Marks & Fleming, 1999). To determine whether the nonlinear effect could be replicated, however, we obtained data for the 1961 birth cohorts and analyzed these data in a way analogous to those presented above. The Australian respondents indicated their life satisfaction ("satisfaction with life as a whole") when they were 18 years old (in 1979). They also reported their gross income in 1994, when they were 33 years old ($N = 1,166$). The Australian data replicated Diener et al.'s (2002) findings. Income in 1994 increases linearly from those reporting to be least satisfied in 1979 to those reporting the average level of satisfaction, peaks at those reporting the moderately satisfied level (4 on the 5-point scale), and then decreases for those at the very high level of satisfaction. In keeping with our prediction and the findings of Diener et al. (2002), "very satisfied" respondents in 1979 did not earn as much money in 1994 as expected from the linear model, $\beta = -0.07, t(1163) = -1.78, p = 0.076$, although this did not reach the 0.05 level of significance (Fig. 2).

Respondents from the Australian Youth in Transition Study also reported the number of years of schooling they completed beyond primary education in 1987, when they were 26 years old. Similar to the income findings, the highest levels of education were reported by those individuals who had moderate levels of satisfaction in 1979. The individuals who reported that they were very satisfied in 1979 did not obtain as much education as would be expected based on the linear model, $\beta = -0.19, t(776) = -3.52, p < 0.01$. Respondents also reported the length of their current intimate relationship in 1994. In contrast to the income and education findings, individuals from the very satisfied group in 1979 were involved in longer intimate relationships in 1994 than were individuals from the second and third most-satisfied groups (see Fig. 3). Indeed, although the linear trend was again significant $\beta = 0.14, t(1468) = 3.91, p < 0.01$, the nonlinear parameter was not, $\beta = -0.03, t(1468) = -0.88, p = 0.38$. In short, the Australian Youth in Transition study supports the prediction that the optimal level of happiness is not the highest level of happiness in the domains of educational achievement and income later in life. However, the highest level of satisfaction may in fact be optimal in terms of relationship stability.

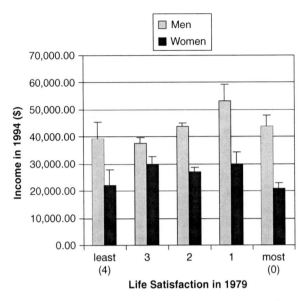

Fig. 2 Australian Longitudinal Study: Life satisfaction and income. Data are from men and women surveyed in 1979 (for life satisfaction) and again in 1994 (for income). *Error bars* represent standard error

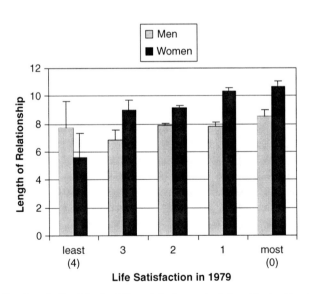

Fig. 3 Australian Longitudinal Study: Life satisfaction and relationship duration. Data are from men and women first surveyed in 1979. *Error bars* represent standard error

German and British Panel Data

The two longitudinal data sets that we analyzed above relied on a single-item measure assessed at a single time point. To address the weaknesses associated with
these data sets, we next analyzed data from two long-running panel studies, the
German Socio-Economic Panel Study (GSOEP; for details see Haisken-De New &
Frick, 2005) and the British Household Panel Study (BHPS; for details see Taylor, Brice, Buck, & Prentice-Lane, 2005; University of Essex Institute for Social
and Economic Research, 2006), which allowed us to aggregate a single-item life
satisfaction item across multiple assessment points. The GSOEP study began in
1984 and initially included a nationally representative sample of households in West
Germany. Twenty waves of data were available for this analysis. The BHPS began
in 1991 and, again, a nationally representative sample of household was selected for
participation. In both studies, participants answered a single-item life satisfaction
item, and this question was administered in every year of the GSOEP and in 7 out
of the last 8 years of the BHPS.

For each study, we constructed an aggregate life-satisfaction measure by averaging across multiple waves. For the longer GSOEP, we aggregated across the first
4 years; for the shorter BHPS, we aggregated across the first 3 years. We then
predicted respondents' income in the most recent waves of the study from these
initial life satisfaction measures. These two data sets clearly support our hypothesis regarding happiness and future earning, as the pattern of declining income
among the happiest people again emerges (see Figs. 4 and 5). Individuals with
moderately high levels of satisfaction reported higher incomes than did individuals
with low levels of life satisfaction. However, as predicted, after this point, salary
levels drop for the happiest individuals. Regression analyses (reflected in the regression lines in Figs. 4 and 5) show that this drop-off is significant: $B_{Quadratic} =$
-481.84, $SE = 92.49$, $\beta = -0.08$, $t(4906) = -5.21$, $p < 0.001$, for the GSOEP,
and $B_{Quadratic} = -70.42$, $SE = 15.91$, $\beta = -0.09$, $t(2844) = -4.43$, $p < 0.001$, for
the BHPS. Furthermore, this effect is still significant even after controlling for salary
in the first 4 years of the survey (i.e., controlling for initial success), $B_{Quadratic} =$
-312.98, $SE = 88.17$, $\beta = -0.05$, $t(4905) = -3.55$, $p < 0.001$, for the GSOEP, and
$B_{Quadratic} = -30.25$, $SE = 13.79$, $\beta = -0.04$, $t(2273) = -2.19$, $p < 0.05$, for the
BHPS. The fact that the drop-off in income occurs not just among those individuals
who consistently use the topmost (10) response option suggests that the suboptimal
effect of a very high level of happiness on future income that we identified is not
due to the way that people use response scales.

Discussion

The findings from our analyses of a very large cross-sectional survey, an intense
data collection project with college students, and four large longitudinal data sets
revealed a consistent pattern of results. As expected, the optimal level of happiness

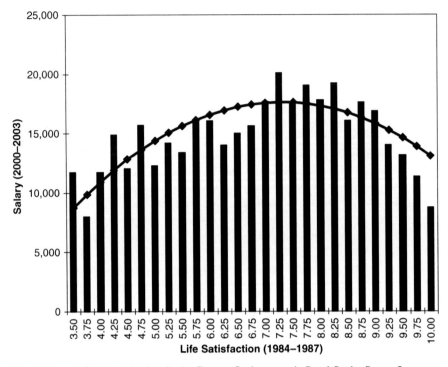

Fig. 4 Life satisfaction and salary in the German Socioeconomic Panel Study. *Bars* reflect average income at the listed life satisfaction level. The *line* reflects the estimated quadratic effect of life satisfaction on salary. Values lower than 3.50 are not shown because of the small number of participants (< 10) per cell

varies across domains and contexts. The optimal level of happiness in the domains of volunteer work and relationships is the highest possible level of happiness. In contrast, the optimal level of happiness for achievement outcomes including income and education is a moderate (but still high) level of happiness. Before discussing our main findings further, we would like to make clear what we are not saying. We are not saying that it is bad to be very happy. We are also not saying that it is desirable to be unhappy. The results reported in this article do not support either of these views. Although it is true that the very happy people tend to be worse off than the moderately happy in certain domains, they still tend to report more successful functioning than do those individuals who are at the midpoint of the distribution, and they are usually better off than are those at the lowest ends.

Fully functioning individuals are often described as those who have loving relationships and contribute to society via work, family, volunteer work, and political engagement (e.g., Keyes & Haidt, 2002; Peterson & Seligman, 2004; Ryan & Deci, 2001; Ryff & Singer, 1998; Sheldon, 2004). Given that no specific level of happiness is associated with all of these positive outcomes, there is no single level

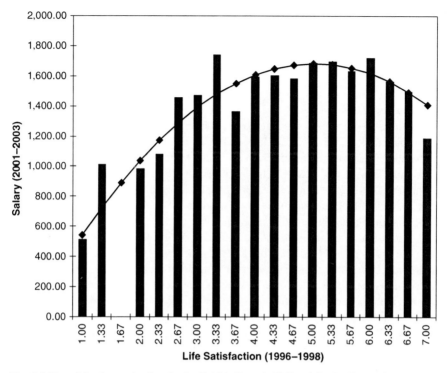

Fig. 5 Life satisfaction and salary in the British Household Panel Study. *Bars* reflect average income at the listed life satisfaction level. The *line* reflects the estimated quadratic effect of life satisfaction on salary

of happiness that is optimal for every individual and every activity. The optimal level of happiness is likely to vary across individuals, depending on their value priorities (cf. Oishi, Diener, Suh, & Lucas, 1999). For those whose primary values center on achievement, moderately high levels of happiness may be optimal; for those individuals whose values give priority to close relationships and volunteer work, it is the highest level of happiness that appears to be optimal. In addition, functional levels of happiness might vary across individuals, depending on their personality dispositions. Tamir (2005), for instance, found that neurotics were more likely than were nonneurotics to choose to increase their levels of worry when performing a demanding task. Furthermore, Tamir offered preliminary evidence that this might have been beneficial for their performance. Thus, the benefit of happy mood might be moderated by individuals' values and personality (see also Norem & Illingworth, 1993). In addition, the optimal level of happiness is likely to differ across cultures, as individuals from different cultures seek different types of positive emotions (e.g., Eid & Diener, 2001; Kitayama, Markus, & Kurokawa, 2000; Tsai, Knutson, & Fung, 2006) and the consequence of positive affect differs across cultures (e.g., Oishi & Diener, 2003).

Why Do Optimal Levels of Happiness Differ in Various Domains?

Complete satisfaction with current conditions might prevent individuals from energetically pursuing change in achievement domains such as education and income. After all, the defining characteristics of need for achievement are high standards of excellence and constant striving for perfection (McClelland, 1961). Similarly, if individuals are completely satisfied with the current political situation, they might be less likely to actively participate in the political process. Whereas wanting more may be an important motivation for income, education, and political participation, in the domain of intimate relationships, wanting more might be detrimental because it prompts individuals to search for alternative partners (e.g., Rusbult, 1980) and to more readily see the faults of others. Indeed, Murray and her colleagues repeatedly found that the idealization of partners and positive illusions about partners are beneficial to relationship quality and stability (see Murray et al., 2003, for review). Individuals who are fully satisfied with their current lives are more likely to view their partner in an idealistic fashion than are others who are not fully satisfied with their lives. In contrast to the achievement situation in which hard work (and wanting more) is usually essential, in the social situation, it may be the case that being content is most beneficial. Thus, the optimal mindset for an intimate relationship might be to see mostly the positive aspects of the partner and relationship, whereas the optimal mindset for income, education, and political participation might be to simultaneously consider the empty part of the glass as well as the fullness of it.

Whereas the patterns of optimal happiness levels for the various outcomes discussed above were consistent with our theoretical predictions, the optimal level of happiness for volunteer work was, unexpectedly, the highest possible level of happiness. Our expectation that above-average happiness would prove optimal was based on the assumption that individuals are motivated to engage in volunteer work in order to make the world a better place and that individuals completely satisfied with their lives and the world might not engage in these activities as much as others who are moderately satisfied. However, there are many motivations for volunteer work, from humanitarian values to self-esteem to social networking (Omoto & Snyder, 1995). Previous research has shown that volunteer work is associated with sociability and agreeableness (Graziano & Eisenberg, 1997), which in turn are positively associated with life satisfaction (e.g., Schimmack, Oishi, Furr, & Funder, 2004). The level of happiness is linearly associated with volunteer work perhaps because it is also linearly associated with agreeableness and sociability. In short, volunteer work might be more similar to close relationships than to achievement domains in terms of its motivational mechanism.

Optimal Variability in Happiness and Other Remaining Issues

Our analyses and discussion so far have focused exclusively on the optimal mean level of happiness. It is important to explore the optimal variability in happiness in the future, as humans are expected to act in accordance with highly variable contexts and there might be an optimal level of variability in happiness. Some might believe that our arguments suggest that flexibility in feelings of positive and negative moods and emotions is the key to effective functioning. Although this is undoubtedly true, as being locked into any specific emotion would be dysfunctional, Eid and Diener (1999) found that people with a large range in their emotions tended to be neurotic. It is interesting that people who were variable on positive emotions were also variable on negative emotions. Thus, variability by itself is probably not sufficient for optimal functioning, and a tendency to experience primarily positive emotions seems functional, at least in many circumstances in the modern world. However, there may also be an optimal level of flexibility in one's emotions, with extreme values in either direction being dysfunctional.

Our analysis has treated subjective well-being as a single entity, whereas there are in fact clearly separable components of happiness (Lucas et al., 1996; Ryan & Deci, 2001; Ryff, 1989). In some of our analyses, we analyzed life satisfaction or cheerfulness, and in other analyses, we used affect balance (the difference between people's experience of positive and negative emotions). We were limited in this endeavour by the subjective well-being variables that were included in the data sets we used. However, it will be important in future research to explore the optimal levels of various types of well-being and discrete emotions. For example, very high levels of purpose and meaning might be beneficial to all kinds of success, whereas very high levels of pleasant emotions, especially intense or aroused ones, may be mixed in their effects. Another important direction for the future is to analyze the combination and interaction of various forms of well-being. For example, most Americans report positive life satisfaction, but a substantial percentage also report being stressed (Pomerantz, Saxon, & Oishi, 2000). Perhaps this combination is functional for a group with American values, in a society where people "want it all" rather than taking a more relaxed view of life. Finally, it is important to identify mediating processes of the connection between a particular level of happiness and success. For instance, the link between the moderate level of happiness and the maximal earning in the future might be mediated by need for achievement, whereas the link between the highest level of happiness and relationship stability might be mediated by variables such as optimism and agreeableness.

Conclusion

Happiness has become a major goal in life around the world (Diener & Oishi, 2006). However, there are dangers involved in searching for ultrahappiness. Because adaptation occurs (Diener, Lucas, & Scollon, 2006; Wilson & Gilbert, 2003) and people's happiness is influenced in part by their temperaments (Lykken & Tellegen, 1996), obtaining continuously high levels of happiness could require risky behaviors such as thrill-seeking activities and the use of drugs. Seeking very high levels of positive affect might also stimulate novelty seeking, in which the person continually seeks new partners and new activities so that aroused levels of positive affect can be maintained. However, this type of search for intense happiness is likely to lead to instability in a person's life.

Ryff (1989) raised the issue of whether subjective well-being has been overemphasized in our conceptions of psychological well-being (see also Ryan & Deci, 2001). In keeping with her analysis, our findings suggest that extremely high levels of happiness might not be a desirable goal and that there is more to psychological well-being than high levels of happiness. It is up to psychologists to educate lay people about optimal levels of happiness and the levels of happiness that are realistic. However, psychologists have not yet been able to give much advice with confidence because no data have existed on these issues. This article represents a first effort to answer the question, "How much happiness is enough?".

As people in modern societies seek higher levels of happiness, a concerted effort is needed to determine the intricate patterns of outcomes resulting from being happy, very happy, or extremely happy. The effects of moods on behavior have been studied by psychologists, but little research has been aimed at uncovering the effects of long-term, more chronic levels of affect and satisfaction on functioning. The optimal levels of happiness are likely to depend on a person's resources, the challenges and dangers they face, the behavioral domain in question, and the type of well-being under consideration. Despite the complexity that is involved, the question of how much happiness is optimal is worth vigorously pursuing because it is a key issue for both scientific and applied psychology.

Acknowledgments Because of the editor's coauthorship, this article was assigned to an outside editor, Christopher Peterson of the University of Michigan. Professor Peterson obtained outside reviewers whose identity was masked from the editor, and he had full editorial authority over the article. We want to thank the guest editor and the reviewers for their work on this article and for their very helpful suggestions.

The data used in this article were made available by the German Institute for Economic Research and by the United Kingdom Data Archive. The British Household Panel Study data were originally collected by the Economic and Social Research Council Research Centre on Micro-Social Change at the University of Essex, now incorporated within the Institute for Social and Economic Research. Neither the original collectors of the data nor the Archive bear any responsibility for the analyses or interpretations presented here.

We would like to thank Gary N. Marks for making the Australian Youth Study data available to us. We would also like to thank Carol Nickerson for her help with the data concerning cheerfulness and later income/unemployment history and Frank Fujita for his help with the Illinois data.

Finally, it should be noted that the descriptive statistics for the World Values Survey and Australian Youth Study reported here are also reported in Oishi and Koo (in press). Shigehiro Oishi was supported by National Institute of Mental Health Grant R01MH066857-01A1 and Richard E. Lucas was supported by National Institute on Aging Grants 1R03AG026028-01 and 1R03AG028744-01 during the preparation of this article.

References

Allport, G. W. (1961). *Pattern and growth in personality*. New York: Holt, Rinehart, & Winston.
Baumeister, R. F., Campbell, J. D., Krueger, J. I., & Vohs, K. D. (2003). Does high self-esteem cause better performance, interpersonal success, happiness, or healthier lifestyles? *Psychological Science in the Public Interest, 4*, 1–44.

Baumeister, R. F., Stillwell, A. M., & Heatherton, T. E. (1994). Guilt: An interpersonal approach. *Psychological Bulletin, 115,* 243–267.

Bodenhausen, G. V., Kramer, G. P., & Süsser, K. (1994). Happiness and stereotypic thinking in social judgment. *Journal of Personality and Social Psychology, 66,* 621–632.

Crocker, J., & Park, L. E. (2004). The costly pursuit of self-esteem. *Psychological Bulletin, 130,* 392–414.

Cropanzano, R., & Wright, T. A. (1999). A 5-year study of change in the relationship between well-being and job performance. *Consulting Psychology Journal: Practice and Research, 51,* 252–265.

Damasio, A. R. (1994). *Descartes' error: Emotion, reason, and the human brain.* New York: Putnam.

Danner, D. D., Snowdon, D. A., & Friesen, W. V. (2001). Positive emotions in early life and longevity: Findings from the nun study. *Journal of Personality and Social Psychology, 80,* 804–813.

Darwin, C. (1872). *The expression of emotions in man and animals.* Chicago: University of Chicago Press.

Diener, E. (2000). Subjective well-being: The science of happiness and a proposal for a national index. *American Psychologist, 55,* 34–43.

Diener, E., & Diener, C. (1996). Most people are happy. *Psychological Science, 7,* 181–185.

Diener, E., Lucas, R., & Scollon, C. N. (2006). Beyond the hedonic treadmill: Revising the adaptation theory of well-being. *American Psychologist, 61,* 305–314.

Diener, E., Nickerson, C., Lucas, R. E., & Sandvik, E. (2002). Dispositional affect and job outcomes. *Social Indicators Research, 59,* 229–259.

Diener, E., & Oishi, S. (2006). *The desirability of happiness across cultures.* Unpublished manuscript, University of Illinois, Urbana-Champaign.

Diener, E., Scollon, C. N., & Lucas, R. E. (2003). The evolving concept of subjective well-being: The multifaceted nature of happiness. *Advances in Cell Aging and Gerontology, 15,* 187–219.

Diener, E., & Seligman, M. E. P. (2004). Beyond money: Toward an economy of well-being. *Psychological Science in the Public Interest, 5,* 1–31.

Diener, E., Suh, E. M., Lucas, R. E., & Smith, H. L. (1999). Subjective well-being: Three decades of progress. *Psychological Bulletin, 125,* 276–302.

Eid, M., & Diener, E. (1999). Intraindividual variability in affect; Reliability, validity, and personality correlates. *Journal of Personality and Social Psychology, 76,* 662–676.

Eid, M., & Diener, E. (2001). Norms for experiencing emotions in different cultures: Inter- and intranational differences. *Journal of Personality and Social Psychology, 81,* 869–885.

Fredrickson, B. L. (2001). The role of positive emotions in positive psychology: The broaden-and-build theory of positive emotions. *American Psychologist, 56,* 218–226.

Fredrickson, B. L., & Losada, M. F. (2005). Positive affect and the complex dynamics of human flourishing. *American Psychologist, 60,* 678–686.

Friedman, H. S., Tucker, J. S., Tomlinson-Keasey, C., Schwartz, J. E., Wingard, D. L., & Criqui, M. H. (1993). Does childhood personality predict longevity? *Journal of Personality and Social Psychology, 65,* 176–185.

Frijda, N. (1988). The laws of emotion. *American Psychologist, 43,* 349–358.

Graziano, W. G., & Eisenberg, N. (1997). Agreeableness: A dimension of personality. In R. Hogan, R. Johnson, & S. Briggs (Eds.), *Handbook of personality psychology* (pp. 795–824). San Diego, CA: Academic.

Haisken-De New, J. P., & Frick, R. (2005). *Desktop companion to the German Socio-Economic Panel Study (GSOEP).* Berlin, Germany: German Institute for Economic Research (DIW).

Isen, A. M. (1999). Positive affect. In T. Dalgleish & M. Powers (Eds.), *The handbook of cognition and emotion* (pp. 75–94). Hillsdale, NJ: Erlbaum.

Janis, I. (1968). When fear is healthy. *Psychology Today, 11,* 46–49, 60–61.

Kahneman, D. (1999). Objective happiness. In D. Kahneman, E. Diener, & N. Schwarz (Eds.), *Well-being: The foundations of hedonic psychology* (pp. 3–25). New York: Russell Sage Foundation.

Kahneman, D., Krueger, A. B., Schkade, D. A., Schwarz, N., & Stone, A. A. (2004). A survey method for characterizing daily life experience: The day reconstruction method. *Science, 306*, 1776–1780.

Kaufman, J. C., & Baer, J. (2002). I bask in dreams of suicide: Mental illness, poetry, and women. *Review of General Psychology, 6*, 271–286.

Keyes, C. L. M., & Haidt, J. (2002). *Flourishing: Positive psychology and the life well-lived*. Washington, DC: American Psychological Association.

King, L.A., & Napa, C.K. (1998). What makes a life good? *Journal of Personality and Social Psychology, 75*, 156–165.

Kitayama, S., Markus, H. R., & Kurokawa, M. (2000). Culture, emotion, and well-being: Good feelings in Japan and the United States. *Cognition and Emotion, 14*, 93–124.

Klandermans, B. (1989). Does happiness soothe political protest? The complex relation between discontent and political unrest. In R. Veenhoven (Ed.), *How harmful is happiness? Consequences of enjoying life or not*. Rotterdam, The Netherlands: Universitaire Pers Rotterdam.

Lorenz, E. N. (1993). *The essence of chaos*. Seattle: University of Washington Press.

Lucas, R. E., Clark, A. E., Georgellis, Y., & Diener, E. (2003). Reexamining adaptation and the set point model of happiness: Reactions to changes in marital status. *Journal of Personality and Social Psychology, 84*, 527–539.

Lucas, R. E., Diener, E., & Suh, E. (1996). Discriminant validity of well-being measures. *Journal of Personality and Social Psychology, 71*, 616–628.

Lykken, D., & Tellegen, A. (1996). Happiness is a stochastic phenomenon. *Psychological Science, 7*, 186–189.

Lyubomirsky, S., King, L., & Diener, E. (2005). The benefits of frequent positive affect: Does happiness lead to success? *Psychological Bulletin, 131*, 803–855.

Marks, G. N., & Fleming, N. (1999). Influences and consequences of well-being among Australian young people: 1980–1995. *Social Indicators Research, 46*, 301–323.

Martin, L. R., Friedman, H. S., Tucker, J. S., Tomlinson-Keasey, C., Criqui, M. H., & Schwartz, J. E. (2002). A life course perspective on childhood cheerfulness and its relation to mortality risk. *Personality and Social Psychology Bulletin, 28*, 1155–1165.

Maslow, A. H. (1971). *The farther reaches of human nature*. New York: Viking.

McClelland, D. C. (1961). *The achieving society*. New York: D. Van Nostrand.

Melton, R. J. (1995). The role of positive affect in syllogism performance. *Personality and Social Psychology Bulletin, 21*, 788–794.

Mowrer, O. H. (1939). A stimulus-response analysis of anxiety and its role as a reinforcing agent. *Psychological Review, 46*, 553–565.

Murray, S. L., Holmes, J. G., & Griffin, D. W. (2003). Reflections on the self-fulfilling effects of positive illusions. *Psychological Inquiry, 14*, 289–295.

Norem, J. K., & Cantor, N. (1986). Defensive pessimism: Harnessing anxiety as motivation. *Journal of Personality and Social Psychology, 51*, 1208–1217.

Norem, J. K., & Illingworth, K. S. S. (1993). Strategy dependent effects of reflecting on self and tasks: Some implications of optimism and defensive pessimism. *Journal of Personality and Social Personality, 65*, 822–835.

Oishi, S., & Diener, E. (2003). Culture and well-being: The cycle of action, evaluation and decision. *Personality and Social Psychology Bulletin, 29*, 939–949.

Oishi, S., Diener, E., Suh, E., & Lucas, R. E. (1999). Value as a moderator in subjective well-being. *Journal of Personality, 67*, 157–184.

Oishi, S., & Koo, M. (in press). Two new questions about happiness: "Is happiness good?" and "Is happier better?". In M. Eid & R.J. Larsen (Eds.), *Handbook of subjective well-being*. New York: Guilford.

Omoto, A. M., & Snyder, M. (1995). Sustained helping without obligation: Motivation, longevity of service, and perceived attitude change among AIDS volunteers. *Journal of Personality and Social Psychology, 68*, 671–687.

Patrick, C. J., Bradley, M. M., & Lang, P. J. (1993). Emotion in the criminal psychopath: Startle reflex modulation. *Journal of Abnormal Psychology, 102*, 82–92.

Peterson, C., & Seligman, M. E. P. (2004). *Character strengths and virtues: A handbook and classification.* Washington, DC: American Psychological Association.

Pomerantz, E. M., Saxon, J. L., & Oishi, S. (2000). The psychological tradeoffs of goal investment. *Journal of Personality and Social Psychology, 79,* 617–630.

Pressman, S. D., & Cohen, S. (2005). Does positive affect influence health? *Psychological Bulletin, 131,* 925–971.

Pressman, S. D., Cohen, S., & Kollnesher, M. (2006, March). *Positive emotion and social word use in autobiography predicts increased longevity in psychologists.* Paper presented at the 64th annual Scientific Meeting of the American Psychosomatic Society, Denver, CO.

Pyszczynski, T., & Cox, C. (2004). Can we really do without self-esteem? *Psychological Bulletin, 130,* 425–429.

Roberts, B. W., Caspi, A., & Moffitt, T. E. (2003). Work experiences and personality development in young adulthood. *Journal of Personality and Social Psychology, 84,* 582–593.

Rogers, C. (1961). *On becoming a person: A therapist's view of psychotherapy.* Boston: Houghton Mifflin.

Rusbult, C. E. (1980). Commitment and satisfaction in romantic associations: A test of the investment model. *Journal of Personality and Social Psychology, 38,* 172–186.

Ruvolo, A. P. (1998). Marital well-being and general happiness of newlywed couples: Relationships across time. *Journal of Social and Personal Relationships, 15,* 470–489.

Ryan, R. M., & Deci, E. L. (2001). On happiness and human potentials: A review of research on hedonic and eudaimonic well-being. *Annual Review of Psychology, 52,* 141–166.

Ryff, C. D. (1989). Happiness is everything, or is it? Explorations on the meaning of psychological well-being. *Journal of Personality and Social Psychology, 57,* 1069–1081.

Ryff, C. D., & Singer, B. (1998). The contours of positive human health. *Psychological Inquiry, 9,* 1–28.

Schimmack, U. (2006). The co-occurrence of happiness and pleasantness. Unpublished raw data. University of Toronto, Mississauga, Ontario, Canada

Schimmack, U., Oishi, S., Furr, R. M., & Funder, D. C. (2004). Personality and life satisfaction: A facet-level analysis. *Personality and Social Psychology Bulletin, 30,* 1062–1075.

Schwartz, R. M. (1997). Consider the simple screw: Cognitive science, quality improvement, and psychotherapy. *Journal of Consulting and Clinical Psychology, 65,* 970–983.

Schwartz, R. M., & Garamoni, G. L. (1989). Cognitive balance and psychopathology: Evaluation of an information processing model of positive and negative states of mind. *Clinical Psychology Review, 9,* 271–294.

Schwarz, N. (1990). Feelings as information: Informational and motivational functions of affective states. In E. T. Higgins & R. M. Sorrentino (Eds.) *Handbook of motivation and cognition* (pp. 527–561). New York: Guilford.

Schwarz, N. (2002). Situated cognition and the wisdom of feelings: Cognitive timing. In L. Feldman-Barrett & P. Salovey (Eds.), *The wisdom in feelings* (pp. 144–166). New York: Guilford Press.

Semmer, N. K., Tschan, F., Elfering, A., Kälin, W., & Grebner, S. (in press) Young adults entering the workforce in Switzerland: Working conditions and well-being. In H. Kriesi, P. Farago, M. Kohli, & M. Zarin-Nejadan (Eds.), *Contemporary Switzerland: Revisiting the special case.* Houndmills, United Kingdom: Palgrave Macmillan.

Sheldon, K. M. (2004). *Optimal human being: An integrated multi-level perspective.* Mahwah, NJ: Erlbaum.

Sinclair, R. C., & Marks, M. M. (1995). The effects of mood state on judgmental accuracy: Processing strategy as a mechanism. *Cognition and Emotion, 9,* 417–438.

Steinhauser, J. (2006). *For Californians, deadly heat cut a broad swath.* Retrieved August, 11, 2006, from http://www.nytimes.com/2006/08/11/us/11parched.html?ex=1156132800&en=e5c09ce65b66b229&ei=5070

Suh, E. M., & Koo, J. (in press) Comparing subjective well-being across nations: Theoretical, methodological, and practical challenges. In M. Eid & R. J. Larsen (Eds.), *Handbook of subjective well-being.* New York: Guilford.

Sumner, L. W. (1996). *Welfare, happiness, and ethics*. New York: Oxford University Press.

Svanum, S., & Zody, Z. B. (2001). Psychopathology and college grades. *Journal of Counseling Psychology, 48*, 72–76.

Tamir, M. (2005). Don't worry, be happy? Neuroticism, trait-consistent affect regulation, and performance. *Journal of Personality and Social Psychology, 89*, 449–461.

Tatarkiewicz, W. (1976). *Analysis of happiness*. Hague, The Netherlands: Martinus Nijhoff.

Taylor, M. F., Brice, J., Buck, N., & Prentice-Lane, E. (2005). *British household panel survey user manual: Volume A. Introduction, technical report, and appendices*. Colchester, United Kingdom: University of Essex.

Thomson, J. A. K. (1953). *The ethics of Aristotle: The Nicomachean ethics*. London: Penguin Books.

Tsai, J. L., Knutson, B., & Fung, H. H. (2006). Cultural variation in affect valuation. *Journal of Personality and Social Psychology, 90*, 288–307.

University of Essex Institute for Social and Economic Research. (2006). *British Household Panel Survey: Waves 1–14, 1991–2004*. Colchester, United Kingdom: UK Data Archive.

Waterman, A. S. (1990). The relevance of Aristotle's conception of eudaimonia for the psychological study of happiness. *Theory and Philosophy of Psychology, 10*, 39–44.

Wilson, T. D., & Gilbert, D. T. (2003). Affective forecasting. In M.P. Zanna (Ed.), *Advances in experimental social psychology* (Vol. 35, pp. 345–411). San Diego, CA: Academic Press.

Zarinpoush, F., Cooper, M., & Moylan, S. (2000). The effects of happiness and sadness on moral reasoning. *Journal of Moral Education, 29*, 397–412.

Beyond Money: Toward an Economy of Well-Being

Ed Diener and Martin E.P. Seligman

Abstract Policy decisions at the organizational, corporate, and governmental levels should be more heavily influenced by issues related to well-being—people's evaluations and feelings about their lives. Domestic policy currently focuses heavily on economic outcomes, although economic indicators omit, and even mislead about, much of what society values. We show that economic indicators have many shortcomings, and that measures of well-being point to important conclusions that are not apparent from economic indicators alone. For example, although economic output has risen steeply over the past decades, there has been no rise in life satisfaction during this period, and there has been a substantial increase in depression and distrust. We argue that economic indicators were extremely important in the early stages of economic development, when the fulfillment of basic needs was the main issue. As societies grow wealthy, however, differences in well-being are less frequently due to income, and are more frequently due to factors such as social relationships and enjoyment at work.

Important noneconomic predictors of the average levels of well-being of societies include social capital, democratic governance, and human rights. In the workplace, noneconomic factors influence work satisfaction and profitability. It is therefore important that organizations, as well as nations, monitor the well-being of workers, and take steps to improve it.

Assessing the well-being of individuals with mental disorders casts light on policy problems that do not emerge from economic indicators. Mental disorders cause widespread suffering, and their impact is growing, especially in relation to the influence of medical disorders, which is declining. Although many studies now show that the suffering due to mental disorders can be alleviated by treatment, a large proportion of persons with mental disorders go untreated. Thus, a policy imperative is to offer treatment to more people with mental disorders, and more assistance to their caregivers.

Supportive, positive social relationships are necessary for well-being. There are data suggesting that well-being leads to good social relationships and does not

E. Diener (✉)
Department of Psychology, University of Illinois, Champaign, IL 61820, USA
e-mail: ediener@s.psych.uiuc.edu

E. Diener (ed.), *The Science of Well-Being: The Collected Works of Ed Diener*, Social
Indicators Research Series 37, DOI 10.1007/978-90-481-2350-6_9,
© Springer Science+Business Media B.V. 2009

merely follow from them. In addition, experimental evidence indicates that people suffer when they are ostracized from groups or have poor relationships in groups. The fact that strong social relationships are critical to well-being has many policy implications. For instance, corporations should carefully consider relocating employees because doing so can sever friendships and therefore be detrimental to well-being.

Desirable outcomes, even economic ones, are often caused by well-being rather than the other way around. People high in well-being later earn higher incomes and perform better at work than people who report low well-being. Happy workers are better organizational citizens, meaning that they help other people at work in various ways. Furthermore, people high in well-being seem to have better social relationships than people low in well-being. For example, they are more likely to get married, stay married, and have rewarding marriages. Finally, well-being is related to health and longevity, although the pathways linking these variables are far from fully understood. Thus, well-being not only is valuable because it feels good, but also is valuable because it has beneficial consequences. This fact makes national and corporate monitoring of well-being imperative.

In order to facilitate the use of well-being outcomes in shaping policy, we propose creating a national well-being index that systematically assesses key well-being variables for representative samples of the population. Variables measured should include positive and negative emotions, engagement, purpose and meaning, optimism and trust, and the broad construct of life satisfaction. A major problem with using current findings on well-being to guide policy is that they derive from diverse and incommensurable measures of different concepts, in a haphazard mix of respondents. Thus, current findings provide an interesting sample of policy-related findings, but are not strong enough to serve as the basis of policy. Periodic, systematic assessment of well-being will offer policymakers a much stronger set of findings to use in making policy decisions.

Our thesis is that well-being should become a primary focus of policymakers, and that its rigorous measurement is a primary policy imperative. Well-being, which we define as peoples' positive evaluations of their lives, includes positive emotion, engagement, satisfaction, and meaning (Seligman, 2002). Although economics currently plays a central role in policy decisions because it is assumed that money increases well-being, we propose that well-being needs to be assessed more directly, because there are distressingly large, measurable slippages between economic indicators and well-being. In this report, we outline some of these and propose that well-being ought to be the ultimate goal around which economic, health, and social policies are built.

We also argue that current measurement of well-being is haphazard, with different studies assessing different concepts in different ways, and therefore that a more systematic approach to measurement is needed. We propose that a set of national indicators of well-being be adopted and review evidence showing that these indicators will reveal important information not contained in the economic indicators. Finally, we argue that national indicators of well-being are needed not only because well-being is an important outcome in itself, but also because well-being is so often a cause of other valued outcomes, such as worker productivity and rewarding relationships.

In reviewing the evidence for our propositions, we first describe research on the societal contributors to well-being. Although much more research is needed on the societal correlates of well-being, it is clear that rising income has yielded little additional benefit to well-being in prosperous nations, pointing to one limitation of economic indicators. We also review factors in the workplace that influence well-being at work, and show that well-being on the job in turn predicts positive work behaviors and perhaps profitability. Finally, we review evidence showing that supportive social relationships are essential to well-being. Well-being, in turn, has positive effects on social relationships, as well as mental and physical health.[1] We begin our review by discussing the relation between economic indicators and well-being.

Economic Indicators Versus Well-Being

Economics now reigns unchallenged in the policy arena, as well as in media coverage of quality-of-life indicators. News magazines and daily newspapers have a section devoted to money, and the *Wall Street Journal* covers economic issues on a daily basis. Economists hold prominent positions in the capitals of the world. When politicians run for office, they speak at length about what they will do, or have done, for the economy. Television presents frequent reports about unemployment, the Dow Jones average, and the national debt. Rarely do the news media report on how depressed, engaged, or satisfied people are. In part, policy and media coverage stems from the fact that economic indicators are rigorous, widely available, and updated frequently, whereas few national measures of well-being exist.

Money, however, is a means to an end, and that end is well-being. But money is an inexact surrogate for well-being, and the more prosperous a society becomes, the more inexact a surrogate income becomes. The measurement of well-being has advanced sufficiently that it is time to grant a privileged place to people's well-being in policy debates, a place at least on a par with monetary concerns. After all, if economic and other policies are important because they will in the end increase well-being, why not assess well-being more directly? The main argument for using only a surrogate, such as money, is that well-being cannot be measured with the same exactitude as money. However, scientists now have good tools with which to index the well-being of societies with considerable precision. Therefore, it is possible to use measurable outcomes to create policies to enhance well-being.

---

[1] For additional scholarly work that broadly covers findings on well-being, the reader is referred to Argyle (2001); Diener (1984); Diener and Suh (1999); Diener, Suh, Lucas, and Smith (1999); Frey & Stutzer (2002a); Kahneman, Diener, and Schwarz (1999); and Seligman (2002).

Media attention should spotlight how a society is progressing in terms of well-being, and politicians should base their campaigns on their plans for reducing distress, increasing life satisfaction and meaning, enhancing marital and leisure satisfaction, and optimizing engagement at work. Our proposed system of well-being indicators would not supplant economic or other current social indicators, but would supplement and enhance their value by placing them within an overarching framework of well-being, underscoring the shortcomings of economic indicators.

Modern economics grew as a handmaiden to the industrial revolution, and together they produced an explosion in the production of goods and services. Since the time of Adam Smith's *Wealth of Nations*, governments have taken an active role in steering economies, for example, by adopting monetary controls, employment and wage laws, trade tariffs, banking and investment laws, antitrust laws, and income taxes. In recent decades, governments have become increasingly involved in the economies of the developed nations, and virtually all nations now have systems for measuring national production and consumption.

In microeconomics (the study of economics at the level of individual areas of activity), the standard assumption is that, other things being equal, more choices mean a higher quality of life because people with choices can select courses of action that maximize their well-being (Kahneman, 2003; Schwartz, 2004; Varian, 1992). Because income correlates with number of choices, greater income is equivalent to higher well-being. This formulation is standard in economics, where income is seen as the essence of well-being, and therefore measures of income are seen as sufficient indices to capture well-being.

At the time of Adam Smith, a concern with economic issues was understandably primary. Meeting simple human needs for food, shelter, and clothing was not assured, and satisfying these needs moved in lockstep with better economics. However, subsequent industrial developments made these goods and services so widely available that in the 21st century, many economically developed nations, such as the United States, Japan, and Sweden, experience an abundance of goods and services (Easterbrook, 2003). Furthermore, although the industrial revolution led to an explosion of goods and services, it also included elements, such as rising aspirations, that to some degree canceled the benefits to well-being that come with economic growth (Easterlin, 1996).

Because goods and services are plentiful and because simple needs are largely satisfied in modern societies, people today have the luxury of refocusing their attention on the "good life"—a life that is enjoyable, meaningful, engaging, and fulfilling—and using economic and other policies in its service. Such a refocus is justified because there is evidence that as societies become wealthier, they often experience an increase in mental and social problems and a plateau in life satisfaction. People rank happiness and satisfaction ahead of money as a life goal (Diener & Oishi, in press). The purpose of the production of goods and services and of policies in areas such as education, health, the environment, and welfare is to increase well-being. Therefore, well-being is the common desired outcome, and it follows directly that society should measure this outcome to provide a common metric for evaluating policies. Although economic progress can enhance the quality

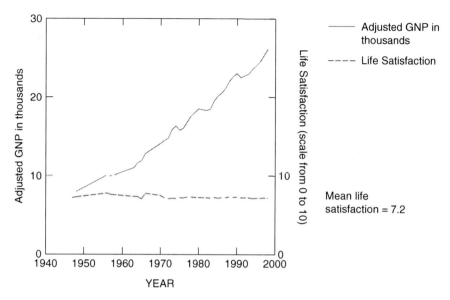

Fig. 1 US gross national product (GNP) and mean life satisfaction from 1947 to 1998

of life even in industrialized nations, it no longer serves as a strong barometer of well-being because there are substantial discrepancies between economic indices and other measures.

Economic measures have seriously failed to provide a full account of quality of life. Later in this monograph (see A System of National Indicators), we review some of the shortcomings of national economic accounts in capturing even the production and consumption of goods and services in nations. However, we want to emphasize here the divergence of economic indicators from indices of well-being. For example, over the past 50 years, income has climbed steadily in the United States, with the gross domestic product (GDP) per capita tripling, and yet life satisfaction has been virtually flat. As can be seen in Fig. 1, since World War II there has been a dramatic divergence between real income (after taxes and inflation) and life satisfaction in the United States, and a similar pattern can be seen in the data from other nations, such as Japan.

Even more disparity shows up when ill-being measures are considered. For instance, depression rates have increased 10-fold over the same 50-year period, and rates of anxiety are also rising (Twenge, 2000). Indeed, Twenge reported that the average American child in the 1980s reported greater anxiety than the average child receiving psychiatric treatment in the 1950s. There is a decreasing level of social connectedness in society, as evidenced by declining levels of trust in other people and in governmental institutions (Putnam, 2001a). Because trust is an important predictor of societal stability and quality of life (Helliwell, 2003a), the decreases are of considerable concern.

We predict that psychology will play a central role in measuring national well-being. Both scientists and practitioners will be required to determine how to rigorously assess well-being and how to intervene to change it. Moreover, other behavioral sciences, such as sociology, anthropology, and neuroscience, will paly important roles. Furthermore, economists will also be involved. They have recently turned their attention to understanding and monitoring well-being. Economists now examine surveys of happiness and life satisfaction to uncover the effects of factors such as unemployment, income equality, commuting, and smoking. Recent conferences on well-being have been attended as much by economists as by psychologists. The European Union nations now monitor psychological well-being with the Eurobarometer, and the German Socioeconomic Panel Survey provides policymakers with information on income, employment, life satisfaction, and related variables in a large sample of respondents that are being assessed repeatedly over time. Organizations such as the Pew Foundation assess well-being in nations around the globe, and the World Value Survey has assessed happiness and life satisfaction in about 70 nations.

Thus, the beginnings of worldwide monitoring of well-being are evident, and economists and sociologists have been heavily involved in this effort. Psychologists are in an ideal position to develop and improve relevant measures and to design interventions that would be maximally effective in increasing well-being.

The Unsystematic Nature of Current Findings and Measures

In the next section, we review many policy-relevant findings that illustrate the divergence between economic indicators and well-being indicators. First, though, we want to discuss some of the shortcomings of the research. It is our contention that a much more systematic approach to the measurement of well-being is needed in order to provide leaders with the best possible well-being indicators. Current findings are based almost entirely on the work of individual researchers, who address their own questions, usually using relatively small, accidental samples of respondents. Furthermore, different investigators measure different concepts (e.g., happiness, stress, distress, life satisfaction, or depression), and it is rare for a broad range of concepts to be assessed in a single study.

In order to examine the number of studies that include multiple well-being concepts, we scanned a large database of publications in psychology journals, PsychLit. Our search found 94,650 publications on "depression" and 4,757 on "life satisfaction" in January 2004, but only 701 of these mentioned both constructs. There were 2,158 publications that discussed "positive affect," but only 93 of these mentioned "life satisfaction." Of the 3,520 publications mentioning "negative affect," only 107 also mentioned "life satisfaction." Current researchers usually assess one or two well-being variables, but rarely measure the broad range of concepts that are relevant to well-being. Thus, it is very unusual for a study to include measures of diverse concepts such as pleasant emotions, life satisfaction, unpleasant emotions, and optimism, despite the fact that these constructs are separable and show different patterns (Lucas, Diener, & Suh, 1996). This shortcoming is readily apparent in the studies that we review in the next section.

In addition, many findings are based on respondents' answers to a single question, and such single-item measures can be unreliable and easily influenced by the testing situation. As we progress through our review, readers will notice that in one area of study we base our conclusions on measures of life satisfaction, in another area we draw conclusions from reports of stress, and in yet another area we review measures map onto more widely used concepts. For example, how are reports of stress related to negative emotions? This is the nature of the current data—a haphazard mix of different measures of varying quality, usually taken from nonrepresentative samples of respondents. Rarely are data longitudinal, and few data sets are based on intensive experience-sampling measures. In the experience-sampling technique, people's moods and emotions are recorded "on-line" at random moments in everyday life, using a device such as a handheld computer. A similar method is to have people record their feelings and activities at the end of each day. Both methods have the advantage of reducing memory biases in reporting, and allow for the detailed recording of affect within specific situations.

There are excellent reviews of specific concepts such as stress (Cohen, Kessler, & Gordon, 1997), positive and negative affect (Watson, 2000), happiness (Argyle, 2001), and depression (Basco, Krebaum, & Rush, 1997), but these concepts have not been systematically explored in depth in relation to each other in order to determine which concepts are necessary in a combined battery for measuring well-being. The unsystematic nature of the existing data point to the importance of developing a set of national well-being indicators based on the best science and technology available.

Well-being includes pleasure, engagement, and meaning, and the concept of life satisfaction may reflect all of these (Seligman, 2002). The pleasant life is characterized by positive moods, positive emotions, and pleasures. Positive and negative emotions and moods give a person ongoing feedback about whether things are going well or poorly. Moods and emotions can change rapidly because they reflect current evaluations of events. Pleasant emotions signify to the individual that events and circumstances are desirable, and unpleasant emotions signify that they are undesirable (Ortony, Clore, & Collins, 1988). Engagement involves absorption and what is sometimes referred to as flow, focused attention on what one is doing (e.g., "being one with the music"). Boredom, the opposite of engagement, is a lack of interest combined with negative feelings. Meaning is a larger judgment of belonging to and serving something larger than the self. Finally, life satisfaction is a global judgment of well-being based on information the person believes is relevant. Well-being includes all of the evaluations, both cognitive and affective, that people make of their lives and components of their lives. Thus, a comprehensive assessment of well-being must include several separable concepts.

Development of a rigorous and systematic set of well-being indicators is crucial to our argument that economic indicators should be supplemented with well-being indicators because of the relative advantages and disadvantages of economic and well-being indicators. The main advantage of using money to assess the well-being of nations is that it is exact, that is, it has very high internal validity. The main disadvantage is the central substance of this report—money lacks external validity because it fails to track actual well-being in developed nations. In contrast, the main advantage of measuring well-being more directly is its external validity; that is, well-being itself is the true target of the indicators. But the main disadvantage of measuring well-being concerns the issue of internal validity; that is, whether well-being measures truly reflect the quality of life of societies.

Currently societal well-being is assessed by broad, global questions asking people, for example, how happy and satisfied they are, how satisfied they are with domains of life such as marriage and work, and how much they trust others. Near the end of this report, we make suggestions about the measures that should be included in a national well-being index in order to increase precision of measurement. We propose that a national index should employ the global questions now in use, but supplement them with questions targeted at specific aspects of well-being, such as engagement at work, stress due to commuting, levels of depression (among adolescents), and trust in neighbors. In addition, we propose that the indicator system include both a *panel component* (assessing the same group of individuals repeatedly over time) and an intensive experience-sampling component (assessing individuals on a daily basis for a week or 2; see Kahneman, Krueger, Schkade, Schwarz, & Stone, 2004). Thus, we are proposing a national system that is much broader and deeper than the current surveys, which base their findings on just a few global items.

Selected Findings with Policy Relevance

In order to convince readers that well-being measures have produced important findings with relevance for policy, we review research in six areas related to well-being: societal conditions, income, work, physical health, mental disorders, and social relationships. The findings reveal discrepancies between economic and well-being indicators, and point to conclusions with relevance to policy. Because we believe that social science should be descriptive and not prescriptive, in mentioning specific possible policies we do not mean to advocate them, but rather to give examples of the policies that might follow from the findings.

National and Political Factors Related to Well-Being

Nationwide patterns such as low divorce rates, high rates of membership in voluntary organizations, and high levels of trust are all substantially related to individual well-being. Political characteristics such as democratic institutions, governmental effectiveness, and stability also predict well-being. The wealth of nations substantially correlates with well-being, although there is little effect once income reaches a moderate level. Finally, religious belief appears to buffer people against stressors such as widowhood, unemployment, and low income. The causal direction between societal variables and national well-being is not fully understood, but policymakers would be remiss to ignore the findings until the time in the distant future when causal influences are fully confirmed.

The Wealth of Nations

Studies looking at the relation between average well-being and average per capita income across nations have found substantial correlations, ranging from about 0.50–0.70 (Diener & Seligman, 2002). The correlations indicate that wealthy nations are happier than less wealthy nations, although the correlations drop substantially when factors such as the quality of government are statistically controlled (Helliwell, 2003a).[2]

Diminishing Returns for Higher Income. Across nations, there are diminishing returns for increasing wealth above US$10,000 per captia income (Frey & Stutzer, 2002a); above that level, there are virtually no increases (Helliwell, 2003a) or only small increases (Schyns, 2003) in well-being. Moreover, health, quality of government, and human rights all correlate with national wealth, and when these variables are statistically controlled, the effect of income on national well-being becomes non-significant. Helliwell (2003a), an economist, concluded that people with the highest well-being "are not those who live in the richest countries, but those who live where social and political institutions are effective, where mutual trust is high, and corruption is low" (p. 355). In Fig. 2, we show levels of well-being (based on the World Value Survey) in countries of varying incomes. The pattern of the data is clear, and supports the conclusions of Frey and Stutzer: Above a moderate level of income, there are only small increases in well-being. Using the World Value Survey II, we computed the correlation between average life satisfaction and the GDP per capita of nations, restricting the analysis to nations with per capita GDP above US$10,000. The correlation was only 0.08, confirming the small effect of further income once a moderate level of income is achieved.

National Income Change. What occurs when the income of an entire society rises? Examining 21 nations over time, Hagerty and Veenhoven (2003) found positive significant correlations between changes in income and well-being in 6, and no significant negative correlations. They concluded that the well-being in nations is rising over time, but that the effects of income on well-being are larger in poorer than in richer nations. However, other researchers have concluded that huge increases in income in wealthy nations, often a doubling or even tripling of real income, have often been accompanied by virtually no increases in well-being in these nations (Diener & Seligman, 2002; Easterbrook, 2003; Easterlin, 1995; Oswald, 1997).

---

[2] For reviews of this area, readers are referred to Diener & Seligman (2002), Diener & Oishi (2000), Frey and Stutzer (2003), and Furnham and Argyle (1998).

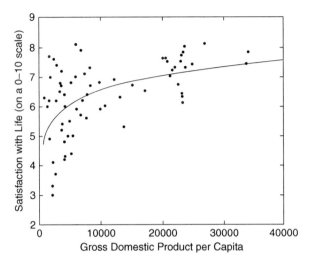

Fig. 2 Satisfaction with life as a function of gross domestic product per capita. Each *circle* represents the gross domestic product and life satisfaction in a nation. The *curve* shows a line that describes the relation between income and life satisfaction in these nations

Donovan & Halpern (2003) discussed the changes in well-being that have occurred in a number of nations, explaining that in some cases well-being has risen, in others it has fallen, and in still others it has zigzagged up and down. Most of these data came from wealthy nations, so it is arguable whether increasing incomes have caused any increases whatsoever in well-being in wealthy nations, in part because income has been rising in most nations and it is difficult to know whether the occasional, slow rises in well-being in wealthy nations are due to noneconomic factors such as increasing rights for women (Schyns, 1998) or increasing democracy (Barro, 1999). What is very clear is that rises in well-being have not been remotely commensurate with increasing wealth. Furthermore, Frey & Stutzer (2002b) reported that the same income in the United States, adjusted for inflation, bought more happiness in 1973 than in 1995. In other words, in rich nations more and more income has been required over time to remain at the same level of well-being.

As we have already noted, increases in income in wealthy societies have been accompanied by smaller (even nonexistent) rises in well-being than have accompanied income increases in poor nations (Hagerty and Veenhoven, 2003). This pattern is consistent with the decreasing marginal utility of money (i.e., the impact of an added dollar decreases as the total amount of money increases). In contrast, there was a strong trend for well-being to drop in the former Soviet bloc nations when communism was forsaken and incomes dropped precipitously (Inglehart and Klingemann, 2000; Schyns, 2003). Losing income may have a greater influence on well-being than gaining income does.

One reason that increasing income does not increase well-being is probably that rising income creates escalating material desires, so that as time passes, the same level of income that once seemed satisfactory results in frustration, and hence less well-being (Frey & Stutzer, 2002b; van Praag & Frijters, 1999). Stutzer (in press) showed that well-being depends to some degree on the gap between income and material aspirations. Graham and Pettinato (2002) found that in poor nations there are "frustrated achievers" who, despite rapid increases in income, become less happy because their aspirations grow even more quickly than their incomes. Unfortunately, there are no studies of whether increases in well-being that stem from noneconomic sources can serve to stimulate economic gains.

Other Economic Factors. Per capita wealth and income are not the only economic variables associated with well-being. For instance, Di Tella, MacCulloch, & Oswald (2001) found that inflation is a negative predictor of the well-being of nations; low inflation also predicts satisfaction with the governing party (Frey & Stutzer, 2002a). High unemployment predicts the ill-being of nations (Frey & Stutzer, 2002a).

Surprisingly, the level of welfare benefits in a nation does not seem to buffer the effects of unemployment on well-being (Ouweneel, 2002), and Veenhoven (2000) found that the level of social-security benefits in nations was not associated with well-being. Alesina, Di Tella, and MacCulloch (2000) reported that in Europe greater inequality of income is associated with lower well-being, but that in the United States only liberals are made less happy by inequality. Thus, the effects of societal characteristics depend to some extent on the ideological views of respondents.

Governance

In 1995 E. Diener, C. Diener, and M. Diener reported that human rights in nations correlated with average well-being. Unfortunately, income was also highly correlated with human rights, so that it was difficult to disentangle the influences from one another. Nations with democratic governments score high on individual well-being (Donovan & Halpern, 2003). Furthermore, Inglehart and Klingemann (2000) reported a very strong correlation of 0.78 between the extent of democracy in nations and their levels of well-being. In a comparison of Swiss cantons, Frey and Stutzer (2000, 2002a) found that those with greater direct democracy (e.g., more referenda and direct voting on initiatives) had higher well-being. They suggested that the benefits of democracy to happiness come from the political process itself, not just from the beneficial outcomes of democracy. Conversely, Inglehart and Klingemann argued that general well-being influences democratic governance, and that a sharp drop in well-being can undermine democratic institutions.

Effective and trustworthy governance also correlates with the well-being of nations, and these effects are over and above those of democracy (Helliwell, 2003b). When there is low corruption and effective rule of law, people report greater life satisfaction (Helliwell, 2003a). Freedom has also been found to have a substantial relation to the well-being of nations (Inglehart and Klingemann, 2000). Veenhoven (2000) found that economic freedom had a stronger effect on well-being in poor nations than in wealthy nations, whereas political freedom was more important in wealthier nations than in poor nations.

Welzel, Inglehart, and Klingemann (2003) argued that socioeconomic develop-ment, "emancipative cultural change" that increases personal freedoms, and democ-ratization develop together in nations. These factors broaden human choice and control by increasing resources and providing legal rights to freedom of choice. These factors in turn are those that E. Diener, C. Diener, and M. Diener (1995) found predict the well-being of nations—income, human rights, and individualism. Although too many choices (Schwartz, 2004) can undermine well-being, it appears that human rights and democracy benefit well-being.

Stable political organization is needed for well-being, and might be even more crucial in the short run than democratic governance. When the former Soviet bloc nations, once stable dictatorships, became unstable democracies, their well-being dropped substantially (Helliwell, 2003a; Inglehart and Klingemann, 2000). Veenhoven (2002) indicated that in the 1990s, out of 68 societies, Russia, Georgia, Armenia, Ukraine, and Moldavia had the lowest enjoyment of life, from 3.0 to 4.2 on a scale from 1 to 10. This suggests that instability is a source of suffering. However, because the massive changes in the former Soviet bloc countries included faltering economies and large drops in real income, a change in the economic and political systems, and abandonment of a pervasive ideology, it is difficult to isolate the causes of their reduced well-being.

A mild decline in well-being occurred in Belgium from the 1970s to the 1990s, perhaps because of economic factors, but also possibly because the nation split into a federation (Inglehart and Klingemann, 2000). The lowest well-being value ever recorded, 1.6 on a 10-point scale of life satisfaction, occurred following the over-throw of the government of the Dominican Republic. Thus, instability in nations seems to result in lowered levels of well-being.

Social Capital

In *Bowling Alone*, Putnam (2001a) suggested that people prosper in neighborhoods and societies where social capital is high, that is, where people trust one another and are mutually helpful. Putnam reviewed evidence showing that communities with high rates of volunteer activity, club membership, church membership, and social entertaining (all thought to be indirect manifestations of social capital) all had higher well-being than communities that were low in these characteristics. Helliwell (2003a) reported that well-being is high and suicide rates are low where trust in others is high, and he also found that well-being is high where memberships in organizations outside of work are at high levels. Thus, there is evidence that individuals are more likely to experience high well-being when they live in nations with high social capital than when they live in nations with low social capital, a finding that dovetails with the results of studies on individuals' social interactions (reviewed later in this section).

Unfortunately, Putnam (2001a) found that social capital, for example, trust and membership in organizations, is declining in the United States. Twenge (2002) con-cluded that rising dysphoria in the United States is in part due to the breakdown of social connectedness. Thus, a factor that appears to enhance societal well-being appears to be declining at the same time that wealth is increasing.

Religion

Extensive data support the idea that religious people tend on average to experience greater well-being than nonreligious people (see Diener et al., 1999). For example, Ferriss (2002) reviewed evidence showing that life satisfaction is higher the more frequently people attend church and that people who have religious beliefs report more life satisfaction than people who say they are atheists, and Clark & Lelkes (2003) reported that having religious beliefs buffers individuals against stressors such as unemployment, low income, and widowhood. Recent evidence now points to the same relation between religion and well-being at the national level. Helliwell (2003b) found that across nations, a higher rate of belief in a god is associated with higher average life satisfaction and lower rate of suicide. In addition to belief, church attendance is associated with higher reports of well-being across nations (Clark & Lelkes, 2003; Helliwell, 2003a). A full discussion of the relation between religion and well-being is beyond the scope of this monograph, but the reader is referred to Baumeister (2002).

Conclusions and Cautions

As the evidence stands now, it appears that nations high in average well-being can be characterized as democracies with effective and stable governments, as well as societies that are high in social capital, are religious, and have strong economies with low rates of unemployment and inflation. The lowered well-being scores in the former Soviet bloc nations strongly suggest that political and economic instability can lead to sharp declines in well-being. Equality and welfare benefits appear not to have a universal positive impact when considered across nations with different ideologies. It is evident that wealth does not tell the whole story when it comes to the well-being of nations. Not only are other factors predictive of well-being, but they may surpass wealth in importance, especially for nations that have already achieved a moderate level of prosperity. Well-being reflects additional factors, such as stability and social capital, that are not entirely captured by economic indicators.

There are data suggesting that well-being in nations increases the likelihood of other beneficial outcomes. For instance, Inglehart and Klingemann (2000) suggested that well-being is a necessary precursor for democratic governance. Vázquez, Hernangómez, and Hervás (2004) found that the well-being of societies predicts their members' longevity, even after statistically controlling for national income and infant mortality. It is possible that the arrow of causality goes from well-being to longevity. However, it is also possible that this relation is due to other, unmeasured factors that influence both well-being and longevity. Much more research on how well-being affects societies is needed, but the limited findings to date suggest beneficial outcomes.

A number of cautions are warranted in interpreting the data on the relations between societal and political factors and well-being. Analyses of the well-being of nations are still sparse, and a number of methodological and conceptual questions remain. For example, data are available primarily from the wealthiest nations, and large areas of the world, such as Africa, are underrepresented. The validity of well-being measures has been demonstrated to some degree at the individual level, but the cross-cultural validity of the measures is largely untested, with a few exceptions (Diener, Suh, Smith, & Shao, 1995; Veenhoven, 1994). Furthermore, why factors such as religiosity affect the well-being of societies is not completely understood, and researchers do not know the conditions that may moderate such effects. It may be that having a coherent belief system that gives meaning to one's life, rather than organized religion per se, is responsible for the higher well-being of religious individuals. It will be important to discover which predictors of well-being might be universal, and which depend on the cultural context in which they occur. Most important, researchers need to determine which characteristics, such as democracy, follow from well-being rather than cause it.

In the next section, we turn to studies of individual income. They show that economic success falls short as a measure of well-being, in part because materialism can negatively influence well-being, and also because it is possible to be happy without living a life of luxury, as long as one's needs are met.

Money and Well-Being

Although high personal income is associated with well-being, the relation between these two variables is intricate. People who report that they are happy subsequently earn higher incomes than people who report that they are not happy, a finding that calls into question the direction of causality between income and well-being. To further complicate matters, as the richer nations have grown in wealth, sometimes dramatically, they have usually experienced only small increases in well-being. Respondents in materially poor societies at times have substantial levels of life satisfaction. Rising expectations and desires to some degree cancel the psychological benefits of greater income. Furthermore, there are negative outcomes related to money, such as the deleterious effects of materialism on happiness and the high stress levels felt by adolescents from rich families. The context in which income is experienced, including ideology and people's material desires and values, moderates its effects on well-being. Individuals may achieve higher happiness for themselves by earning higher incomes, when they move upward relative to their material desires and relative to others. However, as everyone's income rises in affluent societies, rising income does not seem to provide a well-being dividend. Thus, there is a clear divergence between economic and well-being indicators, which points to the need for a system of national well-being indicators to complement the economic indicators already in place.

Income Correlates Positively with Well-Being

Dozens of cross-sectional studies reveal that there is a positive correlation between individuals' incomes and their reports of well-being. However, Veenhoven (1991) found that the within-nation correlations between income and well-being are stronger in poorer than in wealthier societies, and this effect has been replicated by other researchers (E. Diener & M. Diener, 1995; Diener & Oishi, 2000; Schyns, 2003). For example, Diener, Sandvik, Seidlitz and Diener (1993) reported the income and well-being correlation to be 0.13 in the United States, whereas Biswas-Diener and Diener (2001) found that this correlation was 0.45 in the slums of Calcutta. Similarly, E. Diener and M. Diener (1995) discovered a stronger relation between financial satisfaction and life satisfaction in poor than in wealthy countries. Furthermore, as one moves up the income scale in wealthy nations such as Switzerland (Frey & Stutzer, 2002a) and the United States (Diener et al., 1993), there are progressively smaller differences in well-being between successively higher income categories. Helliwell (2003a) found that because of the declining effect of income as one moves up the income ladder, significant variations in well-being occurred in the higher income brackets only in poor nations. In wealthier nations, increases in income were not matched by continuing increases in well-being.

Causal Direction

Researchers attempting to determine the causal influence of income on happiness have examined both lottery winners and participants in negative-income-tax experiments, as well as longitudinal data. (In the negative-income-tax experiments, the federal government supplemented the income of certain low-income people who were randomly assigned to have their income brought up to a certain level. Over time, these people and a control group were tracked for various outcomes.)

Although Brickman, Coates, and Janoff-Bulman (1978) found that a small number of lottery winners were not significantly happier than a matched comparison group, S. Smith and Razzell (1975) found that bettors who won large soccer betting pools in England were significantly more likely to report being very happy than the comparison group. In negative-income-tax studies in which some participants received higher welfare benefits than others, however, greater stress was associated with increased incomes (Thoits & Hannan, 1979). This finding dovetails with one of Smith and Razzell's, because they found that although lottery winners were on average higher in well-being than nonwinners, winners described certain stressors in their lives that resulted from their increased wealth. Thus, the lottery and negative-income-tax studies, which approximate true experiments, present a mixed picture on whether increases in income increase well-being.

If income influences well-being, one would expect that in longitudinal studies, income changes would be followed by changes in well-being. Diener & Seligman (2002) found that this pattern did not occur in the majority of studies they reviewed. In recent analyses of a large panel study in Germany, we found that people with slowly rising incomes show high levels of well-being, and that individuals with comparable mean levels of income but high year-to-year fluctuations show substantially lower levels of life satisfaction. In this study, people with dramatic rises in income showed increasing well-being; although initially they were lower in well-being than the slow-rise group, by the end of the study their well-being had increased to reach the level of the slow-rise group. People experiencing large downward shifts in income showed large declines in life satisfaction.

Income increases might bring costs as well as benefits. For example, Clydesdale (1997) found more divorce in people whose income had risen than among people whose income was stable. Furthermore, substantial increases in one's income are likely to bring disruptions to one's life, and these might be either positive or negative. This might explain, for example, the mixed results of negative-income-tax and lottery studies.

Longitudinal data indicate that part of the typical correlation between income and well-being is due to well-being causing higher incomes, rather than the other way around. Happy people go on to earn higher incomes than unhappy people. Diener, Nickerson, Lucas, and Sandvik (2002) discovered that higher cheerfulness in the first year of college correlated with higher income 19 years or so later, when respondents reached their late 30s; this effect was greatest for those who came from the most affluent families (see Fig. 3). Marks and Fleming (1999) found that well-being predicted later income in an Australian sample of young adults, and Staw, Sutton, and Pelled (1994) uncovered a weak, but significant, tendency of pleasant emotions at an initial assessment to predict pay at a later time, in an analysis that controlled for income at the initial assessment. Finally, Graham, Eggers, and Sukhtankar (in press) found that happiness predicted future income even after they controlled for current socioeconomic and demographic variables. Thus, longitudinal findings indicate that some part of the association between income and happiness is likely due to happy people going on to earn more money than unhappy people. Kenny (1999) has extended this reasoning to the growth rate of the wealth of nations.

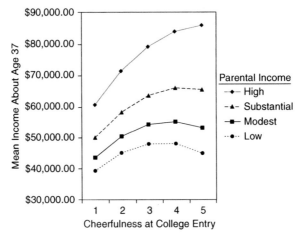

Fig. 3 Mean income at about age 37 as a function of cheerfulness and parents' income at the time of entry into college. Results shown here are for students whose parents' income fell within ranges that can be characterized as low, modest, substantial, or high

Negative Outcomes of Wealth and Materialism

An edited volume by Kasser and Kanner (2004) has detailed the detrimental effects of materialism, defined as placing a high importance on income and material possessions. The authors documented the problems experienced by materialistic individuals relative to less materialistic individuals: lower self-esteem and greater narcissism, greater amounts of social comparison (i.e., comparing oneself with other people, sometimes for the purpose of evaluating oneself) and less empathy, less intrinsic motivation, and more conflictual relationships (Kasser, Ryan, Couchman, & Sheldon, 2004). Nickerson, Schwarz, Diener, and Kahneman (2003) found that materialism predicted later lower well-being, but that this effect was smallest for those people who earned a high income. Across nations, placing a higher importance on money is associated with lower well-being (Kirkcaldy, Furnham, & Martin, 1998). Materialism might lead to lower well-being because materialistic people tend to downplay the importance of social relationships and to have a large gap between their incomes and material aspirations (Solberg, Diener, & Robinson, 2004). In the study by Nickerson et al., it appeared that placing too much value on money had its negative effect in part because it interfered with social relationships.

However, the causal arrow may go the other way: Unhappiness may drive people to focus on extrinsic goals such as material wealth. Srivastava, Locke, and Bartol (2001) found that materialism was damaging to well-being insofar as it arose from a desire to gain power or flaunt wealth, but not if it arose from a desire for freedom or family security. Malka and Chatman (2003) found that intrinsically oriented individuals (i.e., people who enjoy tasks for their own sake) were less happy than extrinsically oriented individuals (i.e., people who enjoy tasks for the external rewards they bring) at higher income levels. Because people who value income tend to earn more money than people who do not, the deleterious effects of materialism can be offset to some degree by the positive experience of a higher income (Nickerson, Kahneman, Diener, & Schwarz, 2004).

Not only materialism, but wealth itself has been found in a few studies to produce negative effects. Hagerty (2000) found that when personal income was statistically controlled, individuals living in higher-income areas in the United States were lower in happiness than people living in lower-income areas. This suggests that wealthy individuals are fortunate if they live in middle-class areas rather than in wealthy enclaves. Similarly, Putnam (2001b) found that higher statewide income was associated with lower well-being once individual income was statistically controlled. The negative effects of wealthy communities might partly be explained by their higher materialism (Stutzer, in press).

In a longitudinal study in which students were followed through high school and beyond, Csikszentmihalyi and Schneider (2000) found that adolescents from affluent suburbs were on average less happy, and reported lower self-esteem, than those from middle-class neighborhoods and inner-city slums. Because the measures were direct, based on recording of moods as they occurred, the results of this study are particularly compelling. The negative effects of affluence on adolescents were reviewed by Luthar (2003), who suggested that high expectations for achievement and relative isolation from adults can both lead to lower well-being among teenagers from financially well-off families. Luthar maintained that aspects of the wealthy lifestyle, such as privacy and competition (which can lead to lack of interpersonal intimacy), can harm the well-being of adults as well. Thus, high income is not an unalloyed benefit.

The Contextual Effects of Income

The effects of income on well-being depend on context, pointing once again to the fact that economic indicators by themselves are insufficient to index the quality of life. Although researchers have usually searched for invariant connections between money and happiness, there is increasing evidence that psychological factors such as values and ideology moderate the connection. So, for example, Clark (2003) reported that the effects of income are smaller among religious believers than among nonbelievers. Di Tella and MacCulloch (1999) reported evidence indicating that unemployment harms the well-being of respondents with a left-wing political orientation more than inflation does. In contrast, inflation harms the well-being of respondents with a right-wing ideology more than unemployment does. Bjørnskov (2003) found that income equality correlates negatively with national well-being, largely because in Latin American nations income is distributed unequally and the people are satisfied.

Malka and Chatman (2003) found that business students who were most motivated by money were happier on the job years later the more income they earned, but that those who were intrinsically motivated were actually lower in life satisfaction and positive affect years later the more income they earned. Research on unemployment also highlights the fact that income alone is not a simple predictor of well-being. Helliwell (2003a) discovered that unemployment had negative effects on well-being in rich and poor nations, but the effects were more severe in wealthier nations. Because welfare benefits are more generous in wealthier nations, the strong negative effects of unemployment in richer societies compared with poorer societies are likely caused not by difficulties in meeting material needs, but by psychological factors such as a decrease in self-respect. In implicating psychological factors, this pattern in the link between well-being and unemployment across nations is consistent with the fact that the effects of income on well-being are stronger for men than for women (e.g., Adelmann, 1987; Ross & Huber, 1985) because both findings point to the importance of identity and values in the effects work and money have on well-being.

Clark and Oswald (1996) found that job satisfaction depends not on absolute pay, but on pay relative to other workers with the same education and job classification. People are more satisfied when they compare themselves with others who have lower income than they do. So, for example, respondents' satisfaction with a given level of income is lower if other people in their household earn more than if other household members earn less (Neumark & Postlewaite, 1998). People's satisfaction with their incomes depends also on the incomes of others in their organization and in their occupation (G. D. A. Brown, Gardner, Oswald, & Qian, 2003). Also suggesting that social comparison is a moderating factor is the finding that unemployment is

Table 1 Life satisfaction for various groups

Group	Rating
Forbes magazine's "richest Americans"	5.8
Pennsylvania Amish	5.8
Inughuit (Inuit people in northern Greenland)	5.8
African Maasai	5.7
Swedish probability sample	5.6
International college-student sample (47 nations in 2000)	4.9
Illinois Amish	4.9
Calcutta slum dwellers	4.6
Fresno, California, homeless	2.9
Calcutta pavement dwellers (homeless)	2.9

Note. Respondents indicated their agreement with the statement "You are satisfied with your life" using a scale from 1 (complete disagreement) to 7 (complete agreement); 4 is a neutral rating.

associated more strongly with lower well-being in regions where unemployment is low than where it is high (Clark, 2001).

In Table 1, we present data on the life satisfaction of a number of groups. Respondents from the Forbes list of the 400 richest Americans are relatively high in well-being (Diener, Horwitz, & Emmons, 1985), yet the Maasai of East Africa are almost equally satisfied (Biswas-Diener, Vittersø, & Diener, 2003). The Maasai are a traditional herding people who have no electricity or running water, and they live in huts made from dung. These results thus underscore the fact that luxury is not necessary for high well-being. Slum dwellers in Calcutta are less satisfied with their lives, although still above the neutral point on the rating scale, perhaps sustained by the pleasures of family, religion, and work. In contrast, homeless people in Fresno, California, report very low levels of well-being. We speculate that meeting one's physical needs and one's desires might be the crucial moderator of the effects of income on well-being. What is clear is that income per se does not directly drive well-being.

Recall that increasing wealth is associated with only a slight rise in well-being once nations have a moderate level of per capita income. A research imperative is thus to determine what contextual factors influence the effects of income on well-being. Whatever these factors turn out to be, it is likely that the effects of income on well-being are strongly moderated by cultural context, and therefore that well-being must be directly assessed to be measured accurately.

Conclusions and Cautions

Many people feel that they would be happier if they had more income and additional material goods, and there is some mixed evidence to support this claim. Within-nation correlations generally do show small positive associations ($\sim$0.15) between income and well-being, and the average reported well-being is higher in wealthy societies than in poor nations. Furthermore, an individual might increase his or her well-being by gaining income relative to other people. In other words, the intuition that one will be happier with more rather than less income might be correct, but this effect occurs only at the individual level and is negated to the extent that everyone's incomes and desires increase. In addition, there have been slight trends upward in well-being in some nations (e.g., Denmark) over the past decades, but not in others (e.g., Japan). But the effects of wealth are not large, and they are dwarfed by other influences, such as those of personality and social relationships.

What might explain the pattern of findings on income and well-being? First, although people's material desires seem to catch up to their incomes and cancel the benefits of higher incomes to some degree, it appears that wealthier individuals have a smaller gap between income and desires than do poor people (Stutzer, in press; van Praag & Frijters, 1999). Rising aspirations seem to nullify only about 70% of increased income (Frey & Stutzer, 2002b). Second, happy people tend to earn higher incomes than unhappy people. Finally, income might correlate with well-being insofar as basic needs are fulfilled, and this explanation is consonant with the evidence showing much stronger effects of income in poorer than in wealthier income groups.

Despite evidence linking income and well-being, economic growth seems to have topped out in its capacity to produce more well-being in developed nations. Thus, although nations will certainly continue to pursue economic growth, in part because of the other benefits besides those that might accrue to well-being (Diener & Diener, 1995), efforts and policies to raise income in wealthy nations are unlikely to increase well-being and might even undermine factors (such as rewarding social relationships or other cherished values) that have higher leverage for producing enhanced well-being.

Thus, when the sciences of economics and of well-being come face-to-face, they sometimes conflict. If the well-being findings simply mirrored those for income and money—with richer people invariably being much happier than poorer people—one would hardly need to measure well-being, or make policy to enhance it directly. But income, a good surrogate historically when basic needs were unmet, is now a weak surrogate for well-being in wealthy nations. What the divergence of the economics and well-being measures demonstrates is that well-being indicators add important information that is missed by economic indicators. Economic development will remain an important priority, but policies fostering economic development must be supplemented by policies that will have a stronger impact on well-being.

Productivity and Well-Being

Job satisfaction and positive mood at work both contribute to the productivity of organizations. Happy employees are better organizational citizens than unhappy employees; they change jobs less frequently, and they shirk less. The costs of unhappy workers to economic productivity are enormous. Policies aimed at producing a happier workforce make sense both because they can enhance well-being in an important realm of life and because they can increase economic productivity and profitability. In an economy of life satisfaction, work should no longer be considered something to be endured in order to obtain income, but rather should be considered a potentially rewarding experience in its own right. When the workplace is properly structured to increase well-being, profits will likely rise. Thus, well-being at work not only is desirable as an end in itself, but also can help to produce greater economic productivity.

Well-Being at Work

Some people consider paid work to be an unpleasant activity that must be suffered in order to earn money. Research, however, indicates that people obtain pleasure from their jobs, even from mundane jobs (Csikszentmihalyi, 1997), and that in many cases they enjoy work activities more than leisure or home life. Dow and Juster (1985) and Juster (1985) found that many working activities are preferred to many nonwork activities. Although Kahneman et al. (2004) found that work was not as pleasant as sex or socializing after work, they did find that it was on average experienced as pleasant. Paid work activities can provide not only enjoyable activities, but also a structure for the day, social contact, a means of achieving respect, and a source of engagement, challenge, and meaning.

A long-standing issue in organizational psychology is the degree to which the happy worker is a good worker. Because early research suggested that the relation between job satisfaction and productivity was small (Iaffaldano & Muchinsky, 1985; Vroom, 1964), many researchers lost interest in the question. In the past decade, however, organizational researchers have altered their conclusions. For one thing, they recognized certain errors in the early reviews, and also realized that seemingly small correlations (e.g., Iaffaldano and Muchinsky reported an average of 0.17 across studies) could amount to huge productivity differences when applied to organizations and to nations. In addition, scientists noticed that certain types of behaviors are consistently related to engagement at work. Job satisfaction is reliably related to organizational citizenship (helping other employees and the organization in ways not specifically related to one's assigned tasks) and the absence of bad citizenship (e.g., stealing from the employer; e.g., Borman, Penner, Allen, & Motowidlo, 2001; Organ & Ryan, 1995). For instance, Bateman and Organ (1983) reported that the more satisfied employees are, the more practical, helpful, and friendly they are, and Miles, Borman, Spector, and Fox (2002) found that the relation between job satisfaction and organizational citizenship can be sizable. Furthermore, studies reveal that experiencing more positive emotions on the job is associated with both better performance and higher levels of organizational citizenship (e.g., Barrick & Mount, 1993; Deluga & Mason, 2000; George, 1990; George & Brief, 1992).

Spector (1997) reviewed evidence showing that satisfied workers have lower turnover and absenteeism than nonsatisfied workers, and are more punctual, cooperative, and helpful to other workers. Carsten and Spector (1987) found that the relation between job satisfaction and turnover can be substantial when unemployment rates are low.

George (1995) found that workers' and managers' positive affect both contributed to performance in the sales staff of a large retail company. In a study in which workers at a technical-support center recorded their moods when prompted as they performed their daily activities, Miner (2001) found that those who were in a pleasant mood performed better than those who were not. He also found that more frequent unpleasant mood was correlated with more withdrawl and lower levels of organizational citizenship (e.g., helping other workers), and that low job satisfaction predicted job absences and turnover. Judge, Thoreson, Bono, and Patton (2001) conducted the most through analysis of the literature on job satisfaction and job performance to date and estimated that the underlying correlation between the two is about 0.30 overall, but higher in relatively complex jobs. Judge et al. maintained that this correlation is large, given the error that is inherent in both satisfaction and performance measures, as well as the organizational benefits of high worker morale. However, a limitation of many studies included in the analysis is that supervisors' ratings were used to measure productivity, and these are subject to several sources of bias.

Well-being of employees also predicts customer satisfaction. Harter, Schmidt, and Hayes (2002) found that the happiness of workers with their jobs correlated with the loyalty of customers, and Fleming (2000) found that customer loyalty and profitability changed together over time. Swaroff (2000) found that the satisfaction of both patients and physicians was correlated with better financial outcomes for a hospital, and Srinivasan and Pugliese (2000) estimated that lack of customer loyalty cost a large bank chain $44 million a year because of customers closing accounts. Thus, one link between employee satisfaction and profitability is that customers are likely to be satisfied when employees are happy in their jobs.

Causality

Could it be that the superior performance of happy workers is due simply to their dispositions, and that workplace characteristics have little or nothing to do with their performance? For example, studies (Diener et al., 2002; Staw, Bell, & Clausen, 1986) have found that measures of dispositional happiness predict people's feelings about their jobs decades later, suggesting that temperament has a long-term influence on job satisfaction. Similarly, after reviewing the literature, Judge and Larsen (2001) reported that the evidence supports the conclusion that dispositions influence job satisfaction. Despite the effects of personality on attitudes toward work, however, it appears that worker satisfaction also depends on characteristics of the work-place (e.g., Roberts, Caspi, & Moffitt, 2003; Watson & Slack, 1993). H. M. Weiss, Nicholas, and Daus (1999) found that positive affect on the job, as well as dispositional happiness, predicts job satisfaction. In a longitudinal study, Spector, Chen, and O'Connell (2000) found that job stressors produce strain in workers beyond the strain explained by temperament. Finally, when outcomes are assessed at the level of organizational work units, benefits are seen. Harter et al. (2002) analyzed a large number of specific divisions within corporations and found that those in which employees were satisfied and engaged were also those with lower turnover and accident rates, and higher productivity and profitability. Because this analysis was based on units, which were aggregates of many workers, individual personality traits are likely to have had less of an influence than in analyses based on individuals. Thus, although personality undoubtedly plays an important role, job satisfaction is influenced by factors in addition to personality.

Causality between well-being on the job and the productivity of the organization is likely to work in both directions (Côté, 1999; Harter, 2000). Among the evidence for causation running from well-being to productivity is a laboratory study by Staw and Barsade (1993). Using an in-basket test (i.e., a test in which participants must quickly handle a large number of standard business situations), they found that happy participants performed better than unhappy participants on interpersonal, managerial, and decision-making tasks. In this case, the happiness could not arise from the "job" because all participants performed the same tasks under the same conditions, and it appears that the happy participants' positive affect was responsible for their superior performance. Second, within-person data showing correlations between mood and performance (e.g., Miner, 2001) suggest that happiness contributes to better performance because they cannot be attributed to the personality of the worker, or to the influence of longterm productivity on mood. In a pioneering study in this area, Hersey (1932) found that workers performed better on days when they were in a good mood than on days when they were in a bad mood, although it is possible in this case that productivity led to better moods.

Longitudinal research provides yet another type of evidence suggesting a causal influence of workplace happiness on productivity. Harter (2000) measured employee engagement using a questionnaire developed by the Gallup Organization (items assessed, e.g., positive relationships with supervisors) and found that employee engagement predicted employee turnover and customer loyalty at a later time period, whereas the association between performance and later engagement was much smaller. The causal path from employee engagement to net sales of the organization went in both directions. Schneider, Hanges, Smith, and Salvaggio (2003) found that financial success of companies and job satisfaction each predicted the other significantly, although the path from financial success to job satisfaction was the stronger one. Koys (2001) found that across time, employees' attitudes predicted organizational effectiveness, but that organizational effectiveness did not predict job attitudes such as work satisfaction at a later time. Kohn and Schooler (1982) found that the nature of the work predicted worker depression over time, and Staw et al. (1994) found that positive affect predicted higher pay and better supervisors' ratings at a later time. In a causal modeling study, Judge (1991) found that job satisfaction predicted lower rates of absenteeism, shirking, and tardiness. Finally, Wright and Bonett (1997) found that emotional exhaustion on the job predicted work performance.

In sum, it is likely that the positive effects of well-being at work on performance go beyond the effects of personality. The well-being of workers results in positive organizational citizenship, customer satisfaction, and perhaps even greater productivity. Because specific workplace variables are known to enhance well-being at work, organizational policies can raise workers' well-being and thereby enhance organizational citizenship and possibly profitability.

Spillover from Work

Feelings about work leak into other realms of life. Rice, Near, and Hunt (1980) reviewed 23 studies and found a reliable association between life satisfaction and work satisfaction for both males and females, with the correlation being stronger for men. Heller, Judge, and Watson (2002) also tested the spillover hypothesis and found that life satisfaction and job satisfaction are correlated, but that this correlation drops when personality variables are statistically controlled. In a 12-year panel study, Rogers and May (2003) found that marital quality and job satisfaction are related over time. Similarly, Kang (2001) found spillover from the job to marriage. In a daily diary study, positive experiences at work reduced conflictual marital interactions that day, and conflictual marital interactions reduced the positivity of work experience the next day (Doumas, Margolin, & John, 2003). In a longitudinal study, Grebner, Semmer, and Elfering (2003) found that employees' evaluations of working conditions produce changes in well-being reported on-line; for example, lack of job control predicts lack of energy on non-workdays. Thus, work satisfaction can spill over into home-life satisfaction and vice versa.

Unemployment

Unemployment so often has deleterious effects on well-being that it deserves a separate discussion. Many researchers have found that the unemployed have lower levels of well-being (e.g., Clark & Oswald, 1994; Di Tella et al., 2001; Helliwell, 2003a) and higher levels of suicide (Kposowa, 2001) than the employed. Shams and Jackson (1994) reported that the longer individuals were unemployed, the lower their well-being, and Viinamaeki, Koskela, and Niskanen (1996) found increasing levels of depression over time in the unemployed. Clark (2001) found that unemployment was associated with more negative effects in communities where unemployment was low than in communities where unemployment was high.

But might unhappy people be more likely to be unemployed than happy people? That is, might unhappiness cause unemployment? Two studies on the same large longitudinal data set (Clark, Diener, Georgellis, & Lucas, 2004; Lucas, Clark, Georgellis, & Diener, 2004) suggest that people who are later unemployed do not start out with low life satisfaction. Rather, their life satisfaction drops dramatically around the time of their layoff. Furthermore, they do not recover to their former levels of life satisfaction even after several years, even after most of them have obtained a new job with pay almost equal to their pay before being laid off. These findings suggest that the unemployed are "scarred" by the experience of losing their jobs. Creed and Macintyre (2001) found that unemployed people experienced lowered well-being because they lacked time structure and feelings of purpose.

Causes of Worker Well-Being

Many possible causes of worker well-being have been investigated, and a host of factors have been implicated, from low noise levels (Raffaello & Maass, 2003) to positive behaviors of the supervisor (Harter, Schmidt, & Killham, 2003). Factors such as workload (Groenewegen & Hutten, 1991), person-job fit (e.g., Bretz & Judge, 1994; De Fruyt, 2002; Rounds, 1990; Rounds, Dawis, & Lofquist, 1987), management's communication style (Dooley, 1996), and the variety of skills used on the job (Glisson & Durick, 1988) also influence job satisfaction. Using a longitudinal design and external ratings of job conditions, Grebner et al. (2003) found that job control (i.e., feelings of control over one's work) correlated with greater well-being on the job, whereas job stressors correlated with lower well-being on the job.

After reviewing the literature on work satisfaction, Warr (1999) concluded that rewarding jobs tend to have the following characteristics:

- Opportunity for personal control
- Opportunity for using skills
- Variety of tasks
- Physical security
- Supportive supervisor
- Respect and high status
- Interpersonal contact
- Good pay and fringe benefits
- Clear requirements and information on how to meet them.

Conclusions and Cautions

The majority of adults spend many waking hours at work. Work policies are often structured to maximize productivity and minimize costs, and issues concerning the quality of work life are usually considered only if they serve one of these goals. However, wealthy societies have now reached such a level of productivity that having engaging, rewarding work is a concern for increasing numbers of workers and can influence their productivity and retention on the job. Recrafting jobs so that they are maximally engaging, rewarding, and meaningful, but still compatible with the mission of the organization, will become a priority of future employers as the top workers are increasingly drawn to organizations that take seriously the goal of producing life satisfaction among their workers.

Well-being at work is likely to interact with other variables in producing its positive effects. Abbott (2003) found that employees working in difficult conditions nevertheless performed well, and that employee morale did not invariably predict the performance of organizations, indicating that the larger motivational context of work will influence the effects of workers' morale. Karasek (2001) suggested that jobs should be redesigned to include well-being as a goal. In a work-redesign experiment, Griffin (1991) altered the tasks of bank tellers to make the job more intrinsically rewarding and professional. Satisfaction and commitment showed short-term increases only, whereas performance increased only later in the 2-year study. Pleasant affect might be most helpful in jobs that involve sales and supervision, because characteristics that are useful in these jobs, such as flexibility and sociability, are enhanced by positive emotions; in contrast, happiness might be less helpful in other types of vocations, such as those requiring vigilance for errors (Lucas & Diener, 2003). Thus, there is a need for more research on how and when positive job attitudes and positive affect on the job lead to better performance. Nevertheless, the preponderance of evidence points to the fact that happy work units tend to be productive work units.

If worker well-being increases productivity, it is important to consider policies that will increase well-being at work. For instance, flextime, on-site day-care facilities, plans for allowing employees to work at home, employee stock options, and generous family-leave policies can all enhance job satisfaction if they are properly implemented. Similarly, training supervisors to give appropriate praise and feedback, facilitating friendships on the job, and providing the tools workers need are likely to enhance job satisfaction (Harter et al., 2003). Finally, selecting workers so that their personality characteristics, strengths, and interests fit the job will likely enhance worker well-being (e.g., Bretz & Judge, 1994).

Physical Health and Well-Being

In general, positive states of well-being correlate with better physical health (e.g., Hilleras, Jorm, Herlitz, & Winblad, 1998; Murrell, Salsman, & Meeks, 2003; Ostir, Markides, Black, & Goodwin, 2000). Correlations between objective physical health (i.e., health as assessed by medical personnel) and well-being are low in broad samples of respondents, in part because people appear to adapt over time to many illnesses and because most people are relatively healthy. However, certain illnesses that interfere with daily functioning produce marked decrements in well-being. In addition, reports of global well-being and ill-being correlate positively and negatively, respectively, with longevity, and subjective health (i.e., how people evaluate their own health) predicts mortality even when differences in objective health are statistically controlled. The intensity of physical pain is magnified by feelings of ill-being. Furthermore, psychosocial interventions can enhance the well-being of ill people, and possibly even increase longevity. Thus, well-being and absence of ill-being predict better later health, but the mixed nature of the data indicates that the association between well-being and physical health is influenced by variables that are not yet understood. Well-being is an important outcome to be considered in studies of and policies regarding physical health because it signifies quality of life, but it also is important because of its implications for health and health care costs.

Physical Health Affects Well-Being

Not surprisingly, self-reported health is related to well-being, as revealed in an analysis of the literature conducted by Okun, Stock, Haring, and Witter (1984), as well as in more recent studies (e.g., Lyubomirsky & Lepper, 2003). Marmot (2003) reported correlations of about 0.60 between low life satisfaction and subjective poor health in the Whitehall samples of people in the British civil service. The relation between objective health and well-being is usually much smaller, however (e.g., Brief, Butcher, George, & Link, 1993; Okun & George, 1984). Nevertheless, severe health problems that interfere with daily functioning can lower well-being, sometimes substantially so, as can lethal illnesses. For example, Verbrugge, Reoma, and Gruber-Baldini (1994) found that the well-being of people with serious illnesses, such as congestive heart failure, declined over 1 year. Even though people with serious illnesses are likely to be above neutral in well-being, their well-being is often lower than that of matched control subjects (e.g., a group of people who are the same age and sex as the ill subjects), and even lower if they have multiple conditions, such as diabetes and heart failure (e.g., Mehnert, Krauss, Nadler, & Boyd, 1990). Furthermore, people with serious illnesses do not invariably adapt to them. In a longitudinal study of patients with congestive heart failure or acute myocardial infarction, mean levels of anxiety and depression remained substantially elevated (compared with levels before the patients became ill) 1 year after diagnosis (van Jaarsveld, Sanderman, Miedema, Ranchor, & Kempen, 2001).

Other illnesses are associated with substantially more negative affect. For example, Stilley et al. (1999) found that nearly half of transplant recipients report clinically significant levels of distress, and more than half of patients with AIDS or cancer are clinically depressed (van Servellen, Sarna, Padilla, & Brecht, 1996). Depression and anxiety are prevalent in women with HIV and often reach clinical levels (van Servellen et al., 1998).

Not only life-threatening diseases, but also illnesses that restrict activities and cause pain can lower well-being. Patients with fibromyalgia and rheumatoid arthritis show more depression and anxiety, and lower life satisfaction, than control subjects (Celiker & Borman, 2001), and Evers, Kraaimaat, Geenen, and Bijlsma (1997) found that lessening of inflammation in arthritis patients was accompanied by lessening in anxiety and depression.

Well-Being Affects Physical Health and Pain

There is also evidence that causality might run from well-being to health. As mentioned earlier, Vázquez et al. (2004) found that longevity is greater in nations where well-being is high, even after controlling statistically for national income and infant mortality; because of the statistical controls in this study, the results suggest the possibility of causation from well-being to health. One study found that patients with end-state renal failure were more likely to survive for 4 years if they were happy than if they were not (Devins, Mann, Mandin, & Leonard, 1990). Conversely, negative emotions often predict worse health outcomes. A study of cardiac patients demonstrated that those with mood disturbances such as depression were particularly likely to show increasingly poor functioning over time and worsening of cardiac symptoms (Clarke, Frasure-Smith, Lespérance, & Bourassa, 2000). In a 4-year longitudinal study of nursing-home residents, patients at the same level of objective physical health lived longer the higher their self-esteem and the lower their levels of depressive symptoms at an initial assessment. In other longitudinal studies, optimism has been associated with longevity. In a Mayo Clinic study of patients in the early 1950s, optimistic patients lived about 8 years longer on average than pessimistic patients (Maruta, Colligan, Malinchoc, & Offord, 2000; Peterson, Seligman, Yurko, Martin, & Friedman, 1998); in another study, hope was associated with increased survival time in cancer patients (Faller, Buelzebruck, Schilling, Drings, & Lang, 1997). Parker, Thorslund, and Nordstrom (1992) found that life satisfaction predicted mortality in old people (i.e., those ages 75–84), but not in the very old (i.e., those over 85), suggesting that well-being might have different effects depending on stage of life or the severity of health problems.

Optimism has consistently been found to predict outcomes in cardiovascular diseases. For example, greater optimism is associated with lowered reports of symptoms of angina in cardiac patients (Fitzgerald, Prochaska, & Pransky, 2000), as well as greater longevity and lowered rates of nonfatal heart attacks (Kubzansky, Sparrow, Vokonas, & Kawachi, 2001). In a longitudinal study, Kubzansky et al. (2002) found that people with an optimistic explanatory style had better pulmonary function than people with a more pessimistic style, and showed a slower decline in health over 8 years. This finding is consistent with evidence showing that pleasant emotions can undo the influence of unpleasant emotions on cardiovascular parameters (Fredrickson & Levenson, 1998; Fredrickson, Mancuso, Branigan, & Tugade, 2000). In a review of studies on coronary heart disease, Carney, Rich, and Jaffe (1995) found that depression (which is reliably related to lack of optimism) predicted increased illness and mortality and attributed this finding to the fact that depressed people do not follow treatment regimens as well as nondepressed people, smoke more, have higher blood pressure, and have poorer physiological functioning. Thus, behavioral as well as physiological pathways are likely to link well-being to health. Other studies have shown that happy people act in healthier ways than unhappy people do. For example, individuals who report high well-being exercise more and engage in more physical activity than people who report low well-being (Audrain, Schwartz, Herrera, Golman, & Bush, 2001; Lox, Burns, Treasure, & Wasley, 1999).

Can well-being affect the course of cancer? Spiegel and Giese-Davis (2003) reviewed the evidence relating depression to cancer and drew several conclusions. First, they concluded that severe depression might raise the risk for cancer, although the data are mixed on this question. Second, they argued that depression may speed up the progression of cancer, as well as reduce longevity, although again, the data are not completely consistent (see also Faller et al., 1997; Naughton et al., 2002). When psychosocial support is given to cancer patients, the support can alleviate pain and depression, and perhaps even increase survival time. Of 10 studies on survival time that Spiegel and Giese-Davis reviewed, 5 showed a benefit from psychosocial interventions, and none showed that such interventions had a detrimental effect on outcomes. Thus, it appears that the reported beneficial effects of psychosocial interventions are not due to chance. Spiegel and Giese-Davis concluded: "There is growing evidence of a relationship between depression and cancer incidence and progression" (p. 278).

In studies of mortality from all causes, well-being predicts longevity. Low life satisfaction was found to predict all-cause mortality in a large and representative sample of adults in the United States (Fiscella & Franks, 1997). Similarly, Danner, Snowdon, and Friesen (2001) found that pleasant emotions expresses at age 22 as women entered a Catholic convent predicted their longevity after age 75. Nuns with high levels of pleasant emotions in young adulthood lived on average more than 9 years longer than nuns with low levels of pleasant emotions in young adulthood. Although this study found that only pleasant affect predicted longevity, and negative affect did not, other studies have found roles for negative affect in a variety of negative health outcomes. For example, a longitudinal study in Scandinavia found that low life satisfaction predicted fatal accidents (Koivumaa-Honkanen, Honkanen, Koskenvuo, Viinamaki, & Kaprio, 2002), and, as already noted, depression has been associated with reduced survival time among patients with cancer and coronary heart disease.

In a large sample of older Americans, Ostir et al. (2000) found that respondents who were high in positive emotions were twice as likely to survive through the 2-year follow-up of the study as those who were low in positive emotions; factors such as chronic health conditions, smoking, diet, and marital status were controlled in the statistical analysis. Ostir et al. also found that high levels of positive emotions were associated with a greatly reduced risk of becoming disabled. In a classic study, Ulrich (1984) studied postoperative patients who were assigned to hospital rooms with a pleasant or unpleasant view. Those who had a view of trees, as opposed to a brick wall, were more rapidly discharged, suggesting that the pleasant view caused faster recovery.

Additional evidence indicates that recovery from diverse health problems is affected by well-being. Kopp et al. (2003) found that preoperative well-being predicted better recovery from surgery. The well-being of people when they entered a whiplash rehabilitation program predicted whether these patients were doing paid work 2 years later (Heikkilä, Heikkilä, & Eisemann, 1998). Patients who had surgery for osteorthritis of the knee reported greater functional improvement at 3 and 12 months after the surgery if they were low in anxiety and depression before the surgery (Faller, Kirschner, & König, 2003).

Does well-being influence pain and whether people seek treatment for pain? People who are low in well-being have a more difficult time coping with pain than people who are high in well-being, and retrospectively overestimate their levels of pain (Keefe, Lumley, Anderson, Lunch, & Carson, 2001). Zelman, Howland, Nichols, and Cleeland (1991) found that people put into a positive mood showed greater pain tolerance than control subjects, and this finding was replicated by Cogan, Cogan, Waltz, and McCue (1987).

People put into a pleasant mood also show lower blood pressure reactivity to a stressor than participants in whom a positive mood was not induced (T. W. Smith, Ruiz, & Uchino, 2001). The number of daily stressors experienced correlates with increases in joint pain in patients with rheumatoid arthritis (Affleck et al., 1997). Zautra et al. (1998) extended this finding by showing that stress is related to changes in the immune system, which are in turn followed by inflammation and increased pain. Patients' indicators of immune activity were higher in a week they experienced high conflict with their spouses than in a baseline week. This pattern was not found, however, in women who had relatively good relationships with their spouses. Although the connection between stress and pain is not direct and is not found in every study, the existing evidence demonstrates that a connection exists.

Experimental evidence reveals that the immune system is influenced by people's well-being; rigorous evidence sometimes points to a beneficial effect of positive emotions and sometimes points to a negative influence for unpleasant emotions. Cohen and his colleagues conducted an impressive set of studies showing that happy people are less susceptible to cold and flu viruses than unhappy people are. For instance, Cohen, Doyle, Turner, Alper, and Skoner (2003) found that people who reported high levels of positive emotions were at a reduced risk of developing cold symptoms when exposed to cold viruses. The least happy third of the participants in this study were 2.9 times more likely to develop a cold than the happiest third, controlling for sex, age, and other factors. In further studies, Cohen and his colleagues found that self-reported stress was associated with increased inflammation following exposure to a flu virus (Cohen, Doyle, & Skoner, 1999), and that both the tendency to chronically experience negative emotions (sometimes referred to as negative affectivity) and exposure to severe or chronic problems resulted in lowered immune response (Cohen, Miller, & Rabin, 2001). The lower immune response due to the experience of problems occurred upon reexposure to the flu virus, and was most pronounced among the elderly. Finally, Marsland, Cohen, Rabin, and Manuck (2001) found a lowered antibody response to the hepatitis virus among people high in negative affectivity.

Other researchers have extended the findings of Cohen and his colleagues. For instance, Solomon, Segerstrom, Grohr, Kemeny, and Fahey (1997) found increases in immune function after positive moods and decreases in immune function after negative moods. Kamen-Siegel, Rodin, Seligman, and Dwyer (1991) reported that optimistic old people had better immune function than pessimistic old people. The results from a within-person longitudinal analysis show that people's immunity is stronger on days when they are in a good mood than on days when they are in a bad mood (Stone, Cox, Valdimarsdottir, Jandorf, & Neale, 1987). Vitaliano et al. (1998) found that among cancer patients, experiencing more daily uplifts (small positive events) and fewer daily hassles (small negative events) was correlated with having more natural killer cells (immune cells that attack invading pathogens), and Lyons and Chamberlain (1994) found that positive events lowered people's incidence of respiratory infections. We view these studies as most likely showing a causal effect of mood because experimental manipulations of moods are followed by similar changes in immune strength (Futerman, Kemeny, Shapiro, & Fahey, 1994; McClelland & Cheriff, 1997).

Conclusions and Cautions

Our review of this extensive literature has not been exhaustive by any means, but instead was designed to give readers a sense of the links that seem to exist between well-being and physical health. It is surprising that people with ill health often adjust so well to their condition and report positive levels of well-being—this is a tribute to human psychological resilience. It does appear, however, that severe health conditions often impair well-being to a degree. In addition, well-being appears to predict future health and longevity, sometimes powerfully. The pathways of this influence are unknown but may involve both psychological (e.g., immune activity) and behavioral (e.g., more exercise) factors. A major task for future research is to explore these pathways. It is very encouraging that psychosocial interventions can in some cases increase the well-being of sick individuals, and perhaps even extend life.

Mental Disorders

Mental disorder is another arena in which historical trends in well-being have been startlingly and strongly opposite the trends in economics: As developed nations have become wealthier, mental health has either dropped sharply or stayed the same. This is an area where governmental and institutional policies can make an enormous difference to well-being. Mental disorders lower well-being, and for many disorders there exist specific treatments, both psychotherapies and medications, that can reduce symptoms and improve well-being. Empirical data have undermined the notion that mental disorders are persistent, unrelievable, and incurable, and it is now realized that people with mental disorders often improve over time and with treatment, and that they can achieve significant improvements in quality of life. Thus, beyond relieving suffering, increasing well-being is becoming an essential part of the treatment and measurement of mental disorders, providing an additional window through which to view the effectiveness of mental health interventions. Although economic indicators can help show the costs of mental disorders, well-being indicators are essential for understanding the full costs of these disorders, as well as the substantial value of treatments and interventions. Furthermore, high well-being is likely to buffer against the incidence of at least some mental disorders.

Mental Disorders are a Major Cause of Low Well-Being

Mental disorders are widespread, and perhaps growing in frequency, in modern society. A structured psychiatric interview was administered to a national sample of adults in the United States just over a decade ago. Almost 50% of the respondents reported having had at least one mental disorder in their lifetime, and nearly 30% reported a disorder during the past year (Kessler et al., 1994). The rate of experiencing a disorder during the past month was an astonishing 18.2% (Kessler & Frank, 1997). Similarly, Jenkins et al. (1997) found that according to standard interpretational criteria, 16% of young adults in a national British sample could be classified as having a "neurotic" disorder during the past week. About half of the disorders were a mix of anxiety and depression (Jenkins et al., 2003). In a study conducted in Ireland, 2.4% of the population had been clinically depressed during the past month, and 6.0% during the past year; 12.2% had experienced a mental disorder of some type during the past year (McConnell, Bebbington, McClelland, Gillespie, & Houghton, 2002).

As medical illnesses have yielded to prevention and treatment in recent decades, mental disorders have risen in the rankings of major causes of suffering. For example, a single mental disorder, depression, is the third leading cause (after arthritis and heart disease) of loss in quality-adjusted life years (a measure of longevity that factors in quality of life), ranking above cancers, stroke, diabetes, and obstructive lung disease (Unutzer et al., 2000). Murray and Lopez (1997) estimated that by 2020 depression will be the second leading cause in the world for disability-adjusted life years (an alternative measure of longevity factoring in loss of ability to do the normal tasks of everyday life), being the first cause of disease burden in the developed societies and the third leading cause in poorer nations.

Not only is mental disorder common, but it almost always causes poor well-being (e.g., Packer, Husted, Cohen, & Tomlinson, 1997). Much research has been conducted on two major forms of mental illness, depression and anxiety, and this work has shown that these disorders lead to significant decrements in well-being. This is not surprising, because these disorders directly worsen people's evaluations of the world, the future, and themselves. Koivumaa-Honkanen, Honkanen, Antikainen, and Hintikka (1999) found that people with depression or anxiety disorders tend to have low life satisfaction. Spitzer et al. (1995) found that people with mood disorders have a lower quality of life than people with arthritis, cardiac disease, pulmonary disease, or diabetes. Although bipolar disorder is sometimes thought to be a pleasant kind of euphoria, this is distinctly false, and individuals with this disorder report significantly lower levels of well-being than other (Arnold, Witzeman, Swank, McElroy, & Keck, 2000).

Other forms of mental disorders, such as schizophrenia, also lower well-being. For example, Koivumaa-Honkanen et al. (1999) found that life satisfaction tends to be low among people with schizophrenia, although they generally have higher life satisfaction than people with depression and anxiety disorders. Suslow, Roestel, Ohrmann, and Arolt (2003) found that schizophrenics reported more fear and disgust than nonschizophrenics, and that anger and guilt increased with the chronicity of the disease. Suicide rates are 20–50 times higher among schizophrenics than in the general population (Pinikahana, Happell, & Keks, 2003). The level of well-being schizophrenics report depends on the overall severity of their symptoms (Bradshaw & Brekke, 1999). Conversely, in one of our studies (Diener & Seligman, 2002), we found that the happiest people showed very low levels of symptoms of mental illness. Our very happy respondents scored low on most pathology scales of the Minnesota Multiphasic Personality Inventory, such as Hysteria, Schizophrenia, and Hypochondriasis.[3]

A significant amount of family suffering also occurs because of mental disorders. Schulz, Visintainer, and Williamson (1990) reviewed evidence showing that the cumulative effects of caring for someone with mental illness increase the caregiver's

---

[3] The Minnesota Multiphasic Personality Inventory (MMPI) is an instrument for measuring personality and psychological adjustment. Most of its scales assess tendencies toward various forms of psychopathology.

chances for a psychological disorder, as well as physical illness. Martens and Addington (2001) found that family members are stressed substantially by having to care for a relative with schizophrenia. The parents of drug addicts experience higher levels of stress compared with other parents (Andrade, Sarmah, & Channabasavanna, 1989). Having a parent with depression or another mental disorder may contribute to the likelihood of depression (Hammen, 2000).

In stark contrast to the improvement in economic statistics over the past 50 years, there is strong evidence that the incidence of depression has increased enormously over the same time period. This is a very revealing paradox. People usually think that depression is intimately related to bad life circumstances, but things have never been better objectively. The hands on the doomsday clock are farther away from midnight than ever before since its debut. Worldwide, there are fewer soldiers dying on the battlefield than at any time in the past hundred years. A smaller percentage of children are now dying of starvation than at any time in human history. There is more purchasing power, more music, more education, more books, worldwide instant communication, and more entertainment than ever before. But contrary to the economic statistics, all the statistics on depression and demoralization are getting worse. These facts indicate that depression is not about poor objective circumstances, and if policymakers rely only on economic statistics, they will completely miss this erosion of well-being.

Four lines of evidence point to a huge increase in depression over the past 50 years: First, the Epidemiological Catchment Area (ECA) study sampled a large and representative group of Americans from catchment areas in the United States and Canada and showed that people born earlier in the 20th century experienced much less depression in their lifetime than people born later (Robins et al., 1984). The data are remarkable. People born around 1910 had only a 1.3% chance of having experienced a major depressive episode, even though by the time of the study they had had at least 75 years to develop the disorder. In contrast, those born after 1960 already had a 5.3% chance, even though they had been alive for only 25 years. Each succeeding cohort in each area had a higher rate of depression than cohorts before it. There were huge differences in the rates of depression across cohorts, suggesting a roughly 10-fold increase in risk for depression across generations.

Second, a massive international study showed similar rises in depression (Cross National Collaborative Group, 1992). In this study, a sample of almost 40,000 adults from the United States, Puerto Rico, Germany, France, Italy, Lebanon, New Zealand, and Taiwan had diagnostic interviews. All national groups showed dramatic increases in risk for depression across the 20th century, despite tremendous economic growth in almost all of these locations.

Third, diagnostic studies of relatives of people who have clinically severe depression show that younger relatives are much more susceptible to depression that older relatives (Klerman et al., 1985). Thousands of relatives of 523 people with affective disorders were given a structured diagnostic interview to determine the prevalence of major depressive disorders in this sample. Consider, for example, women born in 1950 versus women born before 1910. By age 30, about 65% of the women born in 1950 had one depressive episode, whereas fewer than 5% of the women in the 1910 cohort had such an episode by the time they were 30. For almost all age groups, a more recent year of birth conferred more and earlier risk for major depressive disorder. Overall, we estimate the risk increased at least 10-fold across two generations.

Fourth, a study of the Old Order Amish living in Lancaster County, Pennsylvania, showed very low rates of unipolar depression (Egeland & Hostetter, 1983). The Amish are an ultraconservative Protestant sect descended entirely from thirty 18th-century progenitors. No electricity is permitted in their homes, they use horses and buggies for transportation, alcoholism and crime are virtually unknown in this community, and pacifism is absolute. Using diagnostic interviews, researchers found 41 active cases of major depressive disorder in this group for the 5-year period from 1976 to 1980; this is a 5-year prevalence of about 0.5% (there were about 8,000 adult Amish in the area). If we compare this rate with the parallel figures from the ECA study, we can roughly estimate that the Amish have about 1/5 to 1/10 the risk for unipolar depression that neighboring Americans from modern cultures do. In addition, despite the lack of luxury amenities, the Amish are satisfied with their lives (see Table 1).

Sadly, it is young people who are now particularly at risk. Forty years ago, the average age for the first episode of depression was 29.5 (Beck, 1967), and depression was unusual in adolescence. Now it typically attacks its victims for the first time when they are teenagers. For example, Lewinsohn and his colleagues gave diagnostic interviews to 1,710 randomly selected adolescents living in western Oregon and found that by age 14, 7.2% of the youngest adolescents, those born in 1972 through 1974, had experienced a severe depression; in contrast, 4.5% of the older adolescents, those born in 1968 through 1971, had experienced severe depression (Lewinsohn, Rohde, Seeley, & Fischer, 1993). The high percentage of youth experiencing severe depression at such a young age is surprising and dismaying. Depression tends to recur, and a first onset during the teen years typically results in several more episodes in a lifetime than a first onset in middle age.

Is Increasing Depression a Measurement Artifact?

Is the dramatic increase in depression over the past 50 years an artifact? Three possible reasons why this trend might be an artifact are salient: First, perhaps diagnosis has improved, and depression is now better recognized because it is the "flavor of the month." Second, troubles that used to be thought of as an inevitable part of "life" may now be thought of as a disease that ought to be cured, so what people label as depression now may not have been so labeled before. Third, memory of recent events is better than memory of distant events, and depressive episodes from long ago may simply have been forgotten by the respondents in the studies showing rises in the incidence of depression.

The first and second potential reasons are both undercut by the same argument. In the studies investigators did not ask, "Were you ever depressed?" Rather, they asked questions that covered the complete series of symptoms for depression, for example, "Was there ever a time in your life when you cried every day for two weeks?" Then from the answers to these specific symptom questions, a diagnosis was made. So the increasing rates and earlier incidence of depression that were reported were not based on how respondents labeled their experiences, but were based on behaviorally based items. It also seems unlikely that the results are an artifact of memory, because no such fading of memories was found for delusions and hallucinations, or for alcoholic binges; these do not show an increase over time that would indicate that memories of symptoms long ago were systematically forgotten. So the order of magnitude increase in depression over the past 50 years is likely a real phenomenon and not an artifact of the measures.

Many Psychological Interventions are Effective

Although mental disorders are common, are on the rise, and cause significant decrements in well-being, many disorders are treatable. In a large-scale study of psychological treatments, Seligman (1995) found that clients benefit substantially from psychotherapy. Fourteen of the major mental disorders are relievable, and two (blood and injury phobia, panic disorder) are virtually curable by specific forms of medications or psychotherapies. From a review of studies, Tramontana (1981) concluded that about 75% of adolescents improve in psychotherapy, about twice as many as improve without receiving therapy. The benefits of psychotherapy were also demonstrated in a study by Gloaguen, Cottraux, Cucherat, and Blackburn (1998), who found that cognitive therapy is more effective in treating depression than antidepressants, and more likely to prevent long-term relapse (see also Steinbrueck, Maxwell, & Howard, 1983). Westen (2001) reported that treatments for panic disorders are effective and have lasting effects; treatments for depression and generalized anxiety have significant short-term effects, but these might not last over time. Kashdan and Herbert (2001) reviewed the literature on the treatment of social anxiety in children and found that various forms of cognitive behavior therapy are efficacious.

Numerous studies demonstrate that interventions not only reduce symptoms, but also increase well-being. For instance, McCrady, Stout, Noel, Abrams, and Nelson (1991) found that a treatment for alcoholism that involved the spouse led to gradual improvements in abstinence, as well as higher reports of well-being and lower rates of marital separation. Longabaugh et al. (1983) found that two treatments for alcoholism that involved spouses were equally effective in producing abstinence, but that the treatment that allowed patients to go home at nights and on weekends rather than remain hospitalized led to reports of higher well-being. This is but one example of well-being measures providing information beyond what can be gleaned from recovery rates and economic indicators.

It is an important methodological point, however, that the mental illness tradition and the well-being tradition have barely shaken hands. Mental illness investigators only infrequently measure well-being and are content with measures of suffering and its diminution. Such measures almost certainly underestimate the benefits of treatments and miss entirely the likelihood that increased well-being plays a role in the treatment and prevention of mental illness. We strongly recommend the use of both well-being indicators and the usual symptom measures in the future study of mental illness.

Despite the fact that therapy is effective, a large percentage of people with mental problems go untreated, even in wealthy, industrialized societies. For example, McConnell et al. (2002) found that in Ireland, care was provided for only 29% of episodes of mental illness, and care for certain problems, such as anxiety disorders, was provided much less frequently. Kessler et al. (1994) found that in the United States, the majority of individuals with psychological disorders fail to obtain treatment, and even individuals with three or more disorders receive treatment less than half of the time.

Policy Implications

Both economic and well-being analyses of mental disorders lead to the conclusion that these problems are significant and costly. Economic statistics alone, however, completely fail to capture the decrease in well-being caused by mental disorders, particularly because mental disorders have increased substantially over the same period that developed economies have tripled. The two types of statistics are complementary in shedding light on different aspects of the problem, as well as interventions. For instance, an economic analysis shows the monetary costs of mental disorders and the dollar benefits of various forms of treatment, whereas a well-being analysis captures the tremendous suffering caused by mental disorders and the benefits to well-being that treatments provide. It is interesting to note that higher rates of mental illness and ill-being experienced in a society can increase GDP if more money is spent on hospitalization, crime prevention, and imprisonment of individuals with disorders. Paradoxically, a mounting problem in well-being might increase economic indicators, and the increase in GDP does not indicate whether the money is spent effectively.

The most important policy implication of the increased incidence of mental disorders is that people with these disorders should obtain more help in getting treatment. Although such treatment can be expensive, failure to treat individuals can be costly, both in terms of well-being and in terms of losses in productivity, increases in crime, and so forth. Although interventions do not always permanently cure mental disorders, they can nevertheless often boost well-being. A related implication is that all studies on the outcome of treatment ought to include measures of well-being in addition to mere symptom relief, and these should be used in evaluating the effectiveness of interventions (Lehman, 1996).

New policies could help the family members of people with mental problems. For example, policies can establish and support more assisted-living arrangements—board-and-care programs, apartments where support is provided, and group homes (e.g., Nelson, Hall, & Walsh-Bowers, 1999)—in order to reduce the burden on caregivers and increase the well-being and security of the patients. Rimmerman, Treves, and Duvdevany (1999) found that mothers who are caregivers to adult children experience reduced psychological distress if the children participate in day treatment. In a quasi-experimental longitudinal study, Zarit, Stephens, Townsend, and Greene (1998) found that the use of adult day care for people with dementia reduced stress and improved psychological well-being in caregivers. These are but two of many examples showing that aid to caregivers can increase their well-being.

Conclusions About Mental Disorder and Well-Being

Many forms of mental disorder reduce well-being, and there are effective therapies that both alleviate the symptoms of the disorder and increase well-being. Remarkably, mental illness, particularly depression, has increased substantially over the same period that economic statistics have risen substantially. Decreasing the suffering and increasing the well-being of people with mental disorders should be a priority of any society that takes well-being seriously. Because such a high percentage of mental disorder and the attendant suffering goes unrecognized and untreated, we argue that monitoring well-being in addition to rates of disorder in the population as a whole would be very beneficial to a humane society that is committed to enhancing well-being for all citizens. We also urge that mental illness investigators include well-being measures in their studies. Furthermore, it is imperative that researchers uncover the roots of the rising levels of depression and anxiety so that preventive actions can be taken. Finally, research on effective treatments for mental disorders must be a top priority.

Social Relationships

The quality of people's social relationships is crucial to their well-being. People need supportive, positive relationships and social belonging to sustain well-being. Baumeister and Leary (1995) reviewed evidence showing that the need to belong, to have close and long-term social relationships, is a fundamental human need, and that well-being depends on this need being well met. People need social bonds in committed relationships, not simply interactions with strangers, to experience well-being. Economic indicators do not correlate well with the quality of social relationships and hence omit this key contribution to well-being. In some cases, policies based solely on economic analyses can harm social relationships and thereby decrease well-being. Furthermore, high well-being may abet positive social relationships.

Social Relationships are Essential to Well-Being

Numerous studies support the conclusion that social relationships are essential to well-being. In our study of very happy people (Diener & Seligman, 2002), we found that every single respondent in our happiest group had excellent social relationships. Park, Peterson, and Seligman (2003) found that of 24 character strengths, those that best predict life satisfaction are the interpersonal ones. Examining data from both representative surveys of adolescents and adults and focus-group discussions, Lansford (2000) found that high-quality social relationships bolster well-being. Schilling and Wahl (2002) found that the rural elderly in Germany had larger family networks than the elderly people living in cities, and those family networks were partly responsible for the higher life satisfaction of the rural elderly.

People experience more positive emotions when they are with others than when they are alone (Pavot, Diener, & Fujita, 1990); although people have slightly more negative emotions when in social than in nonsocial situations, positive affect is substantially higher on average in social situations. Furthermore, both extraverts and introverts experience a higher amount of pleasant emotions in social situations. Menec (2003) found that frequency of participating in social activities is associated with greater happiness, better functioning, and lower mortality in the elderly.

Thoits and Hewitt (2001) found that people high in life satisfaction and happiness were more likely than others to be community volunteers. Harlow and Cantor (1996) found that older adults' participation in community service and other social activities was associated with greater life satisfaction, after statistically controlling for social support, individual differences in personality variables, health, and prior life satisfaction. Participation in these activities was most important for people who were no longer working. In addition, being married and having contact with one's children and siblings was a significant predictor of life satisfaction, as were congeniality and organizational membership. Social and community service had the strongest relation with life satisfaction (except for prior life satisfaction). Analyses controlling for prior satisfaction showed that organizational membership, congeniality, and social participation all predicted later life satisfaction.

Although receiving social support is often emphasized as a means of coping with stressors, evidence shows that giving support to other people might be at least as important. Fromm (1956) maintained that fully functioning adults not only need to be loved, but also need to love. In a study supporting this thesis, S. L. Brown, Nesse, Vinokur, and Smith (2003) found that giving social support is more important to longevity than receiving social support, and Herzberg et al. (1998) found that difficulties in giving social support to others is a risk factor for interpersonal stress. They measured interpersonal competencies, including the ability to provide emotional support to others, and found that various forms of interpersonal competence inversely predicted interpersonal stress a year later, even when psychopathology and the initial level of interpersonal stress were controlled.

Poor Social Relationships

Not only does companionship predict more positive outcomes, but lack of it predicts diverse problems. Hintikka, Koskela, Kontula, Koskela, and Viinamaeki (2000) found that both men and women with more friends had lower levels of mental distress than men and women with fewer friends. In a national survey on rates of mental illness in Great Britain, Jenkins et al. (1997) found that the highest rates of mental problems were found among unmarried people, single parents, and people living alone. Women with a confidant are less likely to be depressed and are more satisfied with their lives than women who lack a confidant (Antonucci, Lansford, & Akiyama, 2001). Elderly individuals who do not have confidants or companions report lower well-being than those who do, even when demographic, health, and economic factors are controlled (Chappell & Badger, 1989). Although all these correlations might be due to either relationships affecting well-being or the reverse, results we review later suggest that the influences are reciprocal.

Social isolation correlates substantially with low well-being (e.g., Argyle, 1987; Baumeister, 1991). Loneliness stems from a lack of confidants and friends, and in turn increases the risk of psychological problems, physical impairment, and low life satisfaction (Bowling, Edelmann, Leaver, & Hoekel, 1989). People feel lonely when their relationships are severed, and they feel anxious at the prospect of losing important relationships (e.g., Leary, 1990). Negative emotions result when people are excluded from social groups (e.g., Barden, Garber, Leiman, Ford, & Masters, 1985), and individuals with close social bonds suffer if they are separated for long periods of time (Baumeister and Leary, 1995). For example, wives of men who work on submarines often experience increased physical illness and depression during their spouses' absences (Beckman, Marsella, & Finney, 1979). Williams (2001) showed that ostracism from social groups can have a devastating impact on people, and that exclusion even from relatively unimportant groups can create strong negative feelings. Relocating to a new community increases risk for distress and depression among women (Magdol, 2002).

Hammen and her colleagues (e.g., Hammen, 1999; Hammen & Brennan, 2002) suggested that interpersonal problems are a root cause of depression. For example, women who have been depressed, but are not currently so, are less likely than women who have never had depression to be stably married; have more problematic relationships with their children, friends, and family; are more insecure in their beliefs about others; and experience lower marital satisfaction. It appears that the lack of strong and positive interpersonal ties can lead to depression, and that some part of the relationship problems of depressed people might stem from shortcomings in social skills. Hammen (1996) suggested that the majority of depression is caused by interpersonal problems arising from beliefs about others, stressful interpersonal events, dysfunctional social behaviors, and conflictual family relationships. Thus, social relationships constitute another major factor affecting well-being and ill-being that is not captured by economic indicators.

Marriage

Marriage serves as a major vehicle for companionship in Western societies, and marital dissolution is usually accompanied by emotional turmoil, depression, hostility, and loneliness, even when the marriage has become unhappy (Price & McKenry, 1988; R. S. Weiss, 1979). Mental-hospital admissions are highest in separated and divorced individuals, intermediate in the unmarried, and lowest in married individuals (Bloom, White, & Asher, 1979). Happily married individuals are less likely to have physical health problems or psychological difficulties than unmarried persons (DeLongis, Folkman, & Lazarus, 1988), and mortality rates are consistently higher for widowed, single, and divorced individuals than they are for married people

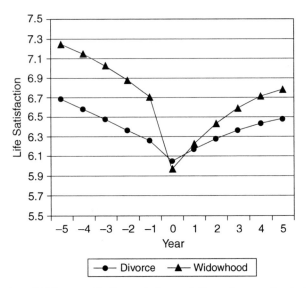

Fig. 4 Satisfaction with life across the 5 years before and after a divorce or the death of a spouse

(Lynch, 1979). People who are happily married experience less unemployment than those with troubled marriages (Forthofer, Markman, Cox, Stanley, & Kessler, 1996).

Research on widows also reveals the importance of social relationships to well-being. Stroebe, Stroebe, Abakoumkin, and Schut (1996) found that widows were more depressed than a comparison group of women who had not lost their husbands, and that depression was higher even several years postbereavement. Longitudinal findings support these cross-sectional data. Lucas, Clark, Georgellis, and Diener (2003) found that widows' life satisfaction dropped substantially prior to and after their husbands' deaths. More important, it took many years for life satisfaction to rise back near former levels, and it never quite returned to those levels.

Figure 4 shows the life satisfaction of individuals in the German Socioeconomic Panel Survey who underwent divorce or widowhood. In most longitudinal studies, participants are lost over time, and the samples at different time points may differ in ways that could affect the results. However, the data shown in the figure are based on changes within individuals, so the results are not affected by such problems. It is clear from the graph that divorce and widowhood both affect life satisfaction for many years. In the case of divorce, problems in the relationship lower life satisfaction for years before dissolution of the marriage, and in the case of both widowhood and divorce, there is decreased life satisfaction for many years afterward.

Causality

The literature supporting a link between supportive social relationships and well-being is strong. Perhaps the most important question is whether the direction of causality goes from social relationships to well-being. Certainly, the idea that high well-being leads to good relationships is also plausible. There is evidence, for example, that compared with people who stay single, people who marry are likely to be more satisfied with life in the first place, long before they marry (Lucas et al., 2003). Also, Cunningham (1988a, 1988b) reported evidence that people put into a pleasant mood became more sociable.

Several lines of evidence, however, point also to a causal arrow going from relationships to well-being. First, there is longitudinal evidence (e.g., Fig. 4) showing that people who lose an important relationship experience lower well-being, and that it takes them years to return near baseline. Second, data from controlled experiments isolate social exclusion or ostracism as causal. Third, a suggestive but interesting finding concerns individuals whose hearing is restored. Nehra, Mann, Sharma, and Verma (1997) found that after people with moderate to high hearing loss acquired hearing aids, their subjective well-being improved, and symptoms of anxiety and depression decreased. These results might have been due to better social involvement, at least in part. Finally, within-person data indicate that it is not just that happy people have better relationships than unhappy people. Rather, the same individuals are happier on average when they are with others than when they are alone (Pavot et al., 1990). These results again suggest that positive social contract causes well-being. Indeed, Kahneman et al. (2004) found that in only 1 of 15 activities of daily living (i.e., praying) was *affect balance* (positive minus negative emotions) greater when people were alone rather than with others. People seemed to enjoy the other 14 activities, such as exercising, resting, commuting, and working around the house, more when others were present than when they were alone.

Watson (2000) concluded that the relation between social relationships and mood is much stronger for positive moods than for negative ones: He found a within-person correlation of 0.24 between pleasant affect and social interaction, but only a -0.08 correlation between unpleasant moods and social interaction. He also reviewed evidence of causality: For example, when people interacted with others in assigned social relationships, their positive affect increased (see also McIntyre, Watson, Clark, & Cross, 1991).

Thus, the causal path from social relationships to well-being moves in both directions. Our focus here, though, is on fostering well-being, and although it is clear that positive social relationships are an important cause of well-being, they are largely missed by economic indicators. Furthermore, it could be that some societal characteristics that foster economic growth in fact interfere with social relationships and therefore lower well-being. Again, it is clear that well-being indicators are a needed complement to current economic and social indicators.

Policy Implications

Current social indicators can capture phenomena such as crime, marriage and divorce, environmental problems (such as pollution), longevity and infant mortality, gender equality in schools, and the amount of land devoted to parks. Thus, social indicators can capture aspects of quality of life that add to the portrait drawn by economic indicators. Nevertheless, these social indicators fail to fully capture the well-being of nations because they do not reflect people's actual experiences—the quality of their relationships, the regulation of their emotions, whether they experience work as engaging, and whether feelings of isolation and depression permeate their daily living. In other words, the social indicators are important, but they do not fully capture well-being.

We do not mean to oversimplify the relation between social contact and well-being. People differ in their need for companions, and social relationships can be controlling and negative rather than rewarding. There are many open questions, such as what the most important aspects of social contact are, and whether the rewarding nature of friendships is absolute or depends on people's expectations. Another question is whether other forms of companionship can take the place of traditional marriage in modern societies. It does appear, however, the social relationships are centrally important to well-being.

Governments cannot solve most problems of social relationships. For example, they cannot prevent widowhood. Nevertheless, because strong social relationships are critical to well-being, there are policies that businesses, governments, and other institutions should consider. For example, the military and corporations should relocate employees and their families only when it is absolutely essential to do so, or when an employee requests it. Automatic moves every few years leave individuals without strong community ties, and with fewer close friends in times of crisis. Also, organizations should respect people's friendship patterns at work, and not try to eliminate friendship opportunities in the mistaken idea that employees will work harder if they are not distracted by the presence of friends. Indeed, research by the Gallup Organization shows that people who work in units where they have a "best friend" perform better than those who do not have a best friend in their unit (Harter et al., 2002). Recognizing the profit in having happy workers, companies are increasingly implementing policies that recognize the family needs of employees, such as their need for bereavement and parental leaves of absence.

School curricula can explicitly educate young people about the importance of long-lasting social relationships and how to increase their chances for a rewarding marriage. Given that not every student will enter a traditional marriage, education about how to develop and nurture supportive and intimate social relationships in general is an educational imperative. Social skills should be a standard component of primary and secondary education.

Mobility is now a hallmark of American society. Yet this mobility has costs in the form of loosened social ties, reduced community involvement, and lower trust. A number of pathologies seem to spring from the lack of a "moral net," the extended family that reinforces and enforces cultural norms (Naroll, 1983). Marginal individuals such as the chronically mentally ill may suffer the most from the lack of strong and extended family ties. Twenge (2002) concluded that increasing levels of dysphoria in modern societies are due not only to environmental stressors, but also to decreasing social connectedness. Thus, policies that encourage long-distance mobility and discourage individuals from forming long-lasting community ties can be dangerous to well-being. Similarly, socialization that emphasizes individual entitlements in lieu of aiding family, friends, and community will likely harm the well-being of society.

A System of National Indicators

There was a time, when many basic needs were unmet, that economic indicators were a very good first approximation of how well a nation was doing. As nations became wealthier and basic needs were largely met, economic indicators increasingly missed their target. We have argued to this point that national economic indicators alone are now "out of sync" with national well-being in the developed nations. While wealth has trebled over the past 50 years, for example, well-being has been flat, mental illness has increased at an even more rapid rate, and data, not just nostalgic reminiscences, indicate that the social fabric is more frayed than it was in leaner times. These inadequacies lead us to advocate that an ongoing system of indicators be instituted by governments and organizations to track well-being over time. It is clear that policymakers now care about well-being, in addition to economics, because policies are being created on the basis of mere guesses and romantic sentiments about what will enhance well-being (e.g., family leave). These guesses are undoubtedly correct in some cases, but they are incorrect in other cases. For this reason, ongoing measurement of well-being in representative samples and in diverse domains of life is required to confirm or disconfirm the efficacy of policies instituted to increase well-being.

The precursors of national well-being measures are in place. These nascent measures are emerging from large-scale national surveys of well-being, surveys of mental health, and many smaller studies focused on particular groups and specific domains of life. For example, the German Socioeconomic Panel, which is a large, ongoing annual survey of life satisfaction in Germany, and the Eurobarometer, which is conducted at regular intervals in the European Union nations, include well-being questions. However, we are proposing something much more ambitious and deep—a full-scale set of measures, including experience sampling of certain subsamples, that will be sensitive to changes of well-being and ill-being in the major domains of life, such as work and health, as well as narrower measures of trust, stress, meaning, and other components of well-being. We can now outline the scope of this project in broad terms. Although large, it will cost only a tiny fraction of what the current system of economic indicators costs. A set of national indicators of well-being should

- Include questions that are relevant to policy
- Broadly and representatively sample various stakeholder groups in a nation
- Include measures of broad facets of well-being, such as life satisfaction, having purpose and meaning in life, trust, engagement, depression, and positive and negative emotions

- Include narrower well-being measures related to different aspects of life, such as work, health, family, community, and leisure
- Include permanent measures that are used in all samples, as well as topical measures and samples that focus on specific current policy issues
- Include in-depth measures over time on subsamples in order to measure experience as it occurs and not rely on people's recall of that experience
- Track subsamples longitudinally to provide a better understanding of changes across time

In our review, we did not systematically discuss the various aspects of well-being (e.g., pleasant emotions vs. engagement or finding meaning and purpose in life) in each domain. Not only would this be beyond the scope of this report, but rarely have studies used a full set of measures. Although we often discussed "life satisfaction," this was primarily because a measure of this global construct is most often included in existing surveys, not because we want to promote life satisfaction as the key well-being variable. A national indicator should include several global indicators, such as life satisfaction, but it should also target positive and negative emotions in specific areas, such as work life, health, social relationships, and mental health, and it should be fine-grained, breaking life satisfaction down into its constituent parts.

What variables should be assessed in a national index? This will require serious discussion among scholars, as well as further research. We (Seligman, 2002) have suggested that well-being includes positive emotions and moods (The Pleasant Life), engagement (The Good Life), and having meaning in life (The Meaningful Life).

Other investigators have outlined well-being components using statistical approaches, such as factor analysis. For example, Lucas et al. (1996) found that life satisfaction, positive affect, and negative affect are separable but related concepts when assessed by multiple methods. There are many additional variables that might be desirable in a set of national well-being indicators, including pleasant emotions within domains such as work and marriage, trust in strangers versus friends, depression and anxiety, and moods during various activities of daily life.

Economic indicators have evolved over many decades through collaborations among many economists. In contrast, there have been very few systematic research projects to refine well-being measures and fully validate their meaning. Thus, we propose not only the implementation of a beginning set of national measures, but also a largescale research program to refine indicators of well-being.

A national system of well-being measures will cost millions of dollars each year. This cost, however, is tiny compared with the cost of economic measures, which are now glaringly inadequate as measures of how developed nations are doing. The benefits promise to be enormous. They will include policy changes that over time will increase most people's well-being. If such a system works even to a small degree in the United States, the total benefits would be large in a nation of 280 million people.

Revisiting the Advantages of Well-Being Measures and Shortcomings of Economic Measures

If a national system of well-being indicators were instituted, what new information would be obtained that is not already captured in economic indicators? After all, mental disorders produce lower productivity as well as lower well-being, and thus perhaps economic indicators suffice to alert policymakers to the problems in this area, as well as in other areas. The most important contribution of a national system of well-being indicators would be that they could focus the attention of policymakers and the public specifically on well-being, and not simply on the production of goods and services; one of the main benefits of well-being measures is that they add a valuable perspective beyond a cost-benefit market analysis in evaluating societal structures and interventions.

Not only would a set of national well-being indicators provide answers to important questions, but they would ensure that certain questions were addressed by policymakers. In Table 2, we show some issues that are addressed by economists

Table 2 Examples of the types of questions stimulated by the economic and well-being approaches

Domain	Economic approach	Well-being approach
Society	How can the government stimulate economic growth?	How does economic growth influence well-being?
	How does central bank policy influence unemployment and inflation?	How does governance influence well-being?
Income	How does income inequality influence economic growth?	Does income inequality influence well-being?
	How do tax rates influence economic growth?	How does unemployment affect well-being?
Work	How does pay influence productivity?	What makes a job enjoyable and engaging?
	What are the causes of unemployment?	Are happy workers more or less productive than unhappy workers?
Physical health	How much is productivity reduced by illness?	Do individuals who report high well-being have better health than those who report low well-being?
	What are the monetary costs and benefits of various treatments for diseases?	What illnesses most interfere with happiness?
Mental disorders	How do mental disorders interfere with productivity?	How much misery do mental disorders cause?
	How costly are mental disorders to society?	Does therapy enhance the well-being of persons with mental disorders?
Social relationships	How do couples jointly determine their participation in the labor market?	Why are married people on average happier than unmarried people?
	How are resources distributed within a household?	How does geographic mobility influence well-being?

in our six domains, and examples of questions that the well-being approach would raise about these same domains. The examples illustrate how national indicators of well-being would draw interest to a new set of questions that complement those issues that are framed by economists. These questions would reframe some policy questions, and in some cases raise new questions.

In the realm of mental health, for example, policymakers would be led by well-being indicators to consider family suffering and burden, as well as the suffering of the individuals involved, when evaluating mental health interventions. Economic analyses focus policymakers on lost workdays and the costs of mental treatment, but do not capture factors such as whether treatments enhance well-being and whether well-being buffers against mental illness. When people continue to work despite their disorders, economic indicators can totally miss the suffering that is present. People with depression or anxiety disorders, for example, sometimes continue to function in the workplace, but are miserable. Furthermore, the economic indicators give no hint as to why the productivity of these individuals might be low. Although an economic analysis suggests that people should use their disposable wealth to alleviate their own suffering, it is likely that many factors besides income determine when people receive mental health services.

The effects of national well-being measures would go beyond the effects on government policymakers. A well-being approach to the assessment of people with mental disorders could lead to strong public sentiment to include adequate treatment for mental disorders in health insurance and health-maintenance organization plans. In focusing attention on the immense suffering and lack of functioning caused by mental disorders, well-being measures would serve to highlight the need for multiple approaches and large-scale interventions to help individuals with mental disorders and perhaps reduce the frequency of such disorders.

Social relationships is an area that shows the importance of a variable that has not been captured by economic indicators. Many people intuitively realize that family and friends are important to happiness, but national attention continually gets focused on economic indicators that are widely reported in the media. In considering what vocation to pursue, for example, students easily can obtain extensive information about potential income, but very little information about how meaningful or engaging particular jobs will be. Indeed, because of the lack of systematic well-being indicators, young adults might not systematically compare professions and consider how engaging the work is or how much stress it involves. If they do consider how engaging, meaningful, or stressful the work is, they are likely to have garnered this information from a favorite television drama series rather than from systematic research findings.

Economic models are built on the assumption that people choose alternatives to maximize their well-being. But one problem with these models is that people do not necessarily realize what might enhance their well-being best; instead, they make choices on the basis of hunches and cultural prescriptions. Thus, a system of well-being indicators would make economic indicators more efficient by providing better information that people could use to make choices. Currently, people have clear information on how to pursue their economic goals. One reason these goals may seem to take on such importance is that it might not be as clear to them how to achieve higher well-being. A set of national indicators could provide information that would make the pursuit of well-being an informed pursuit.

We envision that economic and well-being indicators will often be used in tandem. Economic growth is considered to be very important in most nations. A central question is when, and to what degree, economic growth produces increases in well-being, and when it works against well-being. Only by supplementing economic indices with well-being indicators can one hope to answer such questions.

By understanding some of the limitations of economic indicators, one can better appreciate the complementary role of well-being indicators. In some cases, economic measures are assumed to serve as a proxy for well-being. However, if certain types of consumption enhance well-being and other types of consumption do not, this fact is lost when all goods and services are lumped together. For example, the consumption of certain status goods might not enhance well-being among people who have a competitive nature, because relative position will remain the same despite the growth of these goods; in contrast, the well-being provided by public parks and green spaces might not be constrained by relative position. Direct measures of well-being will allow researchers to examine how various forms of consumption enhance quality of life. For example, it might be that better schools and reduced commuting enhance well-being, whereas status goods, construction of prisons, and cigarette consumption decrease well-being in the long run, but all are given equal weight in national GDP. Direct measures of well-being will allow analysis of these effects.

Well-being indicators can supplement economic indicators, particularly when the economic indicators have large blind spots. For example, GDP is used as a measure of the material well-being of a society because it is designed to capture market production and therefore the goods and services that are produced and consumed in a society. But, for example, GDP substantially underestimates levels of well-being in a society because it does not fully capture production and consumption in some important areas. Housework and other household production (e.g., cooking, laundry, and child care) are not included in these indicators, and are counted in GDP only when they are purchased from outside the home. Thus, a rise in GDP in this sector might not signify an actual rise in material quality of life, but might signify only altered lifestyles (e.g., hiring child care rather than providing it oneself) that might or might not represent improving quality of life (and does not even necessarily indicate that the amount of goods and services produced and consumed has even risen). We are not arguing that household production should be compensated by the government, or that it is necessarily better for well-being than services provided outside the home. What we are describing is the paradox that the very same types of activities and services may or may not count in GDP, depending on who performs them. Because household production can represent as much as 25–50% of an economy (Frey & Stutzer, 2002a), it is widely recognized by economists that this represents a blind spot in the GDP measure. Household production and leisure can add approximately 150% to the conventional GDP measures, although this figure varies dramatically across societies and across time, making it difficult to make comparisons.

Another example of overlooked production in national accounts of GDP are the shadow economies in many nations, the production and exchange of goods and services that are not reported to government agencies (Frey & Stutzer, 2002a). For example, people might pay cash for services to avoid taxes, and these services could then go uncounted by authorities. In some nations, the shadow economy is as large as 75% of the economy reported to officials, making GDP a very inaccurate figure in these instances. Volunteer activity (e.g., in schools and among the poor) is also omitted from the GDP. "Regrettables" such as police protection, prisons, some legal services, mental health services, purchases of cigarettes, gambling, and commuting also are part of GDP even though high expenditures on these things do not necessarily mean a high quality of life. Although a nation's expenditures on regrettables can be salutary in some respects, as is the case for money spent treating mental disorders, money spent on regrettables indexes problems that interfere with well-being.

Non-market goods in general, and social interventions in particular, are not counted in national income, although they can substantially influence well-being. As two economists, Frey & Stutzer (2002a), wrote: "These and other shortcomings of national product are generally known, but the concept is still the center of political, economic, and media attention" (p. 37).

The substantial limitations of GDP make it a measure with a large margin of error when it serves as an index of quality of life. Issues related to household production, volunteer activity, shadow economic activities, and spending on regrettables are known to economists, but not recognized by the public. Other economic indicators, such as the consumer price index, also have nontrivial limitations. The price of goods, for example, is based on marginal demand, so that goods with great value to well-being are given little value if they are plentiful, even though they may contribute substantially to well-being. Furthermore, practical measurement problems, such as how to value new goods, plague economic indicators.

Another limitation of indices of national income such as GDP is that they do not include externalities, side effects of production and consumption that do not result in market transactions. For example, the environmental costs of factories and consumption are not subtracted from national accounts. Another shortcoming of economic measures in terms of their links to well-being is that they rest on models of rational choice, which posit that people follow a set of logical rules when making economic choices. However, recent work (e.g., Kahneman, 1994; Schwartz, 2004; Sunstein & Thaler, in press) in psychology and economics reveals that people do not always make rational choices, and that a surfeit of choices does not necessarily enhance well-being. Furthermore, people are not adept at predicting their future affect in different situations (Gilbert, Pinel, Wilson, Blumberg, & Wheatley, 1998), and therefore economic choices do not necessarily enhance well-being. Thus, measures of well-being are needed because of the inherent limitations of economic measures as reflections of well-being. Furthermore, it is possible that a strong emphasis on economic growth can interfere with well-being (Easterlin, 1996; Lane, 2000).

In sum, well-being measures will add information needed by leaders, as well as by all citizens, to make informed choices in a wealthy society. When people evaluate different possible courses of action—at the individual, corporate, and governmental levels—well-being measures can add a perspective that is not fully captured by existing indicators. In addition, well-being measures will prove important because the psychological Heisenberg principle is at work—what a society measures will in turn influence the things that it seeks. If a society takes great effort to measure productivity, people in the society are likely to focus more attention on productivity, sometimes to the detriment of other values. If a society systematically and regularly assesses well-being, people will focus more of their attention on well-being, and learn more about its causes.

The Desirable Outcomes of High Well-Being

Why is more well-being an important goal for a nation? First, existing evidence indicates that across the board, people high in well-being function more effectively than people low in well-being: They are likely to have more successful relationships, to be more productive at work, to have higher incomes, and to have better physical and mental health. Table 3 summarizes several benefits of high well-being reviewed earlier in this report—advantages that are valued by most individuals. Second, well-being is a meter that tells individuals that their lives are on track, and that they are achieving their goals and accomplishing valued ends. In a democratic society that respects the importance of individual choice, better well-being is an inherent goal—more basic, as the Declaration of Independence contends, than higher income. Finally, national well-being is important because it serves as a global measure of how successful a nation is in fulfilling the needs, the goals, and the values of its citizens.

Table 3 Likely advantages accruing to individuals with high well-being

Domain	Advantages
Society	Well-being of the populace might facilitate democratic governance.
Income	Happy people later earn higher incomes than unhappy people.
Work	Satisfied and happy workers are better organizational citizens than unhappy workers.
	Work units with high satisfaction have more satisfied customers than units with low satisfaction.
	Satisfaction of work units may correlate with productivity and profitability.
Physical health	High well-being may correlate with longevity.
	Individuals low in well-being have compromised immune systems and are more likely to have certain diseases compared with individuals high in well-being.
Mental disorders	The happiest individuals score low in psychopathology.
Social relationships	High well-being is associated with increased probability of marrying and staying happily married. It is also associated with increased numbers of friends and social support.

Are Well-Being Indicators Politically Neutral?

An important question is whether well-being indicators would foster a leftist (or rightist) agenda, and therefore represent a specific political agenda. For example, a number of findings on well-being point to government interventions that might alleviate suffering and increase well-being (e.g., more adequately subsidizing treatment of mental illness), and some interventions requiring government expenditures are associated with a liberal political philosophy. However, many well-being findings point to societal expenditures that are compatible with a conservative viewpoint. For example, market democracies have much more well-being than totalitarian dictatorships, so military expenditures that protect and extend democracy will increase global well-being. Another example is the well-being that rests on strong family and friendship ties. We are not advocating marriage for everyone just because married people on average are happier than unmarried people, but we do argue that government policies should be aimed at cementing strong social ties. This could mean offering tax breaks to married couples (a conservative proposal), and it could mean adopting marriage for gay and lesbian couples (a liberal position). The findings that religious individuals tend to report higher well-being than nonreligious people, that inequality does not invariably result in lower well-being, and that the offspring of unstable and terminated marriages report lower life satisfaction than the offspring of intact marriages (Gohm, Oishi, Darlington, & Diener, 1998) are also congruent with conservative values. Conversely, liberals can take heart in other specific findings, such as that unemployment has lasting negative effects, that certain social-service programs offered by the government are likely to reduce ill-being, and that increased income is likely to raise the well-being of poor people more than it does the well-being of the well-off. Again, we do not mean to imply that governments should directly support religion, or that huge inequalities are fine; we do mean to say that well-being can add another perspective to policy debates in these areas.

So we believe that measures of well-being are—and must be—exactly as neutral politically as are economic indicators. The indicators are descriptive, not prescriptive, and must remain so. They simply yield facts that can be used either by the left or by the right, and therefore they provide an added way to better assess the claims of various political viewpoints by revealing how policies actually influence well-being. Furthermore, well-being is not the only criterion that liberals and conservatives use in deciding which policies to advocate. For instance, liberals might advocate for greater equality in society regardless of whether it increases well-being.

What of the noninterventionist view that the government that governs best governs least? Would this antipaternalism not be hostile to collecting well-being measures on a national level? First, it should be noted that taking economic indicators should be as antithetical or compatible with noninterventionist philosophy as taking well-being indicators. Second, of all people, noninterventionists would be well served by having available measures of well-being. After all, if lack of interventions enhances well-being, this ought to be manifested in the measures. Furthermore, even people who believe that governments should rarely intervene in everyday affairs might nevertheless accept that the measures have value to corporations for making work life more engaging and enjoyable, to local institutions for providing better parks and facilities, and to individuals for making informed choices about their well-being. What is appropriate for individuals and organizations might not be appropriate for central governments; yet measures of well-being can serve a wide constituency at multiple levels, and thus need not be connected with central-government interventions.

One objection to our argument is that the economy interconnects everyone, whereas happiness might be more of a private, individual affair. If so, it could be argued that it is more justifiable for governments to intervene in the economy than in matters related to well-being. However, well-being can be influenced strongly by what other people do, and by the conditions in society. Take the unhappy state of present-day Russia, for example. The loss of stability in that nation substantially depressed the well-being of the society. Although temperament and individual choices can strongly influence well-being, just as they can influence an individual's economic prosperity, community and societal conditions can also substantially influence people's well-being. As in all things political, balancing societal well-being against spending on luxury goods is likely to give rise to tensions, and well-being indicators will yield valuable information to help resolve such debates.

Will Well-Being Replace Money?

We titled this monograph "Beyond Money," not "Instead of Money." It would be sophomoric to believe that people will soon forsake their desires for substantial amounts of goods and services. In the introduction, we suggested that economic models served well when needs went largely unmet, but that these models are less relevant in a time of plenty. However, the money economy has too strong a proven track record for either individuals or nations to quickly abandon it. Not only have capitalism and the industrial revolution at times led to rampant consumerism, but they have allowed large advances in sanitation, education, health, parks, and even, perhaps, virtue (Easterbrook, 2003). At the individual level, the economic model allows people to structure their time in the pursuit of concrete goals, and to readily track progress toward specific goals. It is possible that people derive considerable well-being from goal pursuits related to earning income, and from the activities of consumption, and therefore even a well-being economy will include these activities. Thus, although laments about how economic activity can interfere with family and religion are often heard, it is likely that the economic model will remain dominant for many decades to come. We do not contest this fact of life.

Well-being is not a panacea that will in itself solve all of the world's problems. Even if well-being one day becomes the dominant paradigm, it must be supplemented by other values of societies, and people must be socialized for humane values for the well-being economy to be a desirable concept.

One challenge for a society based on well-being is that individuals do not have ready and concrete models of how to pursue the goal of greater well-being, other than following the economic model. When people are asked what would improve the quality of their lives, the most frequent response is higher income (Campbell, 1981). It is not clear to people how they would achieve greater positive emotions and life satisfaction. Until there are concrete and proven steps toward these noneconomic aims, people are unlikely to abandon the dominant economic paradigm. Thus, psychologists need to demonstrate compellingly the malleable factors that can increase well-being before the well-being paradigm can replace the economic one. In addition, it should not be forgotten that the theoretical models on which the economic model is based are in many cases more sophisticated than current scientific models of well-being. Therefore, although an economy focused on well-being might be an important long-term goal, in the short term it is sufficient to suggest that well-being indicators will complement economic ones.

The Central Place of Psychology in Creating National Well-Being

We reviewed in the previous sections several of the factors that lead to well-being— to frequent pleasant emotions and engagement, to finding meaning and satisfaction in life, and to low levels of stress and depression. The existing findings suggest the following partial formula for high well-being:

- Live in a democratic and stable society that provides material resources to meet needs
- Have supportive friends and family
- Have rewarding and engaging work and an adequate income
- Be reasonably healthy and have treatment available in case of mental problems
- Have important goals related to one's values
- Have a philosophy or religion that provides guidance, purpose, and meaning to one's life

Concluding Remarks

If high well-being is the overarching goal of all nations, national indicators of well-being are crucial to assessing the impact of national and corporate policies. Rudimentary indicators of well-being are now available, and they provide the fascinating findings reviewed here. But much better measures are needed.

Economic indicators have for the most part served society well. However, these indicators have glaring shortcomings as approximations, even first approximations, of well-being. Scientists are now in the position to assess well-being directly, and therefore should establish a system of national measures of well-being to supplement the economic measures. Indeed, it can be argued that the well-being measures should be the central ones, and that the economic indices are best understood in their relation to enhancing well-being. We have reviewed a number of important factors that influence well-being but are not captured by existing indicators, and we have shown the benefits of well-being in producing a successful society. It is time to grant well-being a prominent place in policy discussions.

Acknowledgments Our thanks are extended to the following individuals for their suggestions and comments on ideas and earlier versions of this report: Daniel Kahneman, Howard Tennen, Andrew Clark, Alois Stutzer, Timothy Judge, Paul Spector, and Robert Putnam. Our gratitude is also owed to Christie Scollon and Richard Lucas for their assistance in creating the figures.

References

Abbott, J. (2003). Does employee satisfaction matter: A study to determine whether low employee morale affects customer satisfaction and profits in the business-to-business sector. *Journal of Communication Management, 7,* 333–339.

Adelmann, P. K. (1987). Occupational complexity, control, and personal income: Their relation to psychological well-being in men and women. *Journal of Applied Psychology, 72,* 529–537.

Affleck, G., Urrows, S., Tennen, J., Higgins, P., Pav, D., & Aloisi, R. (1997). A dual pathway model of daily stressor effects on rheumatoid arthritis. *Annals of Behavioral Medicine, 19,* 161–170.

Alesina, A., Di Tella, R., and MacCulloch, R. (2000). *Inequality and happiness: Are Europeans and Americans different?* (National Bureau of Economic Research Working Paper 8198). Cambridge, England: Cambridge University Press.

Andrade, C., Sarmah, P. L., & Channabasavanna, S. M. (1989). Psychological well-being and morbidity in parents of narcotic-dependent males. *Indian Journal of Psychiatry, 31,* 122–127.

Antonucci, T. C., Lansford, J. E., & Akiyama, H. (2001). Impact of positive and negative aspects of marital relationships and friendships on well-being of older adults. *Applied Developmental Science, 5,* 68–75.

Argyle, M. (1987). *The psychology of happiness.* London: Methuen.

Argyle, M. (2001). *The psychology of happiness* (2nd ed.). New York: Routledge.

Arnold, L., Witzeman, K., Swank, M., McElroy, S., & Keck, P. (2000). Healthrelated quality of life using the SF-36 in patients with bipolar disorder compared with patients with chronic back pain and the general population. *Journal of Affective Disorders, 57,* 235–239.

Audrain, J., Schwartz, M., Herrera, J., Golman, P., & Bush, A. (2001). Physical activity in first degree relatives of breast cancer patients. *Journal of Behavioral Medicine, 24,* 587–603.

Barden, R. C., Garber, J., Leiman, B., Ford, M. E., & Masters, J. C., (1985). Factors governing the effective remediation of negative affect and its cognitive and behavioral consequences. *Journal of Personality and Social Psychology, 49,* 1040–1053.

Barrick, M. R., & Mount, M. K. (1993). Autonomy as a moderator of the relationships between the big five personality dimensions and job performance. *Journal of Applied Psychology, 78,* 111–118.

Barro, R. J. (1999). Determinants of democracy. *Journal of Political Economy, 107,* S158–S183.

Basco, M. R., Krebaum, S. R., & Rush, A. J. (1997). Outcome measures of depression. In H. H. Strupp & L. M. Leonard (Eds.), *Measuring patient changes in mood, anxiety, and personality disorders: Toward a core battery* (pp. 191–245). Washington, DC: American Psychological Association.

Bateman, T. S., & Organ, D. W. (1983). Job satisfaction and the good soldier: The relation between affect and employee "citizenship." *Academy of Management Journal, 261,* 587–595.

Baumeister, R. F. (1991). *Meanings of life.* New York: Guilford Press.

Baumeister, R. F. (Ed.). (2002). Religion and psychology [Special issue]. *Psychological Inquiry, 13*(3).

Baumeister, R. F., & Leary, M. R. (1995). The need to belong: Desire for interpersonal attachments as a fundamental human motivation. *Psychological Bulletin, 117*, 497–529.

Beck, A. (1967). *Depression.* New York: Hoeber.

Beckman, K., Marsella, A. J., & Finney, R. (1979). Depression in the wives of nuclear submarine personnel. *American Journal of Psychiatry, 136*, 524–526.

Biswas-Diener, R., & Diener, E. (2001). Making the best of a bad situation: Satisfaction in the slums of Calcutta. *Social Indicators Research, 55*, 329–352.

Biswas-Diener, R, Vittersø, J., & Diener, E. (2003). *Most people are pretty happy, but there is cultural variation: The Inughuit, the Amish, and the Massai.* Manuscript submitted for publication.

Bjørnskov, C. (2003). The happy few: Cross-country evidence on social capital and life satisfaction. *Kyklos, 56*, 3–16.

Bloom, B. L., White, S. W., & Asher, S. J. (1979). Marital disruption as a stressful life event. In G. Levinger & O. C. Moles (Eds.), *Divorce and separation: Context, causes, and consequences* (pp. 184–200). New York: Basic Books.

Borman, W. C., Penner, L. A., Allen, T. D., & Motowidlo, S. J. (2001). Personality predictors of citizenship performance. *International Journal of Selection and Assessment, 9*, 52–69.

Bowling, A. P., Edelmann, R. J., Leaver, J., & Hoekel, T. (1989). Loneliness, mobility, well-being and social support in a sample of over 85 year olds. *Personality and Individual Differences, 10*, 1189–1192.

Bradshaw, W., & Brekke, J. S. (1999). Subjective experience in schizophrenia: Factors influencing self-esteem, satisfaction with life, and subjective distress. *American Journal of Orthopsychiatry, 69*, 254–260.

Bretz, R. D., & Judge, T. A. (1994). Person/organization fit and the Theory of Work Adjustment: Implications for satisfaction, tenure, and career success. *Journal of Vocational Behavior, 44*, 32–54.

Brickman, P., Coates, D., & Janoff-Bulman, R. (1978). Lottery winners and accident victims: Is happiness relative? *Journal of Personality and Social Psychology, 36*, 917–927.

Brief, A. P., Butcher, A. H., George, J. M., & Link, K. E. (1993). Integrating bottom-up and top-down theories of subjective well-being: The case of health. *Journal of Personality and Social Psychology, 64*, 646–653.

Brown, G. D. A., Gardner, J., Oswald, A., & Qian, J. (2003, June). *Rank dependence in pay satisfaction.* Paper presented at the Brookings/Warwick Conference, Washington, DC.

Brown, S. L., Nesse, R. M., Vinokur, A., & Smith, D. M. (2003). Providing social support may be more beneficial than receiving it: Results from a prospective study of mortality. *Psychological Science, 14*, 320–327.

Campbell, A. (1981). *The sense of well-being in America.* New York: McGraw-Hill.

Carney, R. M., Rich, M. W., & Jaffe, A. S. (1995). depression as a risk factor for cardiac events in established coronary heart disease: A review of possible mechanisms. *Annals of Behavioral Medicine, 17*, 142–149.

Carsten, J. M., & Spector, P. E. (1987). Unemployment, job satisfaction and employee turnover: A meta-analytic test of the Michinsky model. *Journal of Applied Psychology, 72*, 374–381.

Celiker, R., & Borman, P. (2001). Fibromyalgia versus rheumatoid arthritis: A comparison of psychological disturbance and life satisfaction. *Journal of Musculoskeletal Pain, 9*, 35–45.

Chappell, N. L., & Badger, M. (1989). Social isolation and well-being. *Journal of Gerontology, 44*, S169–S176.

Clark, A. E. (2001). What really matters in a job? Hedonic measurement using quit data. *Labor Economics, 8*, 223–242.

Clark, A. E. (2003). Unemployment as a social norm: Psychological evidence from panel data. *Journal of Labor Economics, 21*, 323–351.

Clark, A. E., Diener, E., Georgellis, Y., & Lucas, R. E. (2004). *Lags and leads in life satisfaction: A test of the baseline hypothesis.* Manuscript submitted for publication.

Clark, A. E., & Lelkes, O. (2003). *Keep the faith: Is social capital just an instrument?* Unpublished manuscript, Départment et Laboratoire d'Economic Theoretique et Appliquée, Paris, France.

Clark, A. E., & Oswald, A. J. (1994). Unhappiness and unemployment. *Economic Journal, 104*, 648–659.

Clark, A. E., & Oswald, A. J. (1996). Satisfaction and comparison income. *Journal of Public Economics, 61*, 359–381.

Clarke, S. P., Frasure-Smith, N., Lespérance, F., & Bourassa, M. G. (2000). Psychosocial factors as predictors of functional status at 1 year in patients with left ventricular dysfunction. *Research in Nursing & Health, 23*, 290–300.

Clydesdale, T. T. (1997). Family behaviors among early U. S. baby boomers: Exploring the effects of religion and income change, 1965–1982. *Social Forces, 76*, 605–635.

Cogan, R., Cogan, D., Waltz, W., & McCue, M. (1987). Effects of laughter and relaxation on discomfort thresholds. *Journal of Behavioral Medicine, 10*, 139–144.

Cohen, S., Doyle, W. J., & Skoner, D. P. (1999). Psychological stress, cytokine production, and severity of upper respiratory illness. *Psychosomatic Medicine, 61*, 175–180.

Cohen, S., Doyle, W. J., Turner, R. B., Alper, C. M., & Skoner, D. P. (2003). Emotional style and susceptibility to the common cold. *Psychosomatic Medicine, 65*, 652–657.

Cohen, S., Kessler, R. C., & Gordon, L. U. (Eds.). (1997). *Measuring stress: A guide for health and social scientists*. New York: Oxford University Press.

Cohen, S., Miller, G. E., & Rabin, B. S. (2001). Psychological stress and antibody response to immunization: A critical review of the human literature. *Psychosomatic Medicine, 63*, 7–18.

Côté, S. (1999). Affect and performance in organizational settings. *Current Directions in Psychological Science, 8*, 65–68.

Creed, P. A., & Macintyre, S. R. (2001). The relative effects of deprivation of the latent and manifest benefits of employment on the well-being of unemployed people. *Journal of Occupational Health Psychology, 6*, 324–331.

Cross National Collaborative Group. (1992). The changing rate of major depression: Cross national comparisons. *Journal of the American Medical Association, 268*, 3098–3105.

Csikszentmihalyi, M. (1997). *Finding flow*. New York: Basic Books.

Csikszentmihalyi, M., & Schneider, B. (2000). *Becoming adult: How teenagers prepare for the world of work*. New York: Basic Books.

Cunningham, M. R. (1988a). Does happiness mean friendliness? Induced mood and heterosexual self-disclosure. *Personality and Social Psychology Bulletin, 14*, 283–297.

Cunningham, M. R. (1988b). What do you do when you're happy or blue? Mood, expectancies and behavioral interest. *Motivation and Emotion, 12*, 309–331.

Danner, D. D., Snowdon, D. A., & Friesen, W. V. (2001). Positive emotions in early life and longevity: Findings from the nun study. *Journal of Personality and Social Psychology, 80*, 804–813.

De Fruyt, F. (2002). A person-centered approach to P-E fit questions using a multiple-trait model. *Journal of Vocational Behavior, 60*, 73–90.

DeLongis, A., Folkman, S., & Lazarus, R. S. (1988). The impact of daily stress on health and mood: Psychological and social resources as mediators. *Journal of Personality and Social Psychology, 54*, 486–495.

Deluga, R. J., & Mason, S. (2000). Relationship of resident assistant conscientiousness, extraversion, and positive affect with rated performance. *Journal of Research in Personality, 34*, 225–235.

Devins, G. M., Mann, J., Mandin, H., & Leonard, C. (1990). Psychosocial predictors of survival in end-statge renal disease. *Journal of Nervous and Mental Disease, 178*, 127–133.

Di Tella, R., & MacCulloch, R. (1999). *Partisan social happiness* [Mimeograph]. Boston: Harvard Business School.

Di Tella, R., MacCulloch, R. J., & Oswald, A. J. (2001). Preferences over inflation and unemployment: Evidence from surveys of happiness. *American Economic Review, 91*, 335–341.

Diener, E. (1984). Subjective well-being. *Psychological Bulletin, 95*, 542–575.

Diener, E., & Biswas-Diener, R. (2002). Will money increase subjective well-being? A literature review and guide to needed research. *Social Indicators Research, 57*, 119–169.

256 E. Diener and M.E.P. Seligman

256 E. Diener and M.E.P. Seligman
256 E. Diener and M.E.P. Seligman

Diener, E., Diener, C., & Diener, M. (1995). Factors predicting the subjective well-being of nations. *Journal of Personality and Social Psychology, 69,* 851–864.

Diener, E., & Diener, M. (1995). Cross-cultural correlates of life satisfaction and self-esteem. *Journal of Personality and Social Psychology, 68,* 653–663.

Diener, E., Horwitz, J., & Emmons, R. A. (1985). Happiness of the very wealthy. *Social Indicators Research, 16,* 263–274.

Diener, E., Nickerson, C., Lucas, R. E., & Sandvik, E. (2002). Dispositional affect and job outcomes. *Social Indicators Research, 59,* 229–259.

Diener, E., & Oishi, S. (2000). Money and happiness: Income and subjective well-being across nations. In E. Diener & E. M. Suh (Eds.), *Culture and subjective well-being* (pp. 185–218). Cambridge, MA: MIT Press.

Diener, E., & Oishi, S. (in press). Are Scandinavians happier than Asians? Issues in comparing nations on subjective well-being. In F. Columbus (Ed.), *Politics and economics of Asia.* Hauppauge, NY: Nova Science.

Diener, E., Sandvik, E., Seidlitz, L., & Diener, M. (1993). The relationship between income and subjective well-being: Relative or absolute? *Social Indicators Research, 28,* 195–223.

Diener, E., & Seligman, M. E. P. (2002). Very happy people. *Psychological Science, 13,* 80–83.

Diener, E., & Suh, E. (1999). National differences in subjective well-being. In D. Kahneman, E. Diener, & N. Schwarz (Eds.), *Well-being: The foundations of hedonic psychology* (pp. 434–450). New York: Russell Sage Foundation.

Diener, E., Suh, E. M., Lucas, R. E., & Smith, H. E. (1999). Subjective well-being: Three decades of progress. *Psychological Bulletin, 125,* 276–302.

Diener, E., Suh, E. M., Smith, H., & Shao, L. (1995). National differences in reported well-being: Why do they occur? *Social Indicators Research, 34,* 7–32.

Donovan, N., & Halpern, D. (2003, November). *Life satisfaction: The state of knowledge and implications for government.* Paper presented at the Conference on Well-Being and Social Capital, Harvard University, Cambridge, MA.

Dooley, B. (1996). At work away from work. *Psychologist, 9,* 155–158.

Doumas, D. M., Margolin, G., & John, R. S. (2003). The relationship between daily martial interaction, work, and health-promoting behaviors in dualearner couples: An extension of the work-family spillover model. *Journal of Family Issues, 24,* 3–20.

Dow, G. K., & Juster, F. T. (1985). Goods, time and well-being: The joint dependence problem. In F. T. Juster & F. P. Stafford (Eds.), *Time, goods and well-being* (pp. 397–413). Ann Arbor, MI: Institute for Social Research.

Easterbrook, G. (2003). *The progress paradox: How life gets better while people feel worse.* New York: Random House.

Easterlin, R. A. (1995). Will raising the incomes of all increase the happiness of all? *Journal of Economic Behavior and Organization, 27,* 35–47.

Easterlin, R. A. (1996). *Growth triumphant: The twenty-first century in historical perspective.* Ann Arbor: University of Michigan Press.

Egeland, J., & Hostetter, A. (1983). Amish Study: I. Affective disorders among the Amish. *American Journal of Psychiatry, 140,* 56–61.

Evers, A. W., Kraaimaat, F. W., Geenen, R., & Bijlsma, J. W. J. (1997). Determinants of psychological distress and its course in the first year after diagnosis in rheumatoid arthritis patients. *Journal of Behavioral Medicine, 20,* 489–504.

Faller, H., Buelzebruck, H., Schilling, S., Drings, P., & Lang., H. (1997). Do psychological factors influence survival in cancer patients? Findings of an empirical study with lung cancer patients. *Psychotherapie, Psychosomatik, Medizinische Psychologie, 47,* 206–218.

Faller, H., Kirschner, S., & König, A. (2003). Psychological distress predicts functional outcomes at three and twelve months after total knee arthroplasty. *General Hospital Psychiatry, 25,* 372–373.

Ferriss, A. L. (2002). Religion and the quality of life. *Journal of Happiness Studies, 3,* 199–215.

Fiscella, K., & Franks, P. (1997). Does psychological distress contribute to racial and socioeconomic disparities in mortality? *Social Science & Medicine, 45,* 1805–1809.

Fitzgerald, T. E., Prochaska, J. O., & Pransky, G. S. (2000). Health risk reduction and functional restoration following coronary revascularization: A prospective investigation using dynamic stage typology clustering. *International Journal of Rehabilitation and Health, 5*, 99–116.

Fleming, J. H. (2000). Relating employee engagement and customer loyalty to business outcomes in the retail industry. *The Gallup Research Journal, 3*(1), 103–115.

Forthofer, M. S., Markman, H. J., Cox, M., Stanley, S., & Kessler, R. C. (1996). Associations between marital distress and work loss in a national sample. *Journal of Marriage and the Family, 58*, 597–605.

Fredrickson, B. L., & Levenson, R. W. (1998). Positive emotions speed recovery from the cardiovascular sequelae of negative emotions. *Cognition and Emotion, 12*, 191–220.

Fredrickson, B. L., Mancuso, R. A., Branigan, C., & Tugade, M. M. (2000). The undoing effect of positive emotions. *Motivation and Emotion, 24*, 237–258.

Frey, B. S., & Stutzer, A. (2000). Happiness prospers in democracy. *Journal of Happiness Studies, 1*, 79–102.

Frey, B. S., & Stutzer, A. (2002a). *Happiness and economics: How the economy and institutions affect human well-being.* Princeton, NJ: Princeton University Press.

Frey, B. S., & Stutzer, A. (2002b). What can economists learn from happiness research? *Journal of Economic Literature, 40*, 402–435.

Frey, B. S., & Stutzer, A. (2003). *Economic consequences of mispredicting utility.* Unpublished manuscript, University of Zurich, Zurich, Switzerland.

Fromm, E. (1956). *The art of loving.* New York: Harper & Row.

Furnham, A., & Argyle, M. (1998). *The psychology of money.* London: Routledge.

Futerman, A. D., Kemeny, M. E., Shapiro, D., & Fahey, J. L. (1994). Immunological and physiological changes associated with induced positive and negative mood. *Psychosomatic Medicine, 56*, 499–511.

George, J. M. (1990). Personality, affect, and behavior in groups. *Journal of Applied Psychology, 75*, 107–116.

George, J. M. (1995). Leader positive mood and group performance: The case of customer service. *Journal of Applied Social Psychology, 25*, 778–794.

George, J. M., & Brief, A. P. (1992). Feeling good–doing good: A conceptual analysis of the mood at work-organizational spontaneity relationship. *Psychological Bulletin, 112*, 310–329.

Gilbert, D. T., Pinel, E. C., Wilson, T. D., Blumberg, S. J., & Wheatley, T. P. (1998). Immune neglect: A source of durability bias in affective forecasting. *Journal of Personality and Social Psychology, 75*, 617–638.

Glisson, C., & Durick, M. (1988). Predictors of job satisfaction and organizational commitment in human service organizations. *Administrative Science Quarterly, 33*, 61–81.

Gloaguen, V., Cottraux, J., Cucherat, M., & Blackburn, I. M. (1998). A meta-analysis of the effects of cognitive therapy in depressed patients. *Journal of Affective Disorders, 49*, 59–72.

Gohm, C., Oishi, S., Darlington, J., & Diener, E. (1998). Culture, parental conflict, parental marital status, and the subjective well-being of young adults. *Journal of Marriage and the Family, 60*, 319–334.

Graham, C., Eggers, A. & Sukhtankar, S. (in press). Does happiness pay? An exploration based on panel data from Russia. *Journal of Economic Behavior and Organization.*

Graham, C., & Pettinato, S. (2002). Frustrated achievers: Winners, losers and subjective well-being in new market economies. *Journal of Development Studies, 38*(4), 100–140.

Grebner, S., Semmer, N. K., & Elfering, A. (2003). *Working conditions and three types of well-being: A longitudinal study with self-report and rating data.* Manuscript submitted for publication.

Griffin, R. W. (1991). Effects of work redesign on employee perceptions, attitudes, and behaviors: A long-term investigation. *Academy of Management Journal, 34*, 425–435.

Groenewegen, P. P., & Hutten, J. B. (1991). Workload and job satisfaction among general practitioners: A review of the literature. *Social Science and Medicine, 32*, 1111–1119.

Hagerty, M. R. (2000). Social comparisons of income in one's community: Evidence from national surveys of income and happiness. *Journal of Personality and Social Psychology, 78*, 746–771.

Hagerty, M. R., & Veenhoven, R. (2003). Wealth and happiness revisited: Growing wealth of nations does go with greater happiness. *Social Indicators Research, 64,* 1–27.

Hammen, C. (1996). Stress, families, and the risk for depression. In C. Mundt, M. J. Goldstein, K. Hahlweg, & P. Fielder (Eds.), *Interpersonal factors in the origin and course of affective disorders* (pp. 101–112). London: Gaskell/Royal College of Psychiatrists.

Hammen, C. (1999). The emergence of an interpersonal approach to depression. In T. Joiner & J. C. Coyne (Eds.), *The interactional nature of depression: Advances in interpersonal approaches* (pp. 21–35). Washington, DC: American Psychological Association.

Hammen, C. (2000). Interpersonal factors in an emerging developmental model of depression. In S. L. Johnson, A. M. Hayes, T. M. Field, N. Schneiderman, & P. McCabe (Eds.), *Stress, coping, and depression* (pp. 71–88). Mahwah, NJ: Erlbaum.

Hammen, C., & Brennan, P. A. (2002). Interpersonal dysfunction in depressed women: Impairments independent of depressive symptoms. *Journal of Affective Disorders, 72,* 145–156.

Harlow, R. E., & Cantor, N. (1996). Still participating after all these years: A study of life task participation in later life. *Journal of Personality and Social Psychology, 71,* 1235–1249.

Harter, J. K. (2000). The linkage of employee perception to outcomes in a retail environment: Cause and effect? *The Gallup Research Journal, 3*(1), 25–38.

Harter, J. K., Schmidt, F. L., & Hayes, T. L. (2002). Business-unit-level relationship between employee satisfaction, employee engagement, and business outcomes: A meta-analysis. *Journal of Applied Psychology, 87,* 268–279.

Harter, J. K., Schmidt, F. L., & Killham, E. A. (2003). *Employee engagement, satisfaction, and business-unit-level outcomes: A meta-analysis.* Princeton, NJ: Gallup Organization.

Heikkilä, H., Heikkilä, E., & Eisemann, M. (1998). Predictive factors for the outcome of a multidisciplinary pain rehabilitation programme on sick-leave and life satisfaction in patients with whiplash trauma and other myofascial pain: A follow-up study. *Clinical Rehabilitation, 12,* 487–496.

Heller, D., Judge, T. A., & Watson, D. (2002). The confounding role of personality and trait affectivity in the relationship between job and life satisfaction. *Journal of Organizational Behavior, 23,* 815–835.

Helliwell, J. F. (2003a). How's life? Combining individual and national variables to explain subjective well-being. *Economic Modelling, 20,* 331–360.

Helliwell, J. F. (2003b). *Well-being and social capital: Does suicide pose a puzzle?* Unpublished manuscript, University of British Columbia, Vancouver, British Columbia, Canada.

Hersey, R. B. (1932). *Worker's emotions in shop and home: A study of individual workers from the psychological and physiological standpoint.* Philadelphia: University of Pennsylvania Press.

Herzberg, D. S., Hammen, C., Burge, D., Daley, S. E., Davila, J., & Lindberg, N. (1998). Social competence as a predictor of chronic interpersonal stress. *Personal Relationships, 5,* 207–218.

Hilleras, P. K., Jorm, A. F., Herlitz, A., & Winblad, B. (1998). Negative and positive affect among the very old: A survey on a sample age 90 years or older. *Research on Aging, 20,* 593–610.

Hintikka, J., Koskela, T., Kontula, O., Koskela, K., & Viinamaeki, H. (2000). Men, women and friends: Are there differences in relation to mental well-being? *Quality of Life Research, 9,* 841–845.

Iaffaldano, M., & Muchinsky, P. (1985). Job satisfaction and performance: A meta-analysis. *Journal of Applied Psychology, 97,* 251–273.

Inglehart, R., & Klingemann, H.-D. (2000). Genes, culture, democracy, and happiness. In E. Diener & E. M. Suh (Eds.), *Culture and subjective well-being* (pp. 165–184). Cambridge, MA: MIT Press.

Jenkins, R., Bebbington, P., Brugha, T., Farrell, M., Lewis, G., & Meltzer, H. (2003). British Psychiatric Morbidity Survey. *International Review of Psychiatry, 15,* 14–18.

Jenkins, R., Lewis, G., Bebbington, P., Brugha, T., Farrell, M., Gill, B., et al. (1997). The National Psychiatric Morbidity Surveys of Great Britain—initial findings from the household survey. *Psychological Medicine, 27,* 775–789.

Judge, T. A. (1991). Job satisfaction as a reflection of disposition: Investigating the relationship and its effect on employee adaptive behaviors. *Dissertation Abstracts International A: Humanities and Social Sciences, 52*(3), 996. (UMI No. AAT 9114284)

Judge, T. A., & Larsen, R. J. (2001). Dispositional affect and job satisfaction: A review and theoretical extension. *Organizational Behavior and Human Decision Processes, 86*, 67–98.

Judge, T. A., Thoreson, C. J., Bono, J. E., & Patton, G. K. (2001). The job satisfaction-job performance relationship: A qualitative and quantitative review. *Psychological Bulletin, 127*, 376–407.

Juster, F. T. (1985). Preferences for work and leisure. In F. T. Juster & F. P. Stafford (Eds.), *Time, goods, and well-being*. Ann Arbor, MI: Institute for Social Research.

Kahneman, D. (1994). New challenges to the rationality assumption. *Journal of Institutional and Theoretical Economics, 150*, 18–36.

Kahneman, D. (2003, January). *Puzzles of well-being*. Paper presented at the annual meeting of the American Economics Association, Washington, DC.

Kahneman, D., Diener, E., & Schwarz, N. (Eds.). (1999). *Well-being: The foundations of hedonic psychology*. New York: Russell Sage Foundation.

Kahneman, D., Krueger, A. B., Schkade, D. A., Schwarz, N., & Stone, A. A. (2004). A survey method for characterizing daily life experience: The Day Reconstruction Method. *Science, 306*, 1776–1780.

Kamen-Siegel, L., Rodin, J., Seligman, M. E., & Dwyer, J. (1991). Explanatory style and cell-mediated immunity in elderly men and women. *Health Psychology, 10*, 229–235.

Kang, S. N. (2001). The relationship between job and marital satisfaction: Overall and facet satisfaction among professionals. *Dissertation Abstracts International B: Sciences and Engineering, 62*(6), 2958. (UMI No. AAI 3017289)

Karasek, R. (2001). Toward a psychosocially healthy work environment: Broader roles for psychologists and sociologists. In N. Schneiderman, M. A. Speers, J. M. Silva, H. Tomes, & J. H. Gentry (Eds.), *Integrating behavioral and social sciences with public health* (pp. 267–292). Washington, DC: American Psychological Association.

Kashdan, T. B., & Herbert, J. D. (2001). Social anxiety disorder in childhood and adolescence: Current status and future directions. *Clinical Child and Family Psychology Review, 4*, 37–61.

Kasser, T., & Kanner, A. D. (Eds.). (2004). *Psychology and consumer culture: The struggle for a good life in a materialistic world*. Washington, DC: American Psychological Association.

Kasser, T. Ryan, R. M., Couchman, C. E., & Sheldon, K. M. (2004). Materialistic values: Their causes and consequences. In T. Kasser & A. D. Kanner (Eds.), *Psychology and consumer culture: The struggle for a good life in a materialistic world* (pp. 11–28). Washington, DC: American Psychological Association.

Keefe, F. J., Lumley, M., Anderson, T., Lunch, T., & Carson, K. L. (2001). Pain and emotion: New research direction. *Journal of Clinical Psychology, 57*, 587–607.

Kenny, C. (1999). Does growth cause happiness, or does happiness cause growth? *Kyklos, 52*, 3–26.

Kessler, R. C., & Frank, R. G. (1997). The impact of psychiatric disorders on work loss days. *Psychological Medicine, 27*, 861–873.

Kessler, R. C., McGonagle, K. A., Zhao, S., Nelson, C. B., Hughes, M., Eshleman, S., et al. (1994). Lifetime and 12-month prevalence of DSM-III-R psychiatric disorders in the United States: Results from the National Comorbidity Survey. *Archives of General Psychiatry, 51*, 8–19.

Kirkcaldy, B. D., Furnham, A., & Martin, T. (1998). National differences in personality, socioeconomic, and work-related attitudinal variables. *European Psychologist, 3*, 255–262.

Klerman, G. L., Lavori, P. W., Rice, J., Reich, T., Endicott, J., Andreasen, N. C., et al. (1985). Birth cohort trends in rates of major depressive disorder among relatives of patients with affective disorder. *Archives of General Psychiatry, 42*, 689–693.

Kohn, M. L., & Schooler, C. (1982). Job conditions and personality: A longitudinal assessment of their reciprocal effects. *American Journal of Sociology, 87*, 1257–1286.

Koivumaa-Honkanen, H. T., Honkanen, R., Antikainen, R., & Hintikka, J. (1999). Self-reported life satisfaction and treatment factors in patients with schizophrenia, major depression and anxiety disorder. *Acta Psychologica Scandinavica, 95,* 377–384.

Koivumaa-Honkanen, H. T., Honkanen, R., Koskenvuo, M., Viinamaki, H., & Kaprio, J. (2002). Life satisfaction as a predictor of fatal injury in a 20-year follow-up. *Acta Psychiatrica Scandinavica, 105,* 444–450.

Kopp, M., Bonatti, H., Haller, C., Rumpold, G., Söllner, W., Holzner, B., et al. (2003). Life satisfaction and active coping style are important predictors of recovery from surgery. *Journal of Psychosomatic Research, 55,* 371–377.

Koys, D. J. (2001). The effects of employee satisfaction, organizational citizenship behavior, and turnover on organizational effectiveness: A unitlevel, longitudinal study. *Personnel Psychology, 54,* 101–114.

Kposowa, A. (2001). Unemployment and suicide: A cohort analysis of social factors predicting suicide in the US National Longitudinal Mortality Study. *Psychological Medicine, 31,* 127–138.

Kubzansky, L. D., Sparrow, D., Vokonas, P., & Kawachi, I. (2001). Is the glass half empty or half full? A prospective study of optimism and coronary heart disease in the Normative Aging Study. *Psychosomatic Medicine, 63,* 910–916.

Kubzansky, L. D., Wright, R. J., Cohen, S., Weiss, S., Rosner, B., & Sparrow, D. (2002). Breathing easy: A prospective study of optimism and pulmonary function in the Normative Aging Study. *Annals of Behavioral Medicine, 24,* 345–353.

Lane, R. E. (2000). *The loss of happiness in market democracies.* New Haven, CT: Yale University Press.

Lansford, J. E. (2000). Family relationships, friendships, and well-being in the United States and Japan. *Dissertation Abstracts International B: Sciences and Engineering, 61*(3), 1673. (UMI No. AAT 9963831)

Leary, M. R. (1990). Responses to social exclusion: Social anxiety, jealousy, loneliness, depression, and low self-esteem. *Journal of Social and Clinical Psychology, 9,* 221–229.

Lehman, A. F. (1996). Measures of quality of life among persons with severe and persistent mental disorders. *Social Psychiatry and Psychiatric Epidemiology, 31,* 78–88.

Lewinsohn, P., Rohde, P., Seeley, J. R., & Fischer, S. A. (1993). Age-cohort changes in the lifetime occurrence of depression and other mental disorders. *Journal of Abnormal Psychology, 102,* 110–120.

Longabaugh, R., McCrady, B., Fink, E., Stout, R., McAuley, T., Doyle, C., et al. (1983). Cost effectiveness of alcoholism treatment in partial vs. inpatient settings: Six-month outcomes. *Journal of Studies on Alcohol, 44,* 1049–1071.

Lox, C. L., Burns, S. P., Treasure, D. C., & Wasley, D. A. (1999). Physical and psychological predictors of exercise dosage in healthy adults. *Medicine and Science in Sports and Exercise, 31,* 1060–1064.

Lucas, R. E., Clark, A. E., Georgellis, Y., & Diener, E. (2003). Re-examining adaptation and the setpoint model of happiness: Reactions to changes in marital status. *Journal of Personality and Social Psychology, 84,* 527–539.

Lucas, R. E., Clark, A. E., Georgellis, Y., & Diener, E. (2004). Unemployment alters the set point for life satisfaction. *Psychological Science, 15,* 8–13.

Lucas, R. E., & Diener, E. (2003). The happy worker: Hypotheses about the role of positive affect in worker productivity. In M. R. Barrick & A. M. Ryan (Eds.), *Personality and work* (pp. 30–59). San Francisco: Jossey Bass.

Lucas, R. E., Diener, E., & Suh, E. M. (1996). Discriminant validity of well-being measures. *Journal of Personality and Social Psychology, 71,* 616–628.

Luthar, S. S. (2003). The culture of affluence: Psychological costs of material wealth. *Child Development, 74,* 1581–1593.

Lynch, J. J. (1979). *The broken heart: The medical consequences of loneliness.* New York: Basic Books.

Lyons, A., & Chamberlain, K. (1994). The effects of minor events, optimism and self-esteem on health. *British Journal of Clinical Psychology, 33,* 559–570.

Lyubomirsky, S., & Lepper, H. S. (2003). *What are the differences between happiness and self-esteem?* Manuscript submitted for publication.

Magdol, L. (2002). Is moving gendered? The effects of residential mobility on the psychological well-being of men and women. *Sex Roles, 47,* 553–560.

Malka, A., & Chatman, J. A. (2003). Intrinsic and extrinsic orientations as moderators of the effect of annual income on subjective well-being: A longitudinal study. *Personality and Social Psychology Bulletin, 29,* 737–746.

Marks, G. N., & Fleming, N. (1999). Influences and consequences of well-being among Australian young people: 1980–1995. *Social Indicators Research, 46,* 301–323.

Marmot, M. (2003, June). *The social gradient in health and well-being.* Paper presented at the Brookings Warwick Conference "Why inequality matters: Lessons for policy from the economics of happiness," Washington, DC.

Marsland, A. L., Cohen, S., Rabin, B. S., & Manuck, S. B. (2001). Associations between stress, trait negative affect, acute immune reactivity, and antibody response to hepatitis B injection in healthy young adults. *Health Psychology, 20,* 4–11.

Martens, L., & Addington, J. (2001). The psychological well-being of family members of individuals with schizophrenia. *Social Psychiatry and Psychiatric Epidemiology, 36,* 128–133.

Maruta, T., Colligan, R. C., Malinchoc, M., & Offord, K. P. (2000). Optimists vs. pessimists: Survival rate among medical patients over a 30-year period. *Mayo Clinic Proceedings, 75,* 140–143.

McClelland, D. C., & Cheriff, A. D. (1997). The immunoenhancing effects of humor on secretory IgA and resistance to respiratory infections. *Psychology and Health, 12,* 329–344.

McConnell, P., Bebbington, P., McClelland, R., Gillespie, K., & Houghton, S. (2002). Prevalence of psychiatric disorder and the need for psychiatric care in Northern Ireland: Population study in the District of Derry. *British Journal of Psychiatry, 181,* 214–219.

McCrady, B. S., Stout, R., Noel, N., Abrams, D., & Nelson, H. F. (1991). Effectiveness of three types of spouse-involved behavioral alcoholism treatment. *British Journal of Addiction, 86,* 1415–1424.

McIntyre, C. W., Watson, D., Clark, L. A., & Cross, S. A. (1991). The effect of induced social interaction on positive and negative affect. *Bulletin of the Psychonomic Society, 29,* 67–70.

Mehnert, T., Krauss, H. H., Nadler, R., & Boyd, M. (1990). Correlates of life satisfaction in those with disabling conditions. *Rehabilitation Psychology, 35,* 3–17.

Menec, V. H. (2003). The relation between everyday activities and successful aging: A 6-year longitudinal study. *Journals of Gerontology, 58B,* S74–S82.

Miles, D. E., Borman, W. E., Spector, P. E., & Fox, S. (2002). Building an integrative model of extra role work behaviors: A comparison of counterproductive work behavior with organizational citizenship behavior. *International Journal of Selection and Assessment, 10,* 51–57.

Miner, A. G. (2001). *Experience sampling events, moods, behaviors, and performance at work.* Unpublished doctoral dissertation, University of Illinois, Urbana-Champaign.

Murray, C., & Lopez, A. (1997). Alternative projections of mortality and disability by cause 1999–2020: Global Burden of Disease Study. *Lancet, 349,* 1498–1504.

Murrell, S. A., Salsman, N. L., & Meeks, S. (2003). Educational attainment, positive psychological mediators, and resources for health and vitality in older adults. *Journal of Aging and Health, 15,* 591–615.

Naroll, R. (1983). *The moral order: An introduction to the human situation.* Beverly Hills, CA: Sage.

Naughton, M. J., Herndon, J. E., II, Shumaker, S. A., Miller, A. A., Kornblith, A. B., Chao, D., et al. (2002). The health-related quality of life and survival of small-cell lung cancer patients: Results of a companion study to CALGB 9033. *Quality of Life Research, 11,* 235–248.

Nehra, A., Mann, S. B. S., Sharma, S. C., & Verma, S. K. (1997). Psychosocial functions before and after the use of hearing aids in acquired hearing loss patients. *Indian Journal of Clinical Psychology, 24,* 75–81.

Nelson, G., Hall, G. B., & Walsh-Bowers, R. (1999). Predictors of adaptation of people with psychiatric disabilities in group homes, supportive apartments, and board-and-care homes. *Psychiatric Rehabilitation Journal, 22,* 381–389.

Neumark, D., & Postlewaite, A. (1998). Relative income concerns and the rise in married women's employment. *Journal of Public Economics, 70*, 157–183.

Nickerson, C., Kahneman, D., Diener, E., & Schwarz, N. (2004). *Correlates and consequences of wanting money.* Unpublished manuscript, University of Illinois, Urbana-Champaign.

Nickerson, C., Schwarz, N., Diener, E., & Kahneman, D. (2003). Zeroing in on the dark side of the American dream: A closer look at the negative consequences of the goal for financial success. *Psychological Science, 14*, 531–536.

Okun, M. A., & George, L. K. (1984). Physician- and self-ratings of health, neuroticism and subjective well-being among men and women. *Personality and Individual Differences, 5*, 533–539.

Okun, M. A., Stock, W. A., Haring, M. J., & Witter, R. A. (1984). The social activity/subjective well-being relation: A quantitative synthesis. *Research on Aging, 6*, 45–65.

Organ, D. W., & Ryan, K. (1995). A meta-analytic review of attitudinal and dispositional predictors of organizational citizenship behavior. *Personnel Psychology, 48*, 775–802.

Ortony, A., Clore, G. L., & Collins, A. (1988). *The cognitive structure of emotions.* New York: Cambridge University Press.

Ostir, G. V., Markides, K. S., Black, S. A., & Goodwin, J. S. (2000). Emotional well-being predicts subsequent functional independence and survival. *Journal of the American Geriatrics Society, 48*, 473–478.

Oswald, A. J. (1997). Happiness and economic performance. *Economic Journal, 107*, 1815–1831.

Ouweneel, P. (2002). Social security and well-being of the unemployed in 42 nations. *Journal of Happiness Studies, 3*, 167–192.

Packer, S., Husted, J., Cohen, S., & Tomlinson, G. (1997). Psychopathology and quality of life in schizophrenia. *Journal of Psychiatry & Neuroscience, 22*, 231–234.

Park, N., Peterson, C., & Seligman, M. E. P. (2003). *Character strengths and well-being.* Manuscript submitted for publication.

Parker, M. G., Thorslund, M., & Nordstrom, M.-L. (1992). Predictors of mortality for the oldest old: A 4-year follow-up of community-based elderly in Sweden. *Archives of Gerontology and Geriatrics, 14*, 227–237.

Pavot, W., Diener, E., & Fujita, F. (1990). Extraversion and happiness. *Personality and Individual Differences, 11*, 1299–1306.

Peterson, C., Seligman, M. E. P., Yurko, K. H., Martin, L. R., & Friedman, H. S. (1998). Catastrophizing and untimely death. *Psychological Science, 9*, 127–130.

Pinikahana, J., Happell, B., & Keks, N. A. (2003). Suicide and schizophrenia: A review of literature for the decade (1990–1999) and implications for mental health nursing. *Issues in Mental Health Nursing, 24*, 27–43.

Price, S. J., & McKenry, P. C. (1988). *Divorce.* Beverly Hills, CA: Sage.

Putnam, R. (2001a). *Bowling alone: The collapse and revival of American community.* New York: Simon & Schuster.

Putnam, R. D. (2001b). Social capital: Measurement and consequences. In J. F. Helliwell (Ed.), *The contribution of human and social capital to sustained economic growth and well-being* (pp. 117–135). Ottawa, Ontario, Canada: Human Resources Development Canada.

Raffaello, M., & Maass, A. (2003). Chronic exposure to noise in industry: The effects on satisfaction, stress symptoms, and company attachment. *Environment and Behavior, 34*, 651–671.

Rice, R. W., Near, J. P., & Hunt, R. G. (1980). The job-satisfaction/life-satisfaction relationship: A review of empirical research. *Basic and Applied Social Psychology, 1*, 37–64.

Rimmerman, A., Treves, G., & Duvdevany, I. (1999). Psychological distress and well-being of mothers of adults with a psychiatric disability: The effects of day treatment, social support networks, and maternal involvement. *Psychiatric Rehabilitation Journal, 22*, 263–269.

Roberts, B. W., Caspi, A., & Moffitt, T. E. (2003). Work experiences and personality development in young adulthood. *Journal of Personality and Social Psychology, 84*, 582–593.

Robins, L. N., Helzer, J. E., Weissman, M. M., Orvaschel, H., Gruenberg, E., Burke, J. D., et al. (1984). Lifetime prevalence of specific psychiatric disorders in three sites. *Archives of General Psychiatry, 41*, 949–958.

Rogers, S. J., & May, D. C. (2003). Spillover between marital quality and job satisfaction: Long-term patterns and gender differences. *Journal of Marriage and the Family, 65*, 482–495.

Ross, C. E., & Huber, J. (1985). Hardship and depression. *Journal of Health and Social Behavior, 26*, 312–327.

Rounds, J. B. (1990). The comparative and combined utility of work value and interest data in career counseling with adults. *Journal of Vocational Behavior, 37*, 32–45.

Rounds, J. B., Dawis, R. V., & Lofquist, L. H. (1987). Measurement of person-environment fit and prediction of satisfaction in the Theory of Work Adjustment. *Journal of Vocational Behavior, 31*, 297–318.

Schilling, O., & Wahl, H. W. (2002). Family networks and life-satisfaction of older adults in rural and urban regions. *Kolner Zeitschrift für Soziologie und Sozialpsychologie, 54*, 304–317.

Schneider, B., Hanges, P. J., Smith, D. B., & Salvaggio, A. N. (2003). Which comes first: Employee attitudes or organizational financial and market performance? *Journal of Applied Psychology, 88*, 836–851.

Schulz, R., Visintainer, P., & Williamson, G. M. (1990). Psychiatric and physical morbidity effects of caregiving. *Journal of Gerontology, 45*, P181–P191.

Schwartz, B. (2004). *The paradox of choice: Why more is less.* New York: Ecco.

Schyns, P. (1998). Crossnational differences in happiness: Economic and cultural factors explored. *Social Indicators Research, 43*, 3–26.

Schyns, P. (2003). *Income and life satisfaction: A cross-national and longitudinal study.* Delft, The Netherlands: Eburon.

Seligman, M. E. P. (1995). The effectiveness of psychotherapy: The Consumer Reports study. *American Psychologist, 50*, 965–974.

Seligman, M. E. P. (2002). *Authentic happiness: Using the new positive psychology to realize your potential for lasting fulfillment.* New York: Free Press.

Shams, M., & Jackson, P. R. (1994). The impact of unemployment on the psychological well-being of British Asians. *Psychological Medicine, 24*, 347–355.

Smith, S., & Razzell, P. (1975). *The pools' winners.* London: Calibon Books.

Smith, T. W., Ruiz, J. M., & Uchino, B. (2001). Mental activation of supportive ties reduces blood pressure reactivity to stress. *Psychosomatic Medicine, 63*, 114.

Solberg, E. C., Diener, E., & Robinson, M. (2004). Why are materialists less satisfied? In T. Kasser & A. D. Kanner (Eds.), *Psychology and consumer culture: The struggle for a good life in a materialistic world* (pp. 29–48). Washington, DC: American Psychological Association.

Solomon, G. F., Segerstrom, S. C., Grohr, P., Kemeny, M., & Fahey, J. (1997). Shaking up immunity: Psychological and immunologic changes after a natural disaster. *Psychosomatic Medicine, 59*, 114–127.

Spector, P. E. (1997). *Job satisfaction: Application, assessment, cause, and consequences.* Thousand Oaks, CA: Sage.

Spector, P. E., Chen, P. Y., & O'Connell, B. J. (2000). A longitudinal study of relations between job stressors and job strains while controlling for prior negative affectivity and strains. *Journal of Applied Psychology, 85*, 211–218.

Spiegel, D., & Giese-Davis, J. (2003). Depression and cancer: Mechanisms and disease progression. *Biological Psychiatry, 54*, 269–282.

Spitzer, R. L., Kroenke, K., Linzer, M., Hahn, S. R., Williams, J. B., deGruy, F. V., et al. (1995). Health-related quality of life in primary care patients with mental disorders. *Journal of the American Medical Association, 274*, 1511–1517.

Srinivasan, R., & Pugliese, A. (2000). Customer satisfaction, loyalty, and behavior. *The Gallup Research Journal, 3*(1), 79–90.

Srivastava, A., Locke, E. A., & Bartol, K. M. (2001). Money and subjective well-being: It's not the money, it's the motives. *Journal of Personality and Social Psychology, 80*, 959–971.

Staw, B. M., & Barsade, S. G. (1993). Affect and managerial performance: A test of the sadder-but-wiser vs. happier-and-smarter hypothesis. *Administrative Science Quarterly, 38*, 304–331.

Staw, B. M., Bell, N. E., & Clausen, J. A. (1986). The dispositional approach to job attitudes: A lifetime longitudinal test. *Administrative Science Quarterly, 31*, 56–77.

Staw, B. M., Sutton, R. I., & Pelled, L. H. (1994). Employee positive emotion and favorable outcomes at the workplace. *Organization Science, 5*, 51–71.

Steinbrueck, S. M., Maxwell, S. E., & Howard, G. S. (1983). A meta-analysis of psychotherapy and drug therapy in the treatment of unipolar depression with adults. *Journal of Counseling and Clinical Psychology, 51*, 856–863.

Stilley, C. S., Dew, M. A., Stukas, A. A., Switzer, G. E., Manzetti, J. D., Keenan, R. J., et al. (1999). Psychological symptom levels and their correlates in lung and heart-lung transplant recipients. *Psychosomatics, 40*, 503–509.

Stone, A. A., Cox, D. S., Valdimarsdottir, H., Jandorf, L., & Neale, J. M. (1987). Evidence that secretory IgA antibody is associated with daily mood. *Journal of Personality and Social Psychology, 52*, 988–993.

Stroebe, W., Stroebe, M., Abakoumkin, G., & Schut, H. (1996). The role of loneliness and social support in adjustment to loss: A test of attachment versus stress theory. *Journal of Personality and Social Psychology, 70*, 1241–1249.

Stutzer, A. (in press). The role of income aspirations in individual happiness. *Journal of Economic Behavior and Organization.*

Sunstein, C. R., & Thaler, R. H. (in press). Libertarian paternalism is not an oxymoron. *University of Chicago Law Review.*

Suslow, T., Roestel, C., Ohrmann, P., & Arolt, V. (2003). The experience of basic emotions in schizophrenia with and without affective negative symptoms. *Comprehensive Psychiatry, 44*, 303–310.

Swaroff, J. B. (2000). Validating "The Gallup Path": A study of the links between loyalty and financial outcomes in healthcare. *The Gallup Research Journal, 3*(1), 41–46.

Thoits, P., & Hannan, M. (1979). Income and psychological distress: The impact of an income-maintenance experiment. *Journal of Health and Social Behavior, 20*, 120–138.

Thoits, P. A., & Hewitt, L. N. (2001). Volunteer work and well-being. *Journal of Health and Social Behavior, 42*, 115–131.

Tramontana, M. G. (1981). Critical review of research on psychotherapy outcome with adolescents: 1967–1977. In S. Chess & A. Thomas (Eds.), *Annual progress in child psychiatry & child development* (pp. 521–550). New York: Brunner/Mazel.

Twenge, J. M. (2000). The age of anxiety? The birth cohort change in anxiety and neuroticism, 1952–1993. *Journal of Personality and Social Psychology, 79*, 1007–1021.

Twenge, J. M. (2002). Birth cohort, social change, and personality: The interplay of dysphoria and individualism in the 20th century. In D. Cervone & W. Mischel (Eds.), *Advances in personality science* (pp. 196–218). New York: Guilford Press.

Ulrich, R. S. (1984). View through a window may influence recovery from surgery. *Science, 224*, 420–421.

Unutzer, J., Patrick, D., Diehr, P., Simon, G., Grembowski, D., & Katon, W. (2000). Quality adjusted life years in older adults with depressive symptoms and chronic medical disorders. *International Psychogeriatrics, 12*, 15–33.

van Jaarsveld, C., Sanderman, R., Miedema, I., Ranchor, A. V., & Kempen, G. I. J. M. (2001). Changes in health-related quality of life in older patients with acute myocardial infarction or congestive heart failure: A prospective study. *Journal of the American Geriatrics Society, 49*, 1052–1058.

van Praag, B. M. S., & Frijters, P. (1999). The measurement of welfare and well-being: The Leyden Approach. In D. Kahneman, E. Diener, & N. Schwarz (Eds.), *Well-being: The foundations of hedonic psychology* (pp. 413–433). New York: Russell Sage Foundation.

van Servellen, G., Sarna, L., Nyamathi, A., Padilla, G., Brecht, M.-L., & Jablonski, K. J. (1998). Emotional distress in women with symptomatic HIV disease. *Issues in Mental Health Nursing, 19*, 173–189.

van Servellen, G., Sarna, L., Padilla, G., & Brecht, M.-L. (1996). Emotional distress in men with life-threatening illness. *International Journal of Nursing Studies, 33*, 551–565.

Varian, H. R. (1992). *Microeconomic analysis*. New York: Norton.
Vázquez, C., Hernangómez, L., & Hervás, G. (2004). Longevidad y emociones positivas [Longevity and positive emotions]. In L. Salvador, A. Cano, & J. R. Cabo (Eds.), *Longevidad: Tratado integral sobre salud en la segunda mitad de la vida* (pp. 752–761). Madrid, Spain: Panamericana.
Veenhoven, R. (1991). Is happiness relative? *Social Indicators Research, 24*, 1–34.
Veenhoven, R. (1994). *World database of happiness: Correlates of happiness: 7837 findings from 603 studies in 69 nations 1911–1994* (3 vols.). Rotterdam, The Netherlands: RISBO.
Veenhoven, R. (2000). Well-being in the welfare state: Level not higher, distribution not more equitable. *Journal of Comparative Policy Analysis, 2*, 91–125.
Veenhoven, R. (2002). *Average happiness in 68 nations in the 1990s: How much people enjoy their life-as-a-whole*. Retrieved April 12, 2004, from World Database of Happiness Web site: http://www.eur.nl/fsw/research/happiness/hap_nat/nat_fp.htm
Verbrugge, L. M., Reoma, J. M., & Gruber-Baldini, A. L. (1994). Short-term dynamics of disability and well-being. *Journal of Health and Social Behavior, 35*, 97–117.
Viinamaeki, H., Koskela, K., & Niskanen, L. (1996). Rapidly declining mental well-being during unemployment. *European Journal of Psychiatry, 10*, 215–221.
Vitaliano, P. P., Scanlan, J. M., Ochs, H. D., Syrjala, K., Siegler, I. C., & Snyder, E. A. (1998). Psychosocial stress moderates the relationship of cancer history with natural killer cell activity. *Annals of Behavioral Medicine, 20*, 199–208.
Vroom, V. H. (1964). *Work and motivation*. New York: Wiley.
Warr, P. (1999). Well-being and the workplace. In D. Kahneman, E. Diener, & N. Schwarz (Eds.), *Well-being: The foundations of hedonic psychology* (pp. 392–412). New York: Russell Sage Foundation.
Watson, D. (2000). *Mood and temperament*. New York: Guilford Press.
Watson, D., & Slack, A. K. (1993). General factors of affective temperament and their relation to job satisfaction over time. *Organizational Behavior and Human Decision Processes, 54*, 181–202.
Weiss, H. M., Nicholas, J. P., & Daus, C. S. (1999). An examination of the joint effects of affective experiences and job beliefs on job satisfaction and variations in affective experiences over time. *Organizational Behavior and Human Decision Processes, 78*, 1–24.
Weiss, R. S. (1979). The impact of marital separation. In G. Levinger & O. C. Moles (Eds.), *Divorce and separation: Context, causes, and consequences* (pp. 201–210). New York: Basic Books.
Welzel, C., Inglehart, R., & Klingemann, H. D. (2003). The theory of human development: A cross-cultural analysis. *European Journal of Political Research, 42*, 341–379.
Westen, D. (2001). A multidimensional meta-analysis of treatments for depression, panic, and generalized anxiety disorder: An empirical examination of the status of empirically supported therapies. *Journal of Consulting and Clinical Psychology, 69*, 875–899.
Williams, K. D. (2001). *Ostracism: The power of silence*. New York: Guilford Press.
Wright, T. A., & Bonett, D. G. (1997). The role of pleasantness and activationbased well-being in performance prediction. *Journal of Occupational Health Psychology, 2*, 212–219.
Zarit, S. H., Stephens, M. A. P., Townsend, A., & Greene, R. (1998). Stress reduction for family caregivers: Effects of adult day care use. *Journals of Gerontology, 53B*, S267–S277.
Zautra, A. J., Hoffman, J. M., Matt, K. S., Yocum, D., Potter, P. T., Castro, W. L., et al. (1998). An examination of individual differences in the relationship between interpersonal stress and disease activity among women with rheumatoid arthritis. *Arthritis Care & Research, 11*, 271–279.
Zelman, D. C., Howland, E. W., Nichols, S. N., & Cleeland, C. S. (1991). The effects of induced mood on laboratory pain. *Pain, 46*, 105–111.

Conclusion: The Well-Being Science Needed Now

Ed Diener

We have learned much about well-being in the past several decades. Our methods have improved in impressive ways, and we have developed a broader view of who across the globe has high versus low subjective well-being. The articles in this volume review the advances we have made in understanding the causes and consequences of well-being. Importantly, we now have a clearer set of questions to ask. In this chapter, I outline several of the advances in questions asked and methods used that I hope will characterize subjective well-being research in the decades ahead.

In terms of methods, very large-scale surveys of the world now exist, which were not available at the time of Wilson's 1967 review of the field. We also now have many intensive experience-sampling studies of people's feelings of well-being across the diverse activities of everyday life. Longitudinal studies, including very large ones, are no longer rare and have helped enormously to advance our knowledge, for example, in helping shed light on the direction of causality between variables. Although self-reports of well-being remain the dominant type of measure in the field, we also have other methods of assessment such as biological measures and the reports of knowledgeable informants. The sophisticated statistical techniques at our disposal have expanded rapidly, as have the measurement approaches such as Item Response Theory, classification statistics such as latent class analysis, and methods of partitioning variance such as dominance analysis. Moreover, hierarchical linear modeling has been a boon in analyzing data where individuals are nested within larger groupings, such as nations. Therefore, given the advances in methods available to us, it hardly seems worthwhile for contemporary researchers to give a single well-being measure to a small convenience sample and correlate the responses with other subjective predictors that are also taken from self-report measurement. We need to move beyond this simple level of data collection, which is currently overused. Instead, we need to expend our research resources by asking better questions in more sophisticated ways rather than conducting studies relying on methods simply because they are quick and easy.

Advances in science can be judged by the level of sophistication of the questions that are asked. For example, we should no longer ask whether people do or do not adapt to circumstances, but should ask instead, when, to what degree, and why they adapt. We should no longer debate whether people's baseline levels of happiness can change, but should inquire about the conditions that can change them

E. Diener (ed.), *The Science of Well-Being: The Collected Works of Ed Diener*, Social Indicators Research Series 37, DOI 10.1007/978-90-481-2350-6_10,

substantially. We should no longer ask only what correlates with "happiness," but we need to inquire about the effects of well-being on future behavior and success. I admonish those who continue to ask the questions of yesterday with the methods of yesterday—we need more now. Not only should we now be asking more sophisticated questions, but we should be using diverse and larger subject samples, often in longitudinal designs, and we should always employ measures of diverse types of well-being.

One way we can be more sophisticated is to go beyond the main effects and the simple questions of what attributes on average are correlated with well-being. For example, we have asked whether married or religious people are happier, and these descriptive inquiries were useful in the early stages of the field. Now, however, we have to go beyond mapping mean differences between groups. Even if married people on average are somewhat higher in subjective well-being than those in other marital categories such as singles and the divorced, we need to inquire whether this is a selection effect due to the fact that happy people get married and stay married at higher rates than less happy individuals. We need to inquire as to the effect-sizes of the differences we uncover and the degree of overlap between the distributions. After all, average differences can be very small and yet statistically significant with the large sample sizes we often use.

We should study the individual differences that moderate the effects of marriage in order to discover who will be happier if married or religious, and who will not be. For example, we need to ask what factors moderate and mediate the relation between marital status and well-being. In addition, we need to inquire whether the effect is uniform across cultures and across different types of well-being. We do not need another simple study on whether married people are happier; we do need more in-depth studies of when, where, and why this occurs, and the effect sizes for different types of well-being, whether it is life satisfaction, positive emotions, or negative emotions. We can inquire into the situations and activities in which married people are happier. There are so many eager young scientists entering the field; it is imperative that they spend their research time in the most productive manner.

There are a number of very important issues in the field that are now ripe for solution. One of those questions is establishing interventions for increasing subjective well-being. However, even here we must recognize different forms of well-being— for example, life satisfaction, positive emotions, low negative emotions, work satisfaction, and engagement—and we should be careful to explore how potential interventions affect each of these, and which of these are most desired. A related issue is how to help people overcome adaptation to the positive conditions in their lives so that they can continue to enjoy and savor good things and not grow completely accustomed to them. Furthermore, the question of whether people adapt when it comes to some types of well-being more than others, for example judgment versus affect, is also of immense importance.

Related to the above questions, we must establish how functional differing levels of well-being are—how beneficial they are in various domains such as health, social relationships, and work. We should not expect simple answers, and we very much need good theories about why well-being could be harmful or helpful at different levels and in different pursuits. Furthermore, we will need to examine whether varying levels of well-being are beneficial, depending on the circumstances in which people find themselves. We have found, for example, that the level of cheerfulness conducive to earning high income varied depending on whether the person came from a poor or a well-off family (Diener, Nickerson, Lucas, & Sandvik, 2002). This hints at the proposition that high levels of "happiness" might be more helpful to individuals who are living in resource-rich and desirable environments, and that some negative affect might benefit those in worse environments if they motivate a desire for change.

Research on the benefits of well-being and its optimal levels is likely to be of great importance in the coming years. If I were starting out as a new researcher, this would be the area on which I would concentrate—I believe it is a research "hot spot" for the upcoming decades. Not only is this area of great theoretical interest, but it is perhaps the most important area in terms of practical interest as well.

An important question is whether well-being has the same effects on behavior regardless of its source, for example whether well-being derives from temperament, success at goal-striving, or from psychoactive drugs. A related question is how the benefits of well-being depend on the interaction of well-being and a person's values and goals. Many scholars have objected to an emphasis on "happiness" as misplaced. Instead, they argue, we ought to focus on achievement, helping others, and the desirable factors that can increase a feeling of well-being rather than focus directly on subjective well-being itself. Of course, many factors that are socially beneficial and might increase well-being are the targets of interventions to increase well-being, such as gratitude interventions. Nevertheless, the critique highlights the need for research on whether well-being interventions of various types not only are effective in raising "happiness," but how success and societal well-being are affected by such interventions.

In our book, *Happiness: Unlocking the Mysteries of Psychological Wealth* (2008), Robert Biswas-Diener and I discuss the reasons why people can be "too happy." We first trace why generally happy people are better off in terms of health, work, and relationships. This serves as the starting point for exploring optimal levels of well-being for effective functioning. After noting the benefits of well-being for success, we also caution that people need not seek continual euphoria and the avoidance of all unpleasant emotions. Thus, we suggest that less than complete happiness might be the ideal. It is likely that the most desirable levels of well-being depend on a whole host of factors: personality, culture, circumstances, the person's goals, and the types of well-being being considered. However, we currently have virtually no empirical knowledge of the factors that determine ideal levels of well-being. Thus, this critically important area is one that is rich with possibilities for theory and research.

Another important area is analysis of the interface between psychological well-being and subjective well-being. In recent years researchers following in the humanistic tradition have offered a model of effective functioning that has been called *psychological well-being*. Carol Ryff (Keyes, Shmotkin, & Ryff, 2002) proposed that there are six basic human needs (for meaning and purpose, relationships, and autonomy, for example) and that having these needs fulfilled is psychological well-being (PWB). She contrasts PWB with subjective well-being, which is based on a person's feelings about his or her life, and suggests that PWB is more important for good health. Similarly, Ryan and Deci (2000) created a theory they label Self-Determination Theory (SDT), which revolves around the fulfillment of intrinsic needs, and in particular, the needs for autonomy, mastery, and social relationships. Some have likened the psychological well-being approaches to the "eudaimonic" happiness of Aristotle. Kashdan, Biswas-Diener, and King (2008) called into question how distinct eudaimonic forms of well-being actually are from subjective well-being, and this currently is an ongoing debate. What is needed here is a theory about how PWB and SWB overlap and are different, as well as the mechanisms that distinguish them. Importantly, we need a more thorough exploration of the outcomes of each. Finally, we need a more careful examination of how meaning and purpose relate to various forms of subjective well-being, such as life satisfaction.

Another very promising area for theoretical advance is the area of happiness forecasting—how people make decisions based on predicted happiness and other outcomes. So far this area has focused on the types of errors people make in certain situations—for example, in underestimating adaptation. Although this research is important, the area of happiness forecasting should be broader. For instance, scientists can inquire into the conditions in which people make good forecasts, not just where they are likely to go wrong. Only then will we have a good estimate of how accurate people are at making happiness forecasts. The current research might inadvertently convey the view that people are very bad at forecasting, whereas we do not have a good assessment of people's accuracy because the research is often designed to examine errors rather than accuracy per se. A related question in the forecasting domain is whether and when accurate forecasts are necessary or helpful. It could be, for example, that overly-positive forecasts can in some cases be desirable because they serve to create self-fulfilling prophecies that are beneficial.

One of the most important questions facing the field is the nature of universal needs that might affect the happiness of all people, versus factors that influence happiness only in a relative way, in comparison to some set of standards such as social comparisons. For instance, all people try to regulate their core body temperature, and find that temperatures that are much lower than ideal for maintaining this temperature are unpleasant, as are temperatures much above this point. Different people might prefer somewhat different ambient temperatures because of their body mass and fat, activity levels, and so forth. But underlying this diversity of preferred temperatures is a universal that characterizes all people, and that is the need to keep their core body temperature at about 37 degrees Centigrade. In contrast, other influences on happiness such as school grades are almost completely dependent on aspirations, and comparisons with the level of others. What we need is better theories and data on the universals versus particulars in happiness, and how even universals might be shaped to some degree by culture and individual differences. We need scientists to begin asking deeper questions about what Chris Hsee (Hsee, Hastie, & Chen, 2008) has called "evaluability"—whether influences on happiness have inherent value or are comparative in nature.

A recent article by Fowler and Christakis (2008) establishes a new and exciting area of research about the effects of people's "happiness" on the subjective well-being of those around them. The authors found in a large longitudinal study that well-being is contagious in that it spreads to neighbors, family, and friends in the social network. This finding has possible implications for explaining cultural differences in happiness, in helping to devise happiness interventions, and in numerous other applied and social areas.

Another area that is likely to take on increasing importance in a world characterized by globalization and the realization that most behavioral science findings are currently built on a narrow base of westernized, industrialized society, is the question of cultural differences in well-being. We can ask several important questions in this area. Are the structure and contents of subjective well-being similar in all cultures? To what degree are the causes of well-being universal versus culture-specific? To what extent do people in various cultures seek and value subjective well-being. And do the benefits of well-being for effective functioning and success differ across cultures? It is to these questions that I turn in Volume 38 of this series: *Culture and Well-Being*.

References

Diener, E., & Biswas-Diener, R. (2008). *Happiness: Unlocking the mysteries of psychological wealth*. Malden, MA: Wiley/Blackwell Publishing.

Diener, E., Nickerson, C., Lucas, R. E., & Sandvik, E. (2002). Dispositional affect and job outcomes. *Social Indicators Research, 59*, 229–259.

Fowler, J. H., & Christakis, N. A. (2008). Dynamic spread of happiness in a large social network: Longitudinal analysis over 20 years in the Framingham Heart Study. *British Medical Journal, 337*, a2338.

Hsee, C. K., Hastie, R., & Chen., J. (2008). Hedonomics: Bridging decision research with happiness research. *Perspectives on Psychological Science, 3*, 224–243.

Kashdan, T., Biswas-Diener, R., & King, L. (2008). Reconsidering happiness: The costs of distinguishing between hedonics and eudaimnoia. *The Journal of Positive Psychology, 3*, 219–233.

Keyes, C. L. M., Shmotkin, D., & Ryff, C. D. (2002). Optimizing well-being: The empirical encounter of two traditions. *Journal of Personality and Social Psychology, 82*, 1007–1022.

Ryan, R. M., & Deci, E. L. (2000). Self-determination theory and the facilitation of intrinsic motivation, social development, and well-being. *American Psychologist, 55*, 68–78.

Wilson, W. (1967). Correlates of avowed happiness. *Psychological Bulletin, 67*, 294–406.

Printed in the United Kingdom by
Lightning Source UK Ltd., Milton Keynes
342UK00003BA/60/P